Healing Our Children

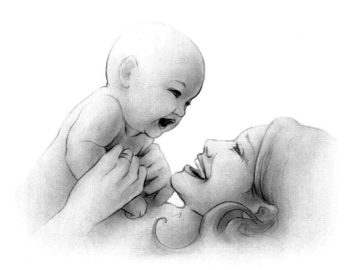

Sacred Wisdom for Preconception,
Pregnancy, Birth and Parenting

For media appearance requests for Mr. Nagel contact: pr@healingourchildren.net

For wholesale orders contact Golden Child Publishing at: orders@goldenchildpublishing.com

For suggestions or corrections for future editions contact: comments@healingourchildren.net

To order copies visit: www.healingourchildren.net

Golden Child Publishing
Post Office Box AG
Los Gatos, CA 95031 U.S.A
goldenchildpublishing.com

ISBN – 13: 978-0-9820213-1-6
ISBN – 10: 0-9820213-1-3
LCCN: 2008933991

Printed and bound in the United States of America

Many Thanks To All Who Have Helped

Editors: Adrian Cousens, Katherine Czapp

Cover Artwork and Interior Illustrations:
Russell Dauterman, russelldauterman.com

Cover Design: Georgia Morrissey
georgi11@optonline.net

Contents

Invocation:

(Please join me if you like.)

I surrender to the divine in all things.

Dear divine mother and father, due to our ignorant ways our children are suffering greatly. Please, let me be a vehicle for your healing grace. Help these children, and these parents, to see the light to a better way for all.

Intention:

The purpose of this book is to ground forgotten knowledge and wisdom of how to create healthy children, and more comfortable pregnancies, into this Earth, in order to support healing, bliss and redemption for all.

Activity:

What is your intention in reading this book? Take a moment to look for it and acknowledge it!

Dedication:

(From Michelle) This book is dedicated to all of Our children, who are a shining light in this world.

An Important Note

Author's Disclaimer

About the Weston A. Price, DDS photos:

Foreword

by
Sally Fallon

Philosophies of child rearing change over the years. We look back with horror at the typical Victorian attitude towards children—one that mandated strict discipline, often by whipping and beating, from an early age, and separation from their mothers, if not at birth, then at the age when the young child was sent away to boarding school.

How will future commentators describe the child-rearing techniques of the 20th and 21st centuries? No doubt we will applaud the progress made in meeting the emotional needs of the child, at least in principle. No one today condones an unnecessarily strict upbringing for children, deprivation of maternal bonding or dangerous corporal punishment.

But how will future generations assess our attitude towards the physical development of the child? Most likely future commentators will point out the egregious errors we are currently making in the physical nourishment of our children, even our complete ignorance of the connection between diet and health. Ramiel Nagel rightly begins *Healing Our Children* with a discussion of responsibility.

He notes that our cultural belief system supports a lack of personal responsibility in the area of the physical development of children. Health problems in children are usually blamed on the two g's—germs and genes. If a child has an acute or infectious illness, we say it is caused by germs—we blame Nature. If a child suffers from a birth defect or chronic disease, we say it is caused by bad genes—we blame God.

This attitude contrasts starkly with the attitude of non-industrialized, so-called primitive peoples described by nutrition pioneer Weston A. Price in his book *Nutrition and Physical Degeneration*. Dr. Price was awestruck by the fact that traditional peoples took full responsibility for the health of their offspring. If a child suffered from disease or was born with a defect, the parents understood that the fault was not Nature's or God's, but their own.

However, this rarely happened because so-called primitive peoples had a profound understanding of the kind of foods needed for the production of healthy children. They understood that both parents required special, nutrient-dense feeding before conception, that mothers required superlative nutrition during pregnancy and lactation, and that growing children required a nutrient-dense diet from their first bite of solid food.

Of course, many scientists and commentators today do acknowledge a connection between diet and health; unfortunately the dietary advice of the vast majority—with their recommendations of lowfat, mostly vegetarian and even salt-free diets for pregnant women and growing children—is appalling, a guaranteed recipe for health problems almost from birth.

Care and attention to the diet during preconception, pregnancy and growth will provide your child with that greatest of gifts—a strong, well-formed healthy physical body and keen, creative mind. But parents need accurate information on how to do this, and there is no better place to start than with the research findings of Dr. Weston A. Price. Ramiel Nagel has done a superlative job of presenting the work of Dr. Weston A. Price and translating those findings into modern terminology and practical guidelines for ensuring the health of your baby.

It is instructive to use the analogy of building a house to underscore the importance of optimal nutrition for the infant. A house that is spacious and strongly built will serve as a pleasant home for many, many years, even if the occupants are less than conscientious about the upkeep. And if such a house falls into disrepair because of poor maintenance, it can be brought back to good condition again with the proper attention. But a house that is poorly built may never be comfortable and will require constant maintenance just to keep it from falling down.

Most children growing up today live in the latter type of house. Throughout life, in order to be healthy, such individuals will need to pay very careful attention to their diets at all times. Their houses will likely be constantly springing leaks—allergies, digestive problems, fatigue, behavior abnormalities, etc.

Those born before the Second World War, when the food most Americans ate was of excellent quality, likely live in a body that is solidly build; these lucky individuals can indulge in junk food, at least for a time, without showing any signs of poor health, and if they are careful to eat a nutrient-dense traditional diet, can count on a long and healthy life.

Providing the information parents need to give their children their birthright of a healthy, well-built body must be our number one priority if humanity is to make any further progress on this earth. The effort parents put into good nutrition for their children, starting even before conception, will return many blessings for the child, the parents and the generations to come.

Healing Our Children will serve as an important tool in reversing the now obvious trend to physical degeneration and restoring vibrant health to all children.

Sally Fallon, President
The Weston A. Price Foundation
October, 2008

Welcome!

Thank you for taking the time, energy, and effort to read my book. In this book, you will learn how to create healthy and vibrant children. You deserve the best for yourself and for your children, and it is my goal to help you achieve that success. That is the purpose of this book. So, welcome…

The Beginning

The world around us is falling apart. We all came into this world on a cloud of hope and inspiration, with a longing to be loved, joyfully received and cared for. Due to the ignorance in this world and in our parents, many of us did not receive this welcoming. Rather than entering a world of peace, joy, love and compassion, we found a world of suffering.

As children, many of us were not well cared for and were not given what we truly longed to receive. Instead of attention and caring, many of us were abused physically, emotionally, and even sexually. We were raised in a generally uncaring world, in which superficial values were given precedence over what really matters — the heart.

Now that we are adults with our own children, we are presented with a new opportunity for hope. With the new generation of our children we can, if we choose, erase many of these pains and sorrows. Rather than raising our children unconsciously, many of us are groping to find a new way.

As a soon-to-be parent, I didn't know how to take care of my coming child. I did not know how to prepare for pregnancy. When I looked to the world around me for answers on how to raise healthy children, I found little or no complete resources for real, natural, healthy parenting.

I did find some good ideas and a few tidbits here and there, but I really felt that I had to carve my own path without the support and concrete guidance I would have liked. In many ways, in fact, I was completely clueless about the effects my lifestyle was having on my child before she was even born, and later as she began to grow. When my daughter was one year old, I started to research natural health care because her teeth started to rapidly decay. This book is the result of that research, of learning the REAL causes of disease and finding REAL cures and treatments to prevent disease.

It is my wish and prayer for your child to be as healthy, happy, and vibrant as my children are, and even healthier.

Nature's Plan for Healthy Children

Can you imagine that the creative force of the Universe, which we see all around us as Nature, which created our DNA and our very existence, has a design and plan for you and your children? There is such a plan — a plan for success and abundance. Throughout this book you will be learning about this plan, and how we as humans, in not following it, mistakenly create unhealthy children. You will learn of many of the ways that we have strayed from this plan. However, you will also be given a view of the beautiful valley of possibilities for aligning with Nature's goal of success: a healthy and content baby.

A Healthy Child

A healthy child is a child who rarely or never gets sick. She may have some minor or **occasional** illnesses, sensitivities or allergies, but these are not chronic and do not affect in any significant way the child's well being. A healthy child does not have Attention Deficit Disorder, does not have autism, and is usually, but not always (that's impossible), well mannered and agreeable. A healthy child has perfect vision of 20/20 or better, has straight teeth without cavities and has a beautiful and well-proportioned face. A healthy child meets and usually exceeds the expectations in terms of intelligence for his or her age group and fulfills his or her developmental potential to the fullest. A healthy child sleeps easily and awakes rested and energized. A healthy child is full of love and compassion. For a healthy child, the world is an engaging playground to live in, learn from, and enjoy. A healthy child is full of vitality and radiates a sense of alertness and aliveness that others can see and feel. Does this child sound like one that you would like to create?

Creating Healthy Children

I know what a healthy child is because this description fits both of my daughter's Sparkle and Yeshe very well. My father has consistently remarked about my older Sparkle's qualities and character. "I don't know what you are doing with your daughter," he says to me, without knowing or even wanting to know, "but I can tell you are doing something right." While you might say I am fortunate or that it is a blessing to have a child like this, I can tell you that as fortunate as I am, it has nothing to do with luck; it happened primarily through my conscious efforts and choices — choices that few parents even are aware of. In this book I aim to guide you to make the best choices for yourself and your child.

Pearls of Wisdom

Interspersed throughout this book are pearls of wisdom from my ~~partner in crime~~ — scratch that — my partner in child creating, living, and child rearing, Michelle. These tidbits add another perspective to the discussion, and we hope will help you, the reader, to drop deeper into yourself and into your longing to create a healthy child.

Michelle Says: "Each one of us has inherent potential to conceive and create a beautiful and healthy child. The first step to this is to know and believe it is true. It may appear that it is easier for some people to have healthy children than it is for others. Nonetheless, it takes effort—both the outer effort of providing proper nutrition, and the inner effort of introspection, of finding that healthy child within ourselves first, so that we can create her in the outer world."

Let's get down to business. We are going to learn all about health. But first, it's time to learn about what really causes disease.

Part I
The Plague

1

The Cause of Disease
Only You Are Responsible
for Your Child's Health

When I was four years old, my knees would hurt frequently at night. I couldn't sleep and sometimes even cried in pain. This seemed only to irritate my parents. In my teenage years, the teeth in the lower half of my mouth grew in crooked; even suffering through braces for two years did not correct the problem. Then, I had to have all of my wisdom teeth surgically removed because they also grew in crooked.

I had other physical problems as well. I would frequently have an upset stomach and I developed poor digestion. My body did not grow properly, and my posture consequently suffered. My vision deteriorated and I had to get glasses, but the glasses were ugly so I tried contact lenses. But the contact lenses burned my eyes so I finally stopped wearing them and had to settle for bad vision. In addition to these ailments, I was excessively shy and afraid to talk with people; I would always try to hide. I was slow to heal as well. I got a sunburn once and developed a rash on my face that has lasted for over twelve years and is now, finally, almost gone. For years, my back would hurt every day for no apparent reason. I saw many doctors and health professionals for my knee problems and skin rashes, but none of them seemed to be able to address the cause of my conditions.

While you may have experienced different symptoms, circumstances and problems while growing up, I share my experience with you because I now know that these conditions are not inherent to the human body. Rather, they are an inherent effect of the modern way in which we live. In the next few chapters, I will demonstrate for you how many of these illnesses and diseases are not natural, but rather are a reaction to the way we live in the modern world. By changing how we live and who we have become, we can prevent and cure modern diseases. By not changing how we live, we will perpetuate modern diseases and as a result our children may suffer.

One last thought here. During my college years, I lacked energy to do anything, and lost most of my will to live because my life was so unfulfilling. I became lazy and despondent. Yet within me was a fire: a "burning for burning," representing the fire of love, of being alive, of action, of doing the right thing, and of everything that represents that burning spark within. This book is a testament to the fire within each of us. It is the phoenix that rises out of the ashes, in all of its glory.

Activity: Take a moment and look for the fire within you. Do you feel a desire to grow, share, and change? Do you feel a longing for oneness with something filled with love, beauty, wholeness and compassion? Do you feel strongly motivated to do something but don't know what it is?

Intention: Due to our laziness, and due to false knowledge perpetuated throughout our culture and family systems, we have given our power away to the "authority." This chapter is dedicated to reclaiming your inner power to create health for yourself and your children.

A Paradigm of Personal Responsibility

Here's something to chew on: If something unfortunate happens in your life, whose fault or responsibility is it? Who or what caused this bad occurrence? What is in your hands, and what is controlled by fate?

Throughout this book, I rely on a set of channeled lectures that are affectionately called the Pathwork®. Without saying more about the precise source of these lectures, I here add some wisdom from this work, adding only that it is powerful and it works.

> *The law of personal responsibility is the guiding principle on the search for the root of one's obstructions. It enables the individual to resolve what-ever problem he may have. It opens up life with all its rich possibilities. It forces him to see things in their true light, and uncomfortable as this may first seem, it leaves him in the end with a lot more self-respect, integrity, and hope than the helpless resignation to the circumstances life is supposed to bring about without one's doing. It makes defeat unnecessary because it also removes, among other things, the childish illusion of one's omnipotence, which is just as unrealistic as the illusion of being life's passive victim. To accept one's own limitations and the limitations of others increases the power to direct one's life meaningfully.* [1]

See what I mean? That's good stuff. So, what does personal responsibility mean? It means you are NOT a passive victim of life or that your life's circumstances are beyond your control. In the end, if you challenge these belief systems, you get a lot more self-respect and integrity (which is something that I assume you want).

Activity: Do you feel like a victim, or feel powerless or helpless in a certain area of your life? If so, just pay attention to those feelings without trying to fix them. Don't blame yourself; just notice how it feels to feel like a victim. It doesn't feel good, so we usually ignore or deny it. Yet change will only happen when we have felt the feeling, no matter how uncomfortable it is.

Our Cultural Belief System Supports a Lack of Personal Responsibility

Let's assume that personal responsibility represents a guiding light, a truthful and more potent way to live. What, then, might life look like when lived from a perspective devoid of personal responsibility? Life would not be full of possibilities, and you would believe that you could never see things in their true form. Defeat would always be around every corner, and you would feel like you were a victim of life's circumstances. Does this sound familiar? If it doesn't, let me remind you of some of the forces influencing your beliefs.

A belief system is a set of ideas that have energy, or feelings, behind them. Beliefs have power, gravity and weight. It is the feelings and emotions beneath the beliefs which give them power over us, and that guide us. We believe in the inherent truth of the system.

Hundreds of years ago, when people were afflicted with various types of ailments and diseases it was a common practice to blame evil spirits (note the lack of personal responsibility in this idea). People around the world still do this today, except that these evil spirits now have a new name. Scientists, doctors, dentists, and government officials have decided that these new "evil spirits" are called micro-organisms (viruses, bacteria, etc). The prevalent modern theory is that these viruses and bacteria are the basic or primary cause of disease.

The germ theory, the modern and accepted theory of disease today, originated with the work of Louis Pasteur (1822–1895), and has become cemented in our minds as the truth. Mr. Pasteur promoted a theory of disease that is now the basis of most forms of modern medicine. This theory projects the idea that pathogenic organisms exist outside the body and that when the body's defenses are lowered, these organisms can invade the body and cause disease.

Modern Medicine/Germ Theory Examples

I am providing here a few examples of the germ theory to make very clear what our culture believes to be the causes of disease and other physical problems. This is important to understand because if you want to have healthy children, you need to have an empowering framework regarding what makes them sick. The following examples are not what I believe, but are the modern beliefs that many people hold:

A cold: A cold is caused when harmful cold viruses touch our eyes, nose or throat. It is caused when we come in contact with someone else who has a cold. They sneeze on us or through some other form of contact transmit their disease to us.

Chicken Pox: This highly contagious disease is caused by the chicken pox virus. You can obtain immunity to chicken pox when you have had the disease. If you do not contract this disease in childhood you could get it in adulthood when its consequences will be worse.

Poor Vision: Poor vision is due to the unlucky combination of genetic material (DNA) you received from your mother and father. Science will soon identify the genes for poor vision and excellent vision and hopefully be able to prevent the former.

Diet: Diet has only a small influence on our health. When you are healthy, you can eat most types of foods without any harm. Be sure to avoid unhealthy saturated fats that cause heart disease, and instead use unsaturated vegetable oils. Eat lean cuts of meat. In general avoid fat —it's bad for you—and make sure to have many servings of grains per day.

Degenerative diseases: Scientists do not understand the cause of cancer, heart disease, diabetes or _____ (name any disease). There is probably not one cause, but many different factors are involved. Family history is

a risk factor. Name any disease, and scientists probably believe that genetics play a role in getting it. There is no known cure for _____ (name any disease), they say, and the secrets to preventing it are not yet known.

Who Is Responsible For Curing Disease?

Based on our current way of thinking, there is one common thread running through the explanation of these examples. It can be summarized as, "You are not responsible for your disease." Just to be clear, if you or a family member has an incurable condition, this doesn't mean it was their fault; but it is their responsibility to take care of.

When you ask the question of who is responsible for curing disease, what answer do you usually get? Well, it's the doctor's responsibility, of course, and the government's and the entire medical establishment—everyone but you, right? Here's the problem: have they succeeded in curing disease? No, they haven't.

If doctors and scientists, the medical establishment and the government do not know how to cure diseases and do not know what causes them, do you want to give the responsibility for treating your disease, or for making you healthy, to them? If **they** are responsible for curing your disease, then what power does that leave you to find solutions and to take action?

If we are to believe in the law of personal responsibility, then we are empowered to reject the role of passive victim in our own lives. Conversely, this means that you will not be able to, or should not listen to, the conventional way of thinking about disease, because doing so makes you a victim to the disease.

Michelle Says: "Nowadays we look towards doctors and other 'professionals' to give us answers, to help us feel better and be healthy, as if we don't know anything about it ourselves. We are supposed to trust these 'professionals,' who are only taught the modern techniques of treating disease with drugs and surgery. They are not taught traditional methods, which have served different cultural groups across the globe in effective ways for thousands of years. Many of these professionals just inject us with chemicals, and then perform mostly needless surgery. What we need to do is relearn traditional methods of healing, and combine them with the modern techniques that are useful and helpful, so we can live healthy and harmonious lives. Very few professionals have spent any time cultivating compassion and love towards another human. How can we really heal ourselves or another without love or compassion?"

Activity: Do you want to be responsible for your health? Ask yourself this question and see what arises. If you listen closely, you'll hear two answers. One that says, yes, I do, and the other that says, no, I don't. Listen to and pay attention to the *yes*, and to the *no*. It is usually our hidden *no* to life that thwarts our efforts. Pay attention to the *no*, and invite in the *yes*.

Germs Don't Cause Disease

We continually breathe in bacteria, viruses, and other micro-organisms.[2] Germs are everywhere. They exist in the soil, water, and on virtually everything we touch. Microbes are also in our bodies, including the beneficial bacteria in our intestines that help us absorb nutrients from our foods. When a person is healthy, germs live within them in a harmonious and positive state.

It is a well accepted fact that many viruses and bacteria such as polio, tuberculosis, and HIV, may be present in many healthy people's bodies in a dormant state, called latency, with the person experiencing no symptoms of disease. In several experiments, different germs from people infected with diseases like diphtheria, could not be passed to healthy subjects no matter what method of infection was tried.[3] Even with our enormous exposure to microbes, most of them don't make us sick. To propose, therefore, that germs do not cause disease seems to provoke a negative reaction in many people; the idea is so contrary to the way we were educated. We were raised to believe that disease is caused by circumstances outside of our control, by the invading evil spirit, back in a new, physical form.

A Paradigm of Personal Responsibility

During the time of Mr. Pasteur, there also lived another French scientist by the name of Antoine Béchamp. He believed . . . yes, hold your breath here . . . **that germs do not cause disease**. Rather, he believed that germs exist and evolve in relationship to the changing conditions of the ecosystem in which they live. In other words, it is the unhealthy environment inside your body that creates sickness by providing the fertile ground on which the germs can mutate into harmful forms. Thus, germs can mutate and take new shapes and forms, and do so in response to their environment. The change occurs in stages, in a progression from simpler to more complex forms. The simplest form of germs are microbes (primitive phase), then bacteria (middle phase), and then fungus (end phase).[4] This idea is similar to a caterpillar morphing into a butterfly, or a tadpole into a frog. It is also similar to what is observed in nature, where only certain plants grow in a particular geographic region. A palm tree grows in the desert; a redwood tree grows in the temperate forest. Redwood trees don't grow in the desert because that climate will not sustain them. Each plant exists in a symbiotic relationship to its geographical location, and only grows when certain conditions are met. But surely, you may be saying, the germ theory must be correct. It has been in application for over a hundred years now, giant corporations make billions off of its tenets, our medical establishment is based on it, and it is taught in schools and reported about in the media. Consider the fact that even Mr. Pasteur is said to have admitted on his death bed that "the microbe is nothing: the terrain is everything."[5] Finally, newer live field microscopes which allow viewing of living samples at high magnifications show clear and irrefutable proof of microscopic forms evolving and changing in response to their terrain in a matter of seconds and minutes.[6] This proves conclusively that pleomorphism is a real phenomenon and a part of our natural world.

There is evidence to suggest that microbes exist within the body to help the body clean and restore itself, and are a condition associated with a diseased state but are *not* the cause of disease per se. For example, tuberculosis is a disease blamed on a bacterium, yet renowned tuberculosis expert Walter R. Hadwen, M.D., states: "Nobody has ever found a tubercle bacillus in the earliest stages of tuberculosis."[7] In several more recent studies, parasites and bacteria such as *E.coli* (stuff we think is really dangerous), have been used to heal conditions in the body with remarkable efficacy.[8]

How Can A "Perfect" Creation Become Sick?

When we look at our human bodies from a biological and chemical viewpoint, we see that they are perfectly created by nature. The various parts of the body such as the heart, the cells, the DNA, all operate as if they had a will of their own. An example of this comes from Nobel Prize winner Alex Carrel (1912), who observed the perfection of a microscopic slice of the heart of a chicken. The slice was kept in a nutrient-rich solution, replaced daily, and lived for 29 years. It only died when an assistant forgot to rinse the cells. Based on the results of this experiment, Dr. Carrel postulated:

> *The cell is immortal. It is merely the fluid in which it floats which degenerates. Renew this fluid . . . and . . . the pulsation of life may go on forever.*[9]

We find this observation confirmed in ordinary anatomy textbooks as well.

> *If the concentration [of fluid outside the cell] changes, so as to contain too much or too little of these [nutrients], the cells will become sick and act abnormally and eventually begin to die.*[10]

Dr. Albert V. Szent-Gyorgyi won the Nobel Prize in 1937 for discovering vitamin C. If the cell is perfect, he wondered, then how or why do we get sick?

> *Should then, man be the only imperfect creature kept alive in the face of all his im-*

perfections only by means created by his own mind? If not, where do all these ailments come from?[11]

In other words, if the cell was created with the potential for immortality, then illness, death and disease may come from somewhere else. Could that source be our own minds, as Dr. Szent-György postulated? Dr. Szent-György is not the only person to allude to some extra-physical source of disease and suffering.

The Yellow Emperor's Classic on Internal Medicine is one of humanity's oldest medical texts in existence. In a translation of this ancient Chinese work, we read of how the Yellow Emperor asked his health minister, Ch'I Po, about the true nature of disease. Why is it, he wonders, that people used to live to an old age with good health, and now people only live to half of that age and become weak and unhealthy?[12] Ch'I Po responds by saying that in ancient times people understood the "Tao" (the way of being) and patterned themselves after the "Yin and Yang," the two divine principles of creation—masculine and feminine—whose existence is reflected in nature. Ch'I Po continues by explaining how people exhaust their vital forces through reckless and overly stimulating behaviors. He gives the example of having sex while intoxicated. Today, excessively stimulating behaviors could be watching too much T.V., eating too many sweet foods, and seeking other forms of worldly stimulation (such as high risk sports and related activities) as a replacement for feeling alive. Ch'I Po further explains that the cravings for gratification of the senses dissipate one's true essence. This happens because people have forgotten how to find contentment within themselves; they devote all their attention to amusement of their mind, thus cutting themselves off from Being, and the real joys of life.[13]

Best-selling author of *The Power of Now* and *A New Earth,* Eckhart Tolle, calls this form of collective dysfunction the *egoic mind.* This is the "me" or the "my" story. It is a mental image and construction of ourselves produced by the mind. It is not real and has evolved out of a pseudo solution to deal with a world in which we didn't receive the love and compassion which we wanted as infants and children. People then live a majority of their lives through this chaotic mind energy and are lost in thought, trying to add more to the story of themselves, and not really living. The human predicament is to be constantly thinking all the time, and not really living. It is almost like some other entity that takes us over. It is this egoic mind which has inflicted suffering on us and the planet. It is this insane mind which starts wars because negativity feeds this false self. The state of being identified with the voice in your head is believed to be a state of suffering. The mind, the voice, creates suffering and is a result of unhealed internal strife and suffering that most people have buried away. If when reading this you hear a voice or thought that says, "There is no such voice," that is exactly the voice, and the energy that is a part of this life-denying self.

The Father of Medicine

Hippocrates, the father of western medicine, understood the principle of the Tao, and could thus heal people with it. He called it *vis medicatrix naturae*—the healing power of nature which cures us from within. Hippocrates defined disease as a combination of Pathos, suffering, and Ponos, toil. Suffering represents the state of disharmony within the ailing person, and toil is the body's response to this suffering as it tries to find stasis and harmony again. In other words, our bodies want health and balance. The Tao or Being—simply existing—is our natural state. Suffering comes from not being rooted in Being, the timeless eternal reality. Nature can heal and cure us from within if we can understand and harmonize with her. Surgery, and medicines, too, can aid nature in a cure, but only if they are used wisely for the purpose of aiding nature, which today they rarely are.

I Resolve To Find the Real Cause of Disease

Thomas Sydenham, considered the English Hippocrates of the seventeenth century, declared that, "Disease is nothing else but an attempt on the part of the body to rid itself of morbific (diseased, toxic) matter." [14]

After years of wandering in the jungles of medical diagnosis, twentieth century American physician, J.H. Tilden, MD, finally became frustrated and declared, "I resolved either to quit the profession or to find the cause of disease."[15] Dr. Tilden observed that in any normal life cycle there is cellular metabolism, and thus waste. Much like cars that produce exhaust, the cells of our body produce minute amounts of waste. When the body cannot eliminate its own waste (or the waste added through contact with toxins in the external environmental), it slowly becomes diseased. Dr. Tilden identified the cause of what prohibits the body from eliminating waste, which he called *habits of enervation*. And it isn't surprising that, likely without ever having seen or known of the *Yellow Emperor's Classic on Internal Medicine,* he came to the same conclusion found in those pages. The conclusion is that disease is caused by habits which excessively stimulate the body. Examples Dr. Tilden gives of these habits are excessive smoking and drinking, eating too much sugar, staying up too late, and over-working. Toxic emotions such as fear or greed also contribute to this over-stimulation.

In this new paradigm for disease there is a common thread. Our behaviors are the cause of disease. If our behaviors can cause or significantly contribute to the disease, then how can one separate the diseased state from the patient who suffers from the disease, as if the patient has nothing at all to do with its creation? Dr. Tilden considers this apparent conundrum and then boldly states:

> *There is no hope that medical science will ever be a science; for the whole structure is built around the idea that there is an object disease—that can be cured when the right drug—remedy, cure—is found.* [16] *(Emphasis added.)*

Usually, a cure for a disease lies in seeing the oneness and symbiotic relationship between the individual, the disease, and the environment in which the sick person lives, which includes the earth under his feet, his food, his home, his family, and his society.

What We Call a Disease Is Really the Symptoms of Disease

When someone sneezes whenever they come into contact with pollen, we say they have allergies. If someone has a fever and a sore throat, we say they have flu. When someone's skin becomes inflamed around a cut, we say they have an infection. When someone's pancreas stops working well, we say they have diabetes, and when someone has a growth of rapidly spreading cells, we say they have cancer. Western medicine takes a magnifying glass and looks at these symptoms of the body, and declares that it has discovered a disease. But sneezing, coughing, irritation, pain, inflammation, fever and so forth are not the disease itself; they represent the body's attempt to cleanse the toxic elements and heal the body. Remember the examples of doctors, like Dr. Carrel with his chicken heart cells, who think disease is caused by dead or otherwise stagnant material or waste in the body? When a collection of this material in the body becomes too great to be eliminated through normal means the body reacts, producing symptoms that we then call a disease. The inflammation on the skin is an attempt to push out toxic material that shouldn't be in the body. The coughing and sneezing are meant to expel toxic material from the body. The fever is meant to burn up dead and harmful matter. Vomiting and diarrhea help rid the body of substances that are making it sick. Tumors are a collection and storage of dead and acrid material that, due to blocked excretion channels in the body, could not escape.

Maverick medical doctor Henry Bieler, author of the best-selling book, *Food Is Your Best Medicine*, writes:

As a practicing physician for over fifty years, I have reached three basic conclusions as to the cause and cure of disease.

1. The first is that the primary cause of disease is not germs.

2. The second conclusion is that in almost all cases the use of drugs in treating patients is harmful. Drugs often cause serious side effects, and sometimes even create new diseases. The dubious benefits they afford the patient are at best temporary.

3. My third conclusion is that disease can be cured through the proper use of correct foods.[17]

Death by Western Medicine

Western medicine has it wrong. Its drugs and surgeries usually, but not always, only suppress the symptoms of disease. Since most Western drugs are toxic by themselves, and cause "side effects" that add to disease, they themselves are a stimulating element to the body. Dr. Bieler explains in *Food is Your Best Medicine* that western drugs like penicillin are so toxic they are eliminated from the body within a few seconds.[18] They work by over-stimulating exhausted glands such as the adrenals. As a result modern drugs drain the body of vital resources and nutrients.

When you consider what is required for healing, in its true light, what comes to mind? Healing requires warmth, compassion, and the awareness of the other as a human being. Western medicine does not usually embody these principles. Western medicine is about power over nature rather than yielding to nature. The body becomes the object whose unfortunate purpose is to be manipulated for a profit. Western medicine is the opposite of Robin Hood. It takes from the poor (the sick, the infirm and the dying) and gives their money to the rich tyrants, the pharmaceutical industry and the medical establishment. In a healthy society, treating disease would not come with such an exorbitant price tag.

According to a compilation of conservative statistics from medical associations and reports from hospitals across the country, the number one cause of death in the United States today is Western medicine. To be exact, the practices of Western medicine result in 783,936 deaths a year, at a cost of $282 billion per year.[19] This research was compiled by medical researchers and doctors, and every count added to this figure came exclusively from published and peer-reviewed scientific studies. [20]

Our medical system is killing us, and reaping huge profits from it.

It is due to this astounding fact, which you won't find in today's newspaper headlines, that Dr. Matthias Rath, a respected physician and scientist who has pioneered many breakthroughs in the treatments of disease, filed a complaint against genocide and other crimes against humanity against the pharmaceutical industry, with the International Criminal Court in Hague. Pfizer Inc., Merck & Co., GlaxoSmithKline PLC, along with senior banking and government officials are named in the complaint. Learn more at www.dr-rath-foundation.org. [21]

Activity: Take a moment to reflect here. You have felt within you that there is something profoundly wrong with life. You couldn't put your finger on what was wrong and since nobody seems to be talking about it, it was easy to just shove the feeling into the closet. But you can feel it, resonate with it, your entire being is filled with this energy telling you something. But what? **Listen to that feeling**. Listen to, or feel what is moving through you right now. By reading this text you may temporarily disconnect from the cultural thought pattern of disease, which believes that disease is separate from us. This thought pattern is really saying that life is separate from you, that you are not a part of life. When you disconnect from these beliefs you start to reconnect to yourself. There is something within you that wants to be born into this world (not just your baby if you are pregnant!). It is the essential you, pure, whole and healthy. When our brains are stuffed with false thinking from childhood on, it becomes easier for us to lose ourselves in the world. This feeling, the burning I mentioned that is the driving force for writing this book, is within you, it is your awakening, the beginning of your return.

Let's Review, Because This Is Important

This chapter began with a brief lesson on personal responsibility. The law of personal responsibility declares that you are not a victim of life, but rather that you can take a stance in facing life with all of the good and bad it has to offer. I then described how our current medical system is predicated on taking personal responsibility away from patients, and on patients submitting their personal responsibility to this system. Meanwhile, even the supposed creator of Western medicine, Hippocrates, believed that it was Nature that healed people, and that the physician's role was to aid Nature in her course. Even ancient Chinese medicine *and* modern physicians and chemists, in search for real cures, have pinpointed the true cause of disease: our lifestyle. It is thus in our realm of responsibility to do something about our health.

Western medicine has become a sick system. While it offers some people good results (usually because of a few good or mindful doctors), for the majority of us, and for the majority of disease conditions, it does more harm than good. The very system that we have put our faith in has betrayed our trust. We are in some ways left floating without a container, without the kind, compassionate embrace of the good healer that we need. The current system is based on disease rather than on health, and is the cause of much suffering. If you place your faith blindly in this system, then what do you think will happen to your children?

Towards A New Paradigm for Health and A Prayer for the True Cause of Disease

Many people want to be healthy and have healthy children. Yet, with so many choices in the world they don't know where to begin or to whom to turn for help. This is where prayer comes in. The words Father and Mother, or Divine Father and Divine Mother may bring up certain positive or negative associations for you depending on your religious beliefs and upbringing. So I urge you, if necessary, to replace those words with other words if it is appropriate for you. For those who are in an atheistic mind set, you can think of the Divine Mother and Father as energies in the Universe. The universal Yin and the universal Yang: the opposite forces that need each other to create.

Consider prayer and asking for help. "Show me, Father, the real reason for my difficulties, so that I can solve them."[22]

Here's another one:

Divine Mother, You who are always close to Your children, guide my every step so that I am always on the right path, thinking positively, never judging anyone or anything. Make me see the Divine always.[23]

So now what? I hope you've asked for help (or maybe you've thrown the book down claiming that I am part of some cult or sect). In any case, there is sweetness, joy, an embrace in just asking for help. To me, it feels so good. I really want to know, great Father, why am I sick? Why are my children sick? Why does disease happen? Show me, so that I can heal them. Show me, so that I can help others to heal themselves.

Disease Is Caused By Stagnant and Blocked Layers of Consciousness

If you try to figure out what the Universe is made of by staring at things with microscopes, or by using giant telescopes, or by looking and listening to the quiet voice within, you'll probably come to the conclusion that this whole thing is quite unfathomable. If you ask a quantum physicist what the Universe is made of, he might point you towards one truth of the Universe: that this world, your body, and life itself are all pulsating fields of energy. And that this pulsating energy is not random, but has order to it and works in a harmonious way. This harmony requires an intelligence, which we call consciousness or aware-

ness. And this intelligence, this awareness, is in our body. We are part of its design.

Consciousness resides in every atom of living matter, in every cell, in every molecule, in every tiniest fraction of living matter. [24]

Traditional Chinese medicine, for example, has identified thousands of points and lines of energy, and has designed systems for stimulating those points with needles (acupuncture); one of many ways whereby you can affect the health of the entire body.

In disease, different layers of our Being, our life force—the energy and consciousness flowing through every fraction of matter, which creates our body—become blocked. So Nature can heal us, when we unblock the life-force.

I share this with you to illustrate one important point. Underlying every disease condition is a layer or block in our consciousness or being. This is an important key to self-responsibility for health. If there is a condition making us sick, then in some way, there is almost always something within us that we probably are not aware of that is making us sick. I'll give you a simple example:

Say you feel unhappy—and most of us feel unhappy at least part of the day—and since you feel unhappy you have the counter thought that you deserve happiness and pleasure. So, you buy yourself a pint of Ben & Jerry's Chocolate Fudge Brownie™ Ice Cream. You eat the entire thing. If a scenario like this happens often enough, you'll start gaining weight, or experiencing digestive distress. Over time you can become sick. In the end, your feeling of unhappiness is what caused you to act in a way that made you sick. Do you see the connections?

It is our feelings that drive us. It is the control of our feelings that suppresses us. Our feelings, collectively, create disease and a culture of disease. In the last analysis, changing our feelings and beliefs is the first step on the path towards health. You can change these beliefs and feelings through acknowledging and accepting them, or merely by taking note of them. Then, it is much easier to make good decisions, and take effective action towards being healthy.

Here are some key feelings and beliefs that make us sick. Notice if any of these resonate with you:

- Self -punishment can create physical disease.
- Self-hatred can cause disease.
- Negative aspects in your personality can weaken you and cause disease.
- Neglecting to take care of yourself and your body can promote disease.
- A denial of pleasure in one's life can create illness.

Physical health and well-being is totally regulated by and dependent upon the state of pleasure a human body is capable of allowing. Health and longevity are results of the capacity for pleasure… Any kind of physical illness or deterioration, therefore also physical death, as it were, is a manifestation of division, conflict, and denial of pleasure.[25]

How the Body Maintains Health on the Physical Level

I may have convinced you that there is something wrong with the Western medical view of disease. This section will help give you a framework of a more holistic medical perspective, which is based on the research of Henry Bieler M.D., who was a practicing physician for more than 50 years.

1. The Digestive System

Health begins with good digestion. The inside of our digestive system, such as the small intestines, is extremely delicate and sensitive. The small intestine protects against the absorption of unnatural and detrimental food elements.[26] You may have seen those online advertisements for intestinal cleansing that claim, "you won't be-

lieve what's inside of you." When, after years and years of eating improper food and taking too many drugs or other substances, our body becomes unhealthy. Then the intestine stops working properly and the bacteria within it, which are meant to help us absorb and utilize our food, come out of balance. The result is an unhappy intestine. If we eat the wrong food, the intestines can get rid of it rapidly (diarrhea) or trap the food (constipation).[27] Diarrhea is your body's attempt to cleanse itself of unhealthy substances that have found their way into the intestine. Over time, eating modern foods destroys the protective mucous lining in the gut. Then, even healthy foods will be absorbed into the bloodstream too rapidly without complete breakdown and become toxic. This is what is known as leaky gut, and is the cause of many allergies and immune dysfunctions.

2. The Liver

Many cultures believe that the liver is the most important organ in the body. [28] The liver performs internal chemistry changes, cleanses poisons and stores fuel. [29] What people don't realize, writes Dr. Bieler, is that our liver hasn't changed for thousands of years, while our diet has.

With civilization came gradual changes. But man's liver didn't change. It remained the old pre-civilization model.[30]

When the liver gets overloaded and overburdened it can no longer clean up and purify the blood. Only then can disease occur.[31] Toxic substances normally cleaned up by the liver thus circulate freely throughout the body via the blood stream, creating an unhealthy environment.

3. The Endocrine Glands

Your glandular system is your body's third line of defense against disease. If the liver is unable to neutralize irritants and toxins entering the body, the endocrine glands kick in. The purpose of the endocrine glands is to secrete hormones, the chemical messengers in our bodies. Three important endocrine glands are the thyroid, pituitary and adrenal glands.

The adrenal glands *lie on top of the kidneys, and are the fire that allows the processes of life to occur.*

The thyroid gland *is at the base of the neck below the Adam's apple. The thyroid helps regulate the reparation of damaged or diseased body tissues; it regulates the heart beat, normal cell growth, and more.*[32]

The pituitary gland *is situated inside the skull at the base of the brain, located directly behind the eyeballs. Its special function is to trigger other members of the endocrine system to produce their particular hormones.*[33]

The pituitary gland has tiny receptors on it that constantly monitor the blood and its chemistry. If the liver begins failing to clean up all the toxic material in the body (including material waste produced through normal metabolic functions of living), signals are sent to the adrenal and thyroid glands. These glands then help eliminate the toxic material through backup mechanisms. The adrenals will direct elimination through the kidneys (urine) and bowels. An example of this type of elimination could be a bladder infection, swelling or bloating, or frequent thirst with urination. The thyroid will direct elimination through the skin and internal smooth membranes within the body; an example of this could be a cough, directing substances out of the body through the throat, or a rash, directing substances out through the skin.

In this short section I hope I can convey to you this perspective of Western medicine treating the symptom and not the disease. If someone has a skin rash, it is very likely the body's attempt to secrete toxic or irritating substances not processed and cleansed by the liver. This, by the way, is also what can cause acne—irritating substances in the blood being eliminated through the skin. If you put an ointment on the skin to stop the irritation you are not addressing the root of the problem, and quite possibly preventing the skin from excreting the toxic material that your body is trying to rid itself of.

The health of our glands, which regulate our entire body, is intimately connected to our emotional, mental, relational and spiritual health. A complex examination of this connection is not appropriate at the moment, but merely holding the concept that *all* of our body's processes are interconnected is an important part of understanding disease. If a part of our body is unhealthy, it is connected to different aspects of our life and personality, on different levels of our being and life experience.

Reclaim Your Health Responsibility

What do you want for your life and your children's lives? Do you want health or disease? Do you want responsibility or lack of responsibility? Usually, how we feel about our health is not totally in one direction or the other, but a mixture of different feelings and influences. That's okay; hardly anybody is 100% aligned with being healthy. If you really feel that excitement to be healthy, then just feel it, even say it, "Yes, yes, I want to be healthy! I want to be free!"

Being healthy is not just about making wise choices in the world. It is about coming into your true self; it is about being who you are. This is the force within us that heals. But it is you, with your active consciousness, who chooses to open the door to this greater reality. Let the love and peace enter your being, and you've made the first step towards reclaiming your responsibility towards health!

David Whyte's poem, "Sweet Darkness," invites us to embrace inner darkness as a path toward light and personal freedom. The poem reminds us that letting go of what is not really ourselves can be a good idea.

SWEET DARKNESS

When your eyes are tired
the world is tired also.

When your vision has gone
no part of the world can find you.

Time to go into the dark
where the night has eyes
to recognize its own.

There you can be sure
you are not beyond love.

The dark will be your home
tonight.

The night will give you a horizon
further than you can see.

You must learn one thing:
the world was made to be free in.

Give up all the other worlds
except the one to which you belong.

Sometimes it takes darkness and the sweet
confinement of your aloneness
to learn

anything or anyone
that does not bring you alive

is too small for you.

2

"Thy Food Shall Be Thy Remedy"

~ Hippocrates

Everyday, a majority of parents in the Western world contribute to the premature death and disease of their children. By unknowingly creating an unhealthy ecosystem in their bodies, they significantly increase the chances of having a difficult pregnancy, a complicated birth, and a child who is not fit for life.

In the previous chapter you learned a bit about what causes disease. Yet I left out a key element to the equation: nutrients. Western medicine has abandoned the premises of its own creator, Hippocrates, who believed that "food shall be thy medicine and medicine shall be thy food."

Intention: If we are to be healthy, we must know why we are sick. Take a moment and align yourself and your thoughts with all of the goodness the world has to offer you.

Improper Nutrition is the Cause of Physical Degenerative Diseases

The late Cleveland, Ohio dentist, Weston Andrew Price, sought an answer to one simple question: why do modern civilizations commonly suffer from dental cavities? In the 1930s, Dr. Price scoured the world to find an answer, and took some remarkable photographs along the way. Dr. Price's studies included the Indians in the far north of Canada, Aborigines of Aus-

tralia, Eskimos, Gaelics in the Outer Hebrides off the coast of Scotland, New Zealand Maori, Polynesians, Melanesians, Coastal and Mountain Indians in Peru, and several agricultural and herding tribes of Africa and central Africa.

Many groups of indigenous people Dr. Price visited exhibited nearly 100% immunity to tooth decay.[34] He also visited areas where the ancestors of the current inhabitants displayed freedom from decay while by contrast most of their modern descendants suffered from dental deformities.[35]

When the skulls of a group of 20,000 persons who were buried in a single valley were exhumed and examined, the teeth showed a remarkable freedom from decay, whereas the people living in that valley today have practically all suffered from dental caries and many of them in its most rampant form. Something has radically changed. [36]

Modern Diseases Were Unknown to Indigenous Groups

The most prevalent and most feared terminal diseases in our country are heart disease and cancer. Yet diseases such as these were nearly unknown and unheard of among indigenous groups living on their native diet. When Dr. Price visited Alaska, he interviewed the well-respected Dr. Joseph Romig, who was also the mayor of Anchorage.

> *[Dr. Joseph Romig] stated that in his thirty-six years of contact with these people he had **never seen a case of malignant disease** among the truly primitive Eskimos and Indians, although it frequently occurs when they become modernized. He found similarly that the acute surgical problems requiring operation on internal organs such as the gall bladder, kidney, stomach, and appendix do not tend to occur among the primitive, but are very common problems among the modernized Eskimos and Indians.[37] (Emphasis added.)*

The term "modernized" used by Dr. Price refers to a way of life that has broken from traditions of the past, characterized especially by a departure from living in harmony with nature — modern living conditions — and the use of the processed foods of commerce. While living the modern way, some native Eskimos became sick. But what happened if they returned to their "primitive" ways?

> *A great majority of the afflicted recover under the primitive type of living and nutrition.[38]*

Similar examples were found in other places Dr. Price visited. For example, isolated Indians in Canada did not have words for "rheumatism" or "arthritis" because these diseases were unknown to them. Yet:

> *At the point of contact with modern civilization where the only apparent important change has been the displacement of the native foods with the foods of modern commerce, I found arthritis and tuberculosis were common. In a group of twenty homes at Telegraph Creek and its vicinity I found ten bedridden cripples. Many of these cases were so hopelessly advanced that nothing could be done.[39]*

In the Torres Straight Islands off the North Coast of Australia, the 4,000 or so native inhabitants never had tumors requiring surgery. Meanwhile, in a group of just 300 white people living on the same island but eating imported modern foods, the local doctor had to perform several dozen surgeries to remove tumors.[40]

These anecdotal stories give us keen insight into something very important. People who don't follow our modern and "civilized" ways of living do not have our modern diseases. On the other hand, when groups of indigenous people changed their diets they developed modern diseases, regardless of their genetic heritage. And when, in the case of the Eskimos, they returned to their primitive diet, they usually recovered from these diseases. What we can conclude from this is if we are to reverse diseases, we need to return to a more primitive diet — the type of diet which our body is designed to eat. Keep this evidence in mind because I am going to apply it to pregnancy, birth and children's health. As we will soon see, diseases of pregnancy and childhood also come with our modern ways of living, so if we want to prevent them, or heal them, then returning to a more natural diet is an important key.

Why Explore The World To Find the Cause Of Cavities?

Dr. Price lost his only son, Donald, to the complications of an infected root canal that he had placed himself.[41] I am going to take a bit of a leap of assumption here and suggest that Dr. Price was driven by the pain of this loss to seek out the cure for tooth decay. This may explain the rigor and extensiveness of Dr. Price's research — that he traveled to the ends of the earth in order to prevent other parents from suffering that which he had to suffer. His work was an expression of a father's love for his son. I am sure that he spent every day of his life, even to the last, seeking every possible method to help people. May his longing to cure disease and his extensive energy for research be a role model of the type of positive motivation that you can bring towards the care and nurturing of yourself and your child-to-be.

Activity: Many other parents faced with the disease and deaths of their children have been motivated to seek cures and educate other parents. Find that part in yourself that would go to the ends of the earth to care for your child if she became gravely ill. Really feel this and imagine what it would be like. This is an immense and generally untapped well of love and compassion that is within each of us, and accessing it can bring a bit of grace into our world.

A Society without Doctors and Prisons!

In 1931 and 1932, Dr. Price, traveled to the remote Loetschental Valley in the Swiss Alps seeking the cause and solution to one of our most prevalent diseases, tooth decay.

To a high degree, the people of the Loetschental Valley lived in harmony with nature, which resulted in a seemingly peaceful existence. Dr. Price describes it eloquently:

> *They have neither physician nor dentist because they have so little need for them; they have neither policeman nor jail, because they have no need for them.* [42]

This harmony is also evident in the production of food.

> *While the cows spend the warm summer on the verdant knolls and wooded slopes near the glaciers and fields of perpetual snow, they have a period of high and rich productivity of milk... This cheese contains the natural butter fat and minerals of the splendid milk and is a virtual storehouse of life for the coming winter.* [43]

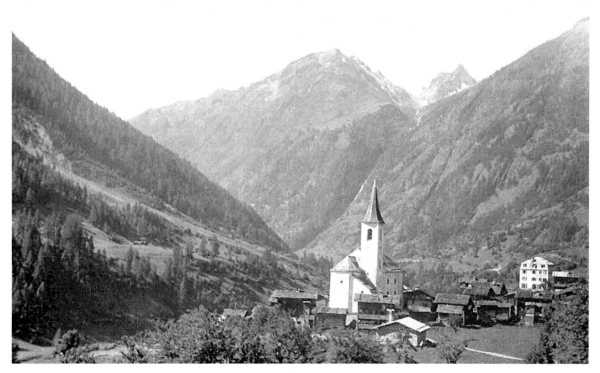

Beautiful Loetschental Valley about a mile above sea level. About two thousand Swiss live here. In 1932 no deaths had occurred from tuberculosis in the history of the valley. [44]

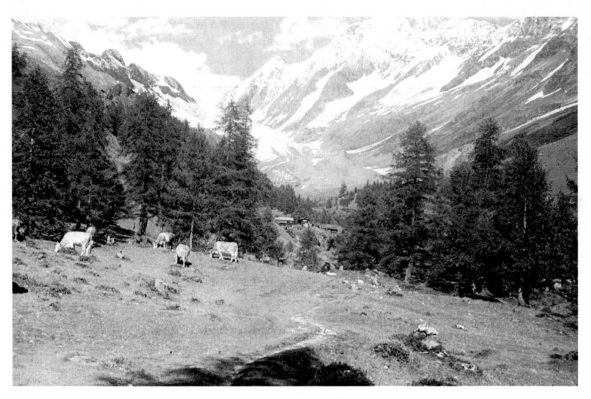

© Price-Pottenger Nutrition Foundation, www.ppnf.org
This shows the cows up near the glacier in the Loetschenthal Valley, Switzerland.[45]

The Presence Of the Divine Masculine (Yang) In Special Foods

Reverend John Siegen, the pastor of the one church in the Valley, tells Dr. Price about the butter from the grazing cattle, made in a high degree of harmony with the land and seasons.

He told me that they recognize the presence of Divinity in the life-giving qualities of the butter made in June when cows have arrived for pasturage near the glaciers. He gathers the people together to thank the kind Father for evidence of his Being in the life-giving qualities of butter and cheese when the cows eat the grass near the snow line... The natives of the valley are able to recognize the superior quality of their June butter, and, without knowing exactly why, pay it due homage.[46]

Does "His" presence in the food lead to a higher standard of living, wonders Dr. Price?

One immediately wonders if there is not something in the life-giving vitamins and minerals of the food that builds not only great physical structures within which their souls reside, but builds minds and hearts capable of a higher type of manhood in which the material values of life are made secondary to individual character.[47]

Sadly, the people of the Loetschental Valley, once isolated from the modern world, now suffer the same common problems faced by the rest of society. I have it on good word that they now have police officers and doctors, when just 70 years ago they didn't have them because they didn't need them.

Sturdy Swiss Children on Their Native Diets

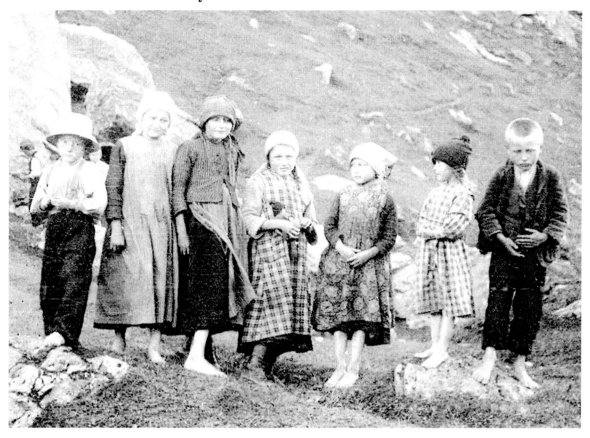

The nutrition of the people of the Loetschental Valley, particularly that of the growing boys and girls, consists largely of a slice of whole rye bread and a piece of the summer-made cheese (about as large as the slice of bread), which are eaten with fresh milk of goats or cows. Meat is eaten about once a week. In the light of our newer knowledge of activating substances, including vitamins, and the relative values of food for supplying minerals for body building, it is clear why they have healthy bodies and sound teeth. The average total fat-soluble activator and mineral intake of calcium and phosphorus of these children would far exceed that of the daily intake of the average American child. The sturdiness of the child life permits children to play and frolic bareheaded and barefooted even in water running down from the glacier in the late evening's chilly breezes, in weather that made us wear our overcoats and gloves and button our collars.[48]

The great Father, or the divine masculine energy of the Universe provides all his symbolic children (us) with great abundance. Through His presence in the butter and cheese, made in the sacred time of year when cows eat the rapidly growing grass, He gives us the gift of life, health, and vitality. I hope that you can begin to see the significant correlations here. A loss of connection with life; a loss of connection with the sacredness of being alive; a loss of connection with the earth and the environment that sustains us; all these lead to disease and suffering. The cause and effect are inseparable. Grassfed dairy products, especially from the time of new growth, are one of the key special foods missing in our modern diet.

Dental Arch

The dental arch is the curve along the row of the teeth. The plural term, dental arches, refers to both the top and bottom curved structures in which the teeth sit. Dr. Price visited residents in several Swiss villages sharing similar Alpine settings. However, in those villages whose inhabitants had abandoned their traditional diet, he found dental imperfections as illustrated in the photos above.

Modern Swiss Children Are Loosing Their Health

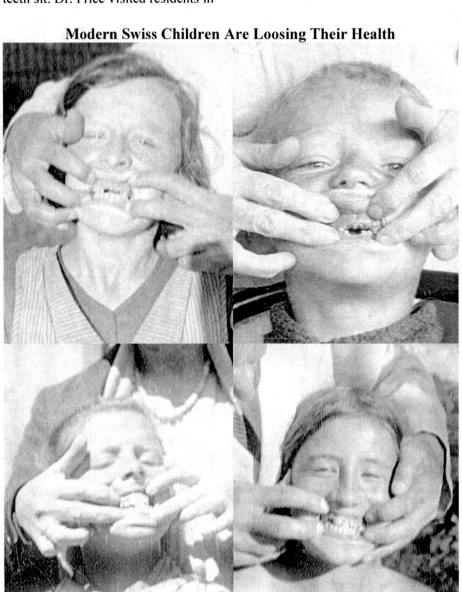

© Price-Pottenger Nutrition Foundation, www.ppnf.org

In the modernized districts of Switzerland tooth decay is rampant. The girl, upper left, is sixteen and the one to the right is younger. They use white bread and sweets liberally. The two children below have very badly formed dental arches with crowding of the teeth. This deformity is not due to heredity.[49]

*St. Moritz [one such typical village] is however, provided with modern nutrition consisting of an abundance of white-flour products, marmalades, jams, canned vegetables, confections, and fruits—all of which are transported to the district. Only a limited supply of vegetables is grown locally. We studied some children here whose parents retained their primitive methods of food selection, and **without exception those who were immune to dental caries were eating a distinctly different food from those with high susceptibility to dental caries.**[50] (Emphasis added.)*

Is Health the Result of Genetic Or Environmental Influences?

Cavities and other physical imbalances are the types of diseases that we are told to believe are based upon a genetic predisposition. And I think "told" is a good word to describe it. It's not an open discussion of facts; it is more of a presentation by the "authorities" of what they think we need to know. Yet Dr. Price's field studies give evidence to the contrary — that both cavities and other degenerative illnesses are primarily a result of our diet.

Dr. Price next visited the Outer Hebrides, rugged islands off the coast of Scotland in which people were still eating their native foods.

Two Brothers, One with Cavities, the Other without Cavities

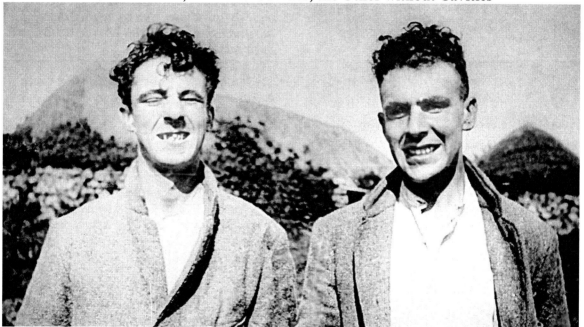

© *Price-Pottenger Nutrition Foundation, www.ppnf.org*

*We found a family on the opposite coast of the island where the two boys shown in the figure resided. One had excellent teeth and the other had rampant caries. These boys were brothers eating at the same table. The older boy, with excellent teeth, was still enjoying primitive food of oatmeal and oatcake and sea foods with some limited dairy products. The younger boy, seen to the left, had extensive tooth decay. Many teeth were missing including two in the front. He insisted on having white bread, jam, highly sweetened coffee and also sweet chocolates. **His father told me with deep concern how difficult it was for this boy to get up in the morning and go to work.**[51] (Emphasis Added.)*

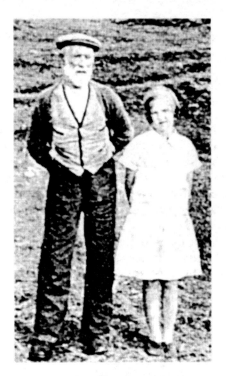

Healthy Grandfather, Unhealthy Granddaughter

The change in the two generations was illustrated by a little girl and her grandfather on the Isle of Skye. He was the product of the old régime, and about eighty years of age. He was carrying the harvest from the fields on his back when I stopped him to take his picture. He was typical of the stalwart product raised on the native foods. His granddaughter had pinched nostrils and narrowed face. Her dental arches were deformed and her teeth crowded. She was a mouth breather. She had the typical expression of the result of modernization after the parents had adopted the modern foods of commerce, and abandoned the oatcake, oatmeal porridge and sea foods. [52]

The Plague of Modernization

Dr. Price found that, time and time again, when "blighted by the touch of modern civilization,"[53] with our foods of commerce, the once robust native person "withers and dies."[54] Let's look at more examples of what our modern foods do to healthy and beautiful people.

The Aborigines - Living With Superb Health in the Harshest of Climates

*Over half of Australia has less than ten inches of rain a year. It is significant that **the natives have maintained a vigorous existence** in districts in which the white population which expelled them is unable to continue to live. **Among the white race there, the death rate approaches or exceeds the birth rate.**[55]*

*It is doubtful if many places in the world can demonstrate so great a contrast in physical development and perfection of body as that which exists between the primitive Aborigines of Australia who have been **the sole arbiters of their fate**, and those Aborigines who have been under the influence of the white man. The white man has deprived them of their original habitats and is now feeding them in reservations while using them as laborers in modern industrial pursuits.[56]*

*I have seldom, if ever, found **whites suffering so tragically** from evidence of physical degeneration, as expressed in tooth decay and change in facial form, as are the whites of eastern Australia. This has occurred on the very best of the land that these primitives formerly occupied and becomes at once a monument to the wisdom of the primitive Aborigines and **a signboard of warning to the modern civilization** that has supplanted them.[57] (Emphasis added.)*

A Cause for Alarm and a Warning to Modern Civilizations

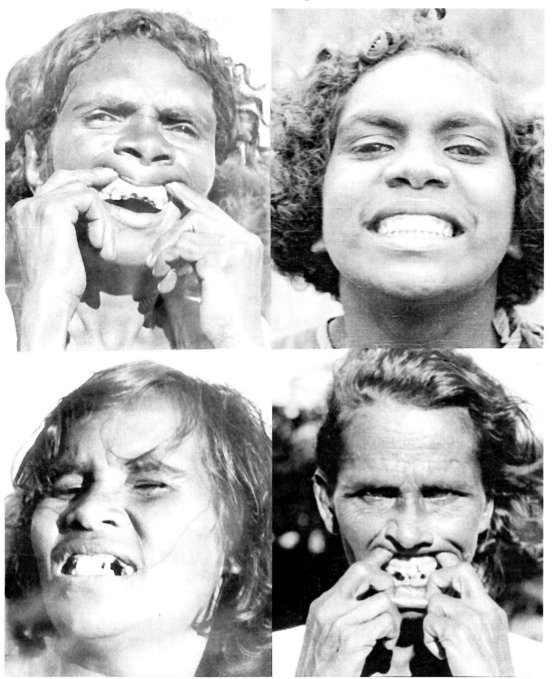

© Price-Pottenger Nutrition Foundation, www.ppnf.org

Wherever the primitive Aborigines have been placed in reservations and fed on the white man's foods of commerce dental caries has become rampant. This destroys their beauty, prevents mastication, and provides infection for seriously injuring their bodies. Note the contrast between the primitive woman in the upper right and the three modernized women. [58]

After Twenty Six Children, No Cavities

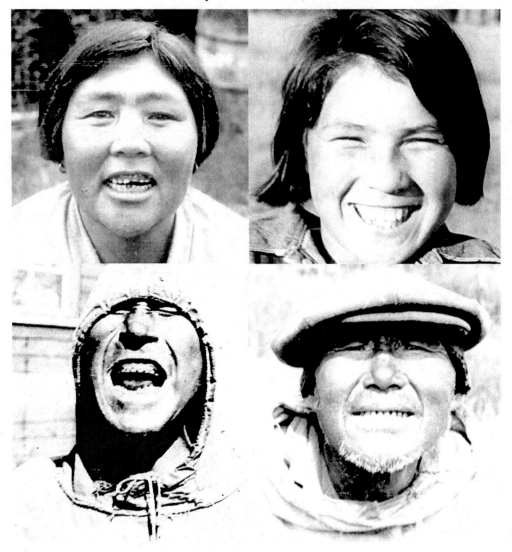

© Price-Pottenger Nutrition Foundation, www.ppnf.org
Typical native Alaskan Eskimos. Note the broad faces and broad arches and no dental caries (tooth decay). Upper left, woman has a broken lower tooth. She has had twenty-six children with no tooth decay. [59]

In the upper left is a picture of a healthy mother who ate the diet typical of Eskimos, which included salmon, caribou, berries and grass preserved in seal oil, organs of large animals of the sea, and layers of the skin of one species of whale.

In each example of native peoples from around the globe, the modern or displacing foods (foods that displaced the primitive diet followed for millennia) that cause the loss of pristine health are nearly identical. These modern foods included large amounts of white flour and sweeteners such as sugar, jams, and syrups, as well as sweetened goods and confections, canned fruits, canned vegetables, polished rice, tea, salt, chocolate, and vegetable fats with a relatively smaller amount of milk, eggs, or meat.

When Eskimos Changed Their Diet They Suffered From Cavities

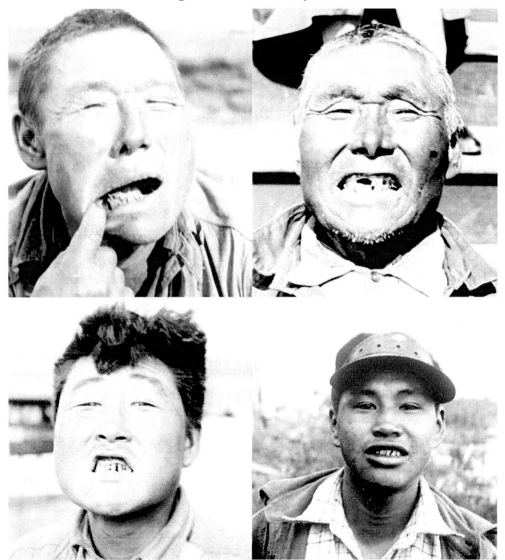

© Price-Pottenger Nutrition Foundation, www.ppnf.org

When the primitive Alaskan Eskimos obtain the white man's foods, dental caries become active. Pyorrhea also often becomes severe. In many districts dental service cannot be obtained and suffering is acute and prolonged.[60]

When these adult Eskimos exchange their foods for our modern foods, they often have very extensive tooth decay and suffer severely.[61]

The mouth is a window into the health of the body. It takes about a 25% imbalance of body chemistry to cause teeth to decay.[62] You might think that images of teeth don't have their place in a pregnancy and child raising book, but they do. The images demonstrate the collapse of the internal health of the body. What happens to the teeth is happening to the entire body.

Serving Others As One Would Wish To Be Served, the Aborigines of Australia

*Their code of ethics is built around the conception of a **powerful Supreme Force** that is related to the sun. They believe that there is an after-existence in which the myriads of stars represent the spirits of the Aborigines that lived before. The boys and girls are taught the names of the great characters that make up the different constellations. These were individuals **who had conquered all of the temptations of life** and had lived so completely **in the interest of others** that they had fulfilled the great motivating principle of their religion, which is **that life consists in serving others** as one would wish to be served.[63] (Emphasis added.)*

Loss of Facial Beauty When Encountering Modern Foods

People across the globe, following their native diets high in fat-soluble and water soluble vitamins (we'll discuss this more in part II), enjoyed vibrant health. In just one generation, after adopting modern foods, their children lost a great deal of their beauty and no longer had developed or fully formed faces. The loss of facial beauty is illustrated in the next images.

Intention: If you want to have beautiful children, with well-proportioned faces, it helps to understand what contributes to future generations *not* maintaining their health or beauty.

The following image shows the typical effects of modernization. On the top are two boys who are following their native diets. On the bottom left we see a boy who is suffering from improper facial bone growth due to his poor diet.

Once you begin to understand the poorly developed facial features that accompany our modern diet, you'll see that most of our modern society suffers from significant facial imbalances. The boys on the top have well-developed faces and wide dental arches. Their bodies are much like fully grown plants blossoming in the spring time, full of life and vitality. The dental arch represents the width of the bone that holds the top and bottom teeth. A wide dental arch represents full facial development and has space to fit all the teeth, even the wisdom teeth, which would come in straight and have lots of space. A narrow dental arch leads to crowded teeth. If you ask around, you'll see that a majority of us modern folks have crowded teeth requiring braces, and even the removal of the wisdom and other teeth. **This is not how our body was designed to develop. It is a result of an inherited defect** — inherited **not through our DNA but through the effects of eating food devoid of His presence, of life-giving substances.** The boy on the bottom left of the figure shows significant effects of modernization. He has a narrow and not fully developed face, a narrow dental arch and pinched nostrils. Pinched or narrow nostrils are common in our society. Yet these are not inherent in our DNA either, but are a result of our poor diet. This is like a plant that was not well cared for, withering in dry and impoverished soils, whose fruit are small and inedible. A modernized diet can also cause deficient bone growth, resulting in mouth breathing from incorrectly formed nasal passages. This, by the way, is a contributing or causal factor of snoring. With a modernized diet, as seen in this image, the middle third, and/or lower third of face has an irregular appearance; it can look elongated, compressed, or narrowed.

Affects of Modernization

Well Developed Facial Features From Native Diet

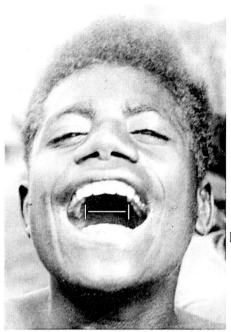

Middle third of face is wide and fully formed

Well developed jaw and lower third of face

Above: Wide dental arch indicated with white lines.

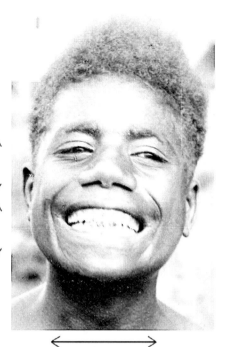

Above: Wide face and jaw.

Poorly Developed Features from Modern Diet

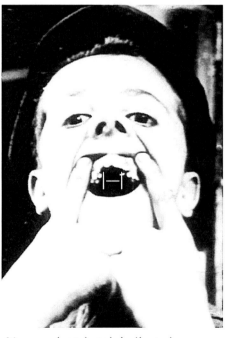

Middle third of face is narrow

Jaw is narrow, some compression of facial features

Narrow dental arch indicated with white lines.

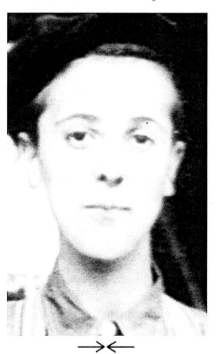

Narrow face and jaw.

Healthy Boys with Well-Proportioned Faces

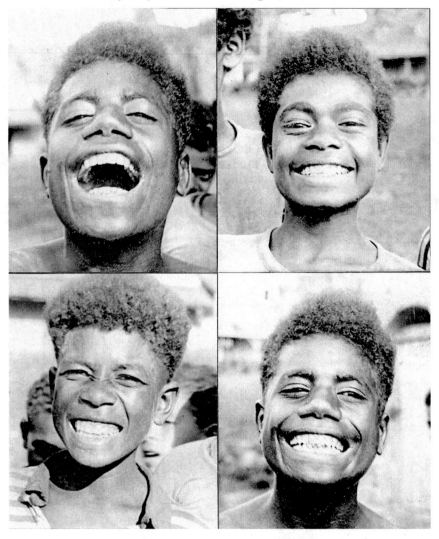

© Price-Pottenger Nutrition Foundation, www.ppnf.org

These four Melanesian boys born on different islands look like brothers but are not blood relations. They illustrate the role of heredity in reproducing racial type. Heredity, however, can only operate normally when the germ cells have not been injured.[64]

Let's look at a few more examples of lost facial beauty so you can really get the idea.

It is most remarkable and should be one of the most challenging facts that can come to our modern civilization that such primitive races as the Aborigines of Australia, have reproduced for generation after generation through many centuries—no one knows for how many thousands of years—without the development of a conspicuous number of irregularities of the dental arches. Yet, in the next generation after these people adopt the foods of the white man, a large percentage of the children developed irregularities of the dental arches with conspicuous facial deformities. The deformity patterns are similar to those seen in white civilizations.[65] *(Emphasis added.)*

Aboriginal Children Develop Facial Abnormalities

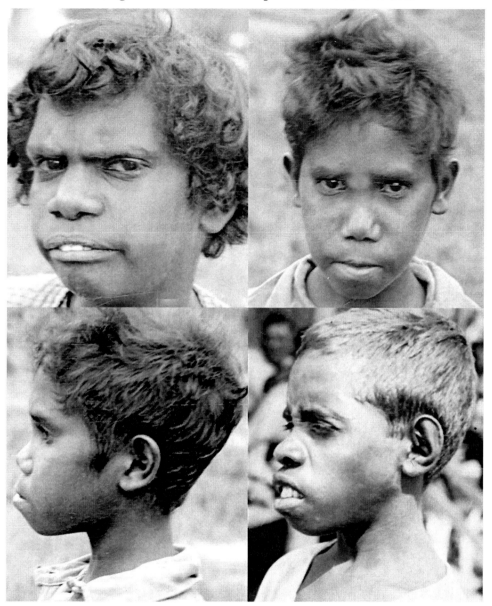

Deformity patterns produced in the modernized Aborigines of Australia by white men's food. Note the undershot mandible, upper left, the pinched nostrils and facial deformity of all four. [66]

Aboriginal children develop patterns of facial deformity similar to the white people, not because of a similarity in their genetic lineage, but because of a similarity in their modern food selection. One can probably correlate certain nutrient imbalances with certain types of ab-normal facial features. Imagine the hundreds of millions of dollars spent yearly on children's orthodontics (which are uncomfortable and rarely correct imbalanced facial features properly), when the problem could have been prevented with nutritional "orthodontics."

The Affects of Modernization are Independent of Genetic Heritage.

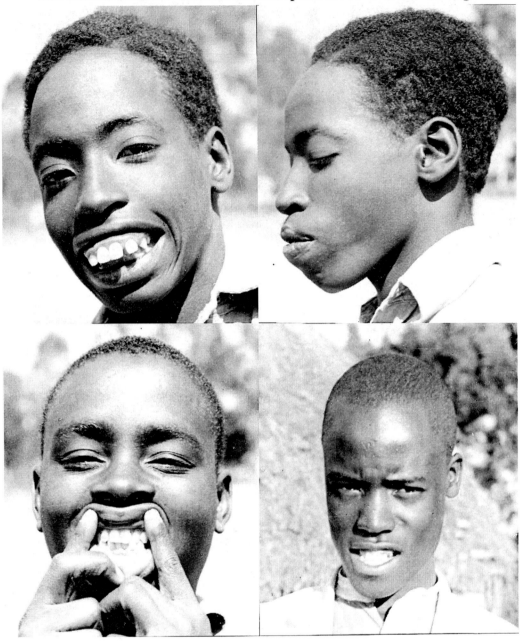

As in our civilization, even the first generation, after the adoption of modernized foods many show gross deformities. Note the extreme protrusion of the upper teeth with shortening of the lower jaw in the upper pictures and the marked narrowing with lengthening of the face in the lower views. The injury is not limited to the visible structures.

Modern White Children Have Lost Their Facial Beauty

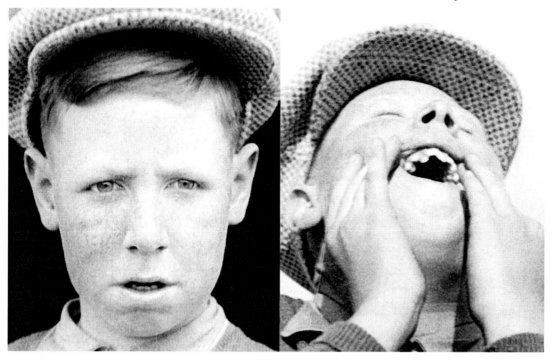

This white boy was born and raised in Alaska on imported foods. His facial deformity includes a lack of development of the air passages, so that he breathes through his mouth. Lack of bone development creates the crowded condition of the teeth. Note his narrow nostrils.[67]

Intercepted Heredity – Blocked Genetic Potential

The cases I have presented to you throughout this chapter are examples of *intercepted heredity.* Understanding the concept of intercepted heredity is a key to understanding health problems that occur frequently in pregnancy, birth, and in young children. The idea of intercepted heredity fits right in with the concept of personal responsibility for health — the idea that we are not "life's passive victim" to circumstances beyond our control. One of the stories taught in schools, reported on television and in newspapers, and upheld by the modern medical establishment is that the causes of important disease conditions like birth defects, miscarriages, or an unhealthy child are NOT KNOWN or, at best, are genetically predetermined. This is a belief system that discourages parents from assuming any responsibility for preventing these difficult conditions.

The truth is that the causes of these disease conditions are KNOWN and KNOWABLE. You will continue to gain in your understanding of intercepted heredity throughout the next two chapters. For now, I want to amplify a core belief that is resonating with me. The Creator— whoever you believe created humans and the earth, whoever created our DNA, whoever created the possibility of the male and female to unite and create children—clothed us in His/Her abundance. For now, let's call this Creator the great nurturing Mother, the divine feminine, and take a few moments to examine the Yin element. The divine feminine creative aspect of the Universe, which we all possess to some degree within us (just as we all possess aspects

Modern Eskimo Children Loose Their Beauty

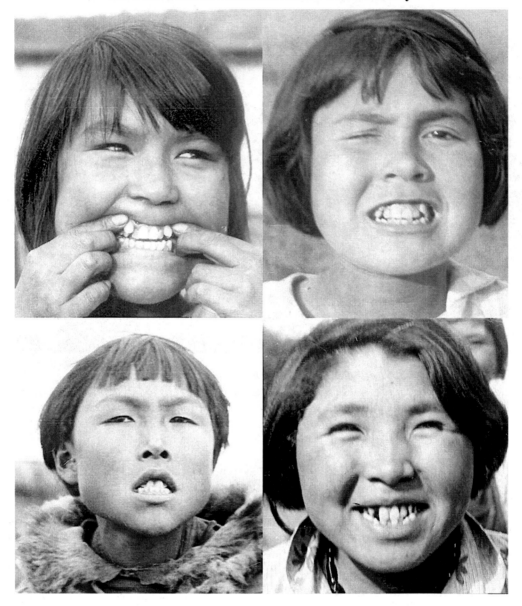

© *Price-Pottenger Nutrition Foundation, www.ppnf.org*

While dental arch deformities or crowded teeth are practically unknown among many of the primitive groups of Eskimos, they occur frequently in the first generation of children born after the parents have adopted the white man's foods. Note the narrow nostrils and changed facial form of these children. This is not due to thumb sucking.[68]

of the divine masculine), wants all of Her children to be healthy. She gave us, each and every one of us, a gift. This gift is stored within the map of our DNA as the potential for perfect health. And we can achieve this potential provided we fulfill the conditions laid forth in this map.

Pay careful attention to this because you may feel its ringing reverberations in your body and soul. She created us with the potential for perfection. Yet our society as a whole believes and has been compelled to believe that we were not made in Her glory, that we were born into a state of suffering in which She did not give us sound DNA. And as a result, we believe we have been cursed with poor health, or birth defects, or miscarriages, for example. Yet this belief, which is based on the concept that human beings are bad and sinful (which we are not) has compelled us to mistakenly blame forces, such as the creative aspects of the universe or the divine masculine and feminine, or a faulty throw of the genetic dice, for our problems. The reality — and this is the gem of intercepted heredity — is that WE are causing our problems. We <u>have not been forsaken</u>; rather, we have forsaken ourselves by forgetting our true place in the Garden of Eden. The Garden is the place of a real embodied feeling that we are loved and cared for by the great Mother and the great Father.

These photographs of Dr. Price are not merely images of what happens when our diet has gone wrong. They are proof that we can be masters of our world. They show us that we have hope for healing and redemption. We can return to our state of grace if we understand how WE have repudiated it and not the other way around. We were not thrown out of the Garden of Eden, represented by good health and a happy life, but rather, we have forgotten how to nurture and maintain that garden, which is a dormant potential within each one of us.

Now is a good time to remind you of a quote that perhaps did not make sense in chapter 1, from Nobel Prize-winning Dr. Albert V. Szent-Gyorgyi.

Should then, man be the only imperfect creature kept alive in the face of all his imperfections only by means created by his

own mind? If not, where do all these ailments come from? [69]

In other words, if the cell and biochemical construction in the human being is perfect, then what could possibly cause humans to suffer if not what is in our own minds? And now you can begin to see that disease and suffering, which we felt powerless to remedy, may very well be our own creations — the creations of our minds, our beliefs, and the results of our unconscious habits.

Here are two pictures that further illustrate intercepted heredity. Many more can be found in *Nutrition and Physical Degeneration* by Weston Price. Here we see how the children's facial health and development were not inherited from their fathers. These facial changes are due to a change in diet, and not due to a genetic flaw.

Can You Hike Carrying 300 pounds?

I was told that an average adult Eskimo man can carry one hundred pounds in each hand and one hundred pounds in his teeth with ease for a considerable distance. This illustrates the physical development of other parts of the body. [70]

Could you imagine how easy parenting would be if you were even half that strong?

Healthy Traits Not Inherited with Modern Diet

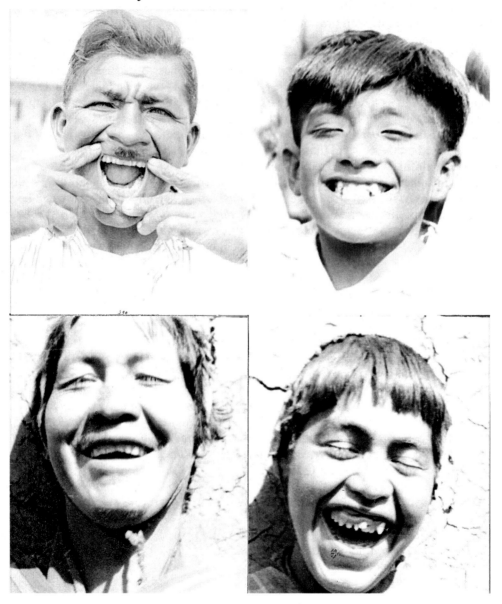

© Price-Pottenger Nutrition Foundation, www.ppnf.org

Above: *A father and son, pure-blooded Coastal Indians of the Chimu tribe of Peru. Even though the son is as pure-blooded as his father, the facial development is very different. Note the regularity of the teeth of the father and the marked deformity of the dental arches of the son. This is intercepted heredity in a single generation.*"[71]

Below: *We see a father and son, pure-blooded Indians of the High Andes. Note again the marked difference in facial design. The fathers in both these cases were the product of the native diets as used by their parents. The sons are the result of the change in diet of the parents from the native foods to the imported foods of commerce.*[72]

Healthy Bodies from Healthy Diets

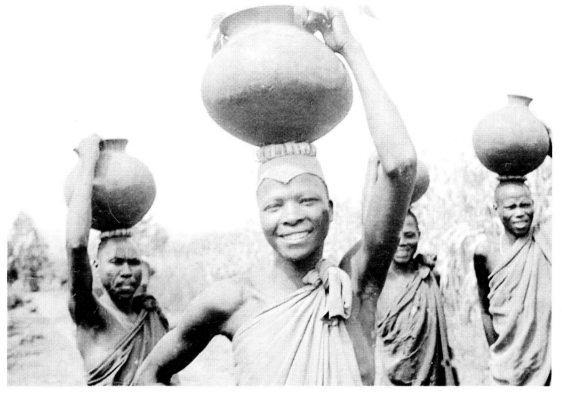

© Price-Pottenger Nutrition Foundation, www.ppnf.org

This illustrates the fine physiques of the women. They carry heavy loads on their heads with apparent ease. This jar with its water probably weights over 40 pounds. Splendidly illustrated here is the strength of their necks of carrying loads.[73] (Central Africa)

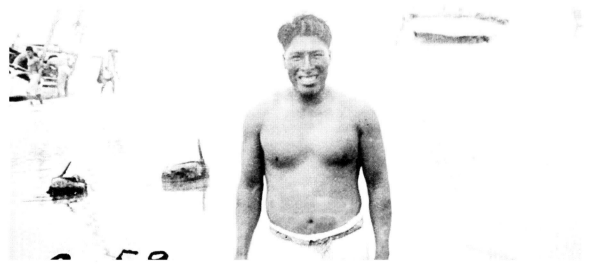

© Price-Pottenger Nutrition Foundation, www.ppnf.org

Note the magnificent physique of the man in the foreground.[74] (Coastal Indians, Peru)

Healthy Mothers and Healthy Babies

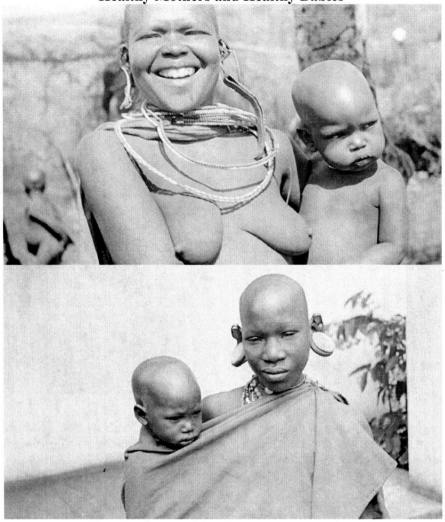

© Price-Pottenger Nutrition Foundation, www.ppnf.org

Above: *We see another splendid illustration of the wisdom of the primitives in the matter of preparation for motherhood by use of special foods. This young mother belongs to the Masai tribe in Central Africa. Their foods are dairy products, milk, meat and blood. In their more primitive condition girls are required to delay marriage until after the drought period in order that she may use the milk products produced after the cows are on the rapidly growing young grass following the rains. It is their belief and practice that by the use of fresh grass milk for three moons, they will prepare their bodies for marriage and reproduction.[75]*

Below: *Here we see a young mother and her child of the Kikuyu tribe. In this agricultural tribe, girls are required to eat special foods for six months before marriage, during which time they must not be required to do* ***hard*** *work.[76]*

By inference, one can assume that if a healthy diet creates a healthy facial structure and a healthy body, the result will be healthy mothers with healthy babies. Here are some images of healthy mothers with their children. See if you can feel or sense the bond between mother and child.

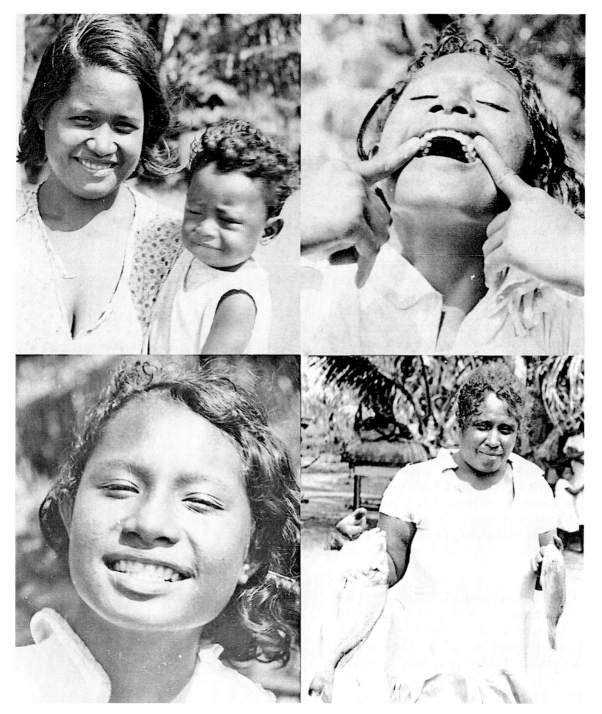

© *Price-Pottenger Nutrition Foundation, www.ppnf.org*

These pictures tell an interesting story. The grandmother shown in the lower right knew the importance of sea food for her children and grandchildren and did the fishing herself. Note the beautiful teeth and well formed faces of her daughters. [77] *(Torres Straight Islanders)* **The young mother shown here is free from tooth decay.** [78]

Are Happiness, Health, Disease and Lifestyle Connected?

Of the Torres Strait Islanders (seen on the opposite page) off the north coast of Australia, Dr. Price wrote:

> *It would be difficult to find a more happy and contented people than the primitives in the Torres Strait Islands as they lived **without contact** with modern civilization. Indeed, they seem to resent very acutely the modern intrusion. They not only have nearly perfect bodies, but an associated personality and character of a high degree of excellence. One is continually impressed with happiness, peace and health while in their congenial presence...Their home life reaches a very high ideal and among them there is practically no crime.* [79] *(Emphasis added.)*

After visiting the Aborigines confined in reservations Dr. Price wrote:

> *As we had found in some of the modernized islands of the Pacific, we discovered that here, too, **discouragement and a longing for death had taken the place of a joy in living in many**. Few souls in the world have experienced this discouragement and this longing to a greater degree.*[80] *(Emphasis added.)*

With the coming of the "white man," for lack of a better term, comes his plague. Beautiful and happy people, who once experienced the joy of living, have had their joy replaced with a longing to die. Clearly, there is a link between the type of food we are eating, the work we are doing, and our feelings towards life.

This longing for death and destruction is inherent in the modern way of living. Our modern culture seeks to exploit nature for a temporary profit and call it good.

With the coming of the *white man* comes his diseases. Let's examine further how our way of living affects our children.

3

Children's Disease
Our modernized ways cause diseases in our children's bodies

Nobody is more affected by our modern nutritional program than our children.

Intention: To learn the essential causes of childhood diseases, so that you can prevent them.

In the last chapter we saw examples of how improper facial growth affected children's beauty and ability to have all of their teeth fit into their mouths. Dr. Price, after his thorough research finds:

> *It is clear that a definite association of abnormal facial patterns with specific disease susceptibilities exists.*[81]

In other words, lost facial beauty in children is only the surface glimpse of a deeper problem. The outer appearances of children have changed due to unseen internal changes in their physiology. These changes increase susceptibility to disease. If you want a healthy child who is highly immune to disease, then they need to have a healthy internal biology, which will be evidenced through healthy and balanced facial proportions.

Modernized Native Populations Decimated

Along with the modern white man came his modern foods and a plague that blighted the existence of indigenous groups. In many groups Weston Price studied, he found societies dying out or being severely affected by tuberculosis, a disease that was only present after the introduction of modernized foods. Tuberculosis usually affects the lungs and can cause fever, chills, and a general weakness. It can spread throughout the body, particularly to the spine, and eventually cause death.

> *Due to susceptibility to tuberculosis and other diseases the average life span of the Eskimo of Alaska is only 20 years and their race is doomed to extinction within a few generations.*[82]

In a school with Eskimo children, even with highly trained dietitians and a medical ward filled with nurses, tuberculosis had taken the lives of 60% of its students.[83]

> *One of the sad stories of the Isle of Lewis has to do with the recent rapid progress of the white plague. The younger generation of the modernized part of the Isle of Lewis is not showing the same resistance to tuberculosis as their ancestors. Indeed a special hospital has been built at Stornoway for the rapidly increasing number of tubercular patients, particularly for girls between twenty and thirty years of age.*[84] *(Outer Hebrides, Scotland)*

Healthy and Modernized Gaelic Children

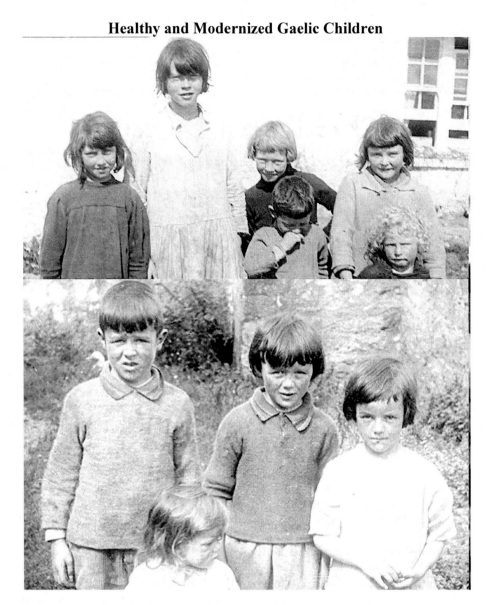

© Price-Pottenger Nutrition Foundation, www.ppnf.org

Above: *Typical rugged Gaelic children, Isle of Harris, living on oats and sea food. Note the breadth of the faces and nostrils. "An examination of the growing boys and girls disclosed the fact that only one tooth out of every hundred examined had ever been attacked by tooth decay. The general physical development of these children was excellent, as may be seen in the upper half of the figure. Note their broad faces."*

Below: *These Tarbert children had an incidence of 32.4 carious teeth out of every hundred teeth examined. The distance between these two points is not over ten miles and both have equal facilities for obtaining sea foods, being on the coast. Only the latter, however, has access to modern foods, since it supports a white bread bakery store with modern jams, marmalades, and other kinds of canned foods... The faces are so badly developed that all are mouth breathers because the air passages are too small to permit normal breathing. They have marked deformities of the dental arches and all have tooth decay.[85]*

Another example Dr. Price witnessed is on the Marquesan islands, about 750 miles northeast of Tahiti. This locale was once thought to be the Garden of Eden, a heavenly place on earth. In a group of seven islands the populations once numbered in the hundreds of thousands; that is, until the plague of modernization arrived.

Probably in few places in the world can so distressing a picture be seen today as is found there. A French government official told me that the native population had decreased to about two thousand, chiefly as a result of the ravages of tuberculosis... In the past some of the natives have had splendid physiques, fine countenances, and some of the women have had beautiful features. They are now a sick and dying primitive group. A trader ship

was in port exchanging white flour and sugar for their copra. They have largely ceased to depend on the sea for food. Tooth decay was rampant.[86]

Our modernized way of living has led to the destruction of indigenous populations throughout the globe. "In Tahiti a population of two hundred thousand had been reduced to less than eight thousand." [87]

Degenerative Diseases Were Found at the Point of Contact with "Modern" Civilization

In the following images we see the contrast between the Canadian Indian children of the forest, full of life and health, eating traditional foods, and the modernized Canadian Indian children eating modern foods of commerce.

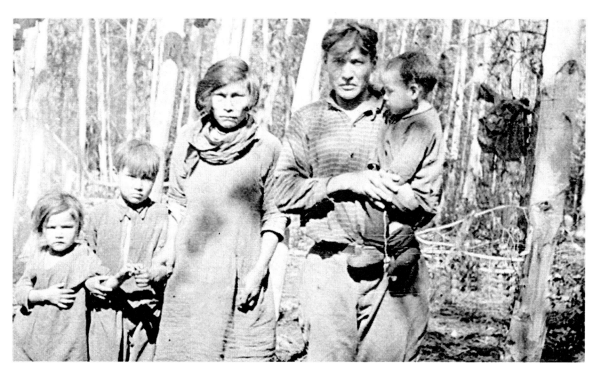

This typical family of forest Indians of Northern Canada presents a picture of superb health. They live amidst an abundance of food in the form of wild animal life in the shelter of the big timber. [88]

Modernized Child Dying of Tuberculosis

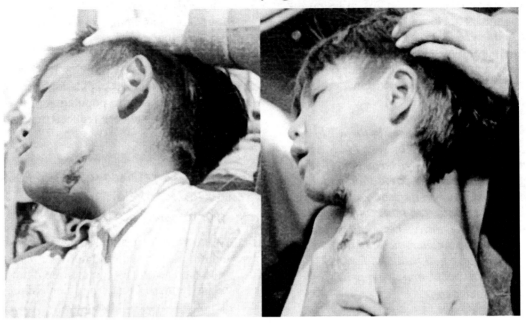

At the point of modernization including the use of the foods of modern commerce, the health problem of the Indians is very different. These modernized Indian children are dying of tuberculosis, which seldom kills the primitives.

In light of our awareness of disease as a response to a set of circumstances in the environment, what we are seeing in this image is vicarious elimination of toxic material through the skin and thyroid gland.

Dr. Price writes, angry at what he has seen:

> *Does our boasting civilization which is so ignorantly but so thoroughly accomplishing the extermination of the American primitives know how to produce as good bodies and maintain as good health and as high a resistance to disease as do the primitive Indians of the isolated interior? Unfortunately, the cost of modernization to the primitives is not limited to pulmonary form of tuberculosis. In the communities in contact with modern civilization the children were often found with suppurating tuberculous glands of the neck which for them was the beginning of almost certain progressive decline and ultimate death as the disease extended throughout the system.[89]*

Worse Than an Animal Imprisoned in a Cage

> *Many families were found in which several children were seen who were either bedridden or coughing. Another disease that was conspicuous there was arthritis. In the interior beyond the mountain range, where we studied the primitive Indians, we did not see a single case of arthritis. **At this point of contact,** however, at Telegraph Creek, we found ten bedridden, or nearly so, cripples with arthritis; several of the individuals were under twenty-five years of age.[90] (Emphasis added.)*

A careful inquiry reveals that Canadian Indians on their native diets did not suffer from arthritis.[91]

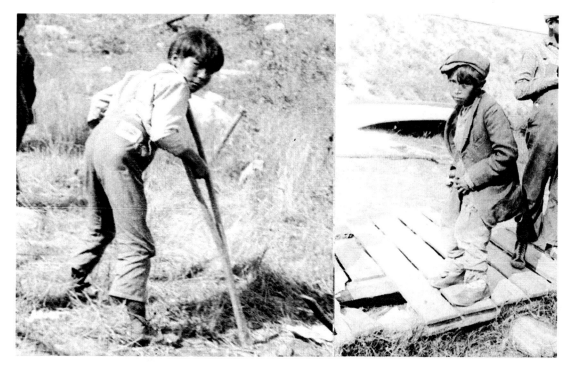

These are typical cripples met at the point of contact of our modern civilization with the primitive Indians. The boy at the left has arthritis in nearly all of his joints. He has several abscessed teeth. The boy at the right has tuberculosis of the spine.[92]

No animals taken from the wilds and placed in cages could suffer more intensely from enforced confinement than these boys and girls of the echoing mountains and multicolored valleys with their great stretches of timber and beckoning streams. One can never forget the pathetic appeal for help of these boys and girls who are progressively becoming crippled and who seem to sense their own doom.[93]

Again, degenerative diseases in Indian children only occurred at the point of contact with modern civilization.[94] In Ketchikan, Alaska the same diseases were commonplace:

In many of the homes individuals were ill with tuberculosis or arthritis. Tuberculosis had robbed many of the homes of one or more of its children.[95]

The modern diet of these children, and the parents of these children, consisted of a variety of foods provided by modern commerce. These included white flour, polished rice, canned goods, sugar, potatoes, syrup, jams, and many other sweets. Modernized diets will be examined more thoroughly in Chapter 5. Today, the symptoms of tuberculosis are less common. It is unclear what has happened to the disease, whether the symptoms are relabeled, or whether the same conditions now produce slightly different diseases, such as autism or juvenile diabetes. Another factor is that many times in the modern world today, our diet appears to be slightly better than the 100% modernized diets that caused significant disease. As a result, there seems to be a slight variation in the diseases produced from our modern lifestyle. But regardless of exactly how today's foods make people sick, the outcome remains the same. With our modern way of living comes disease, suffering, and even death for children.

On The Other Side of the Planet

On the other side of the planet, Aboriginal children suffer the same gruesome fate, due to their contact with the same modern civilization.

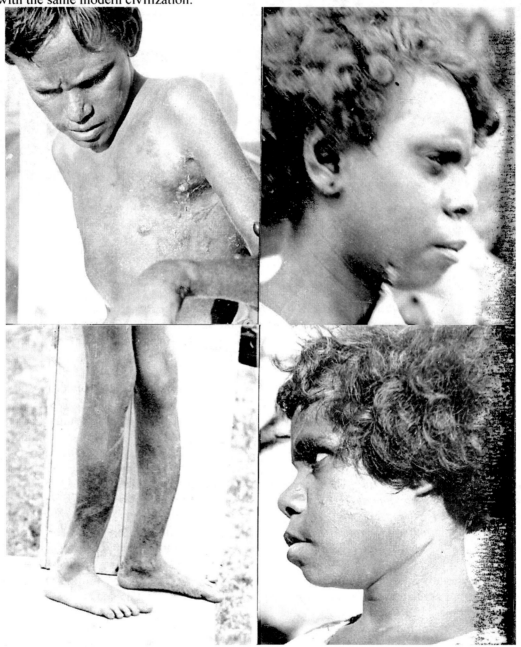

© Price-Pottenger Nutrition Foundation, www.ppnf.org

Aborigines in Australia living on a reservation. *The boy at the upper left has suppurating tubercular axillary glands. The girl at the upper right has pus running to the outside of her face from an abscessed tooth. The boy whose legs are shown at the lower left has a badly deformed body from malnutrition. The girl at the lower right has tubercular glands of the neck.*[96]

The Cruelty of Our "Civilized" Ways

*One can scarcely visualize, without observing it, the distress of a group of primitive people situated as these people are, compelled to live in a very restricted area, forced to live on food provided by the government, while they are conscious that if they could return to their normal habits of life they would regain their health and again enjoy life. Many individuals were seen with abscessing teeth. One girl with a fistula exuding pus on the outside of her face is shown in the upper right (**opposite page**).*

The Monkey with a Modern Diet

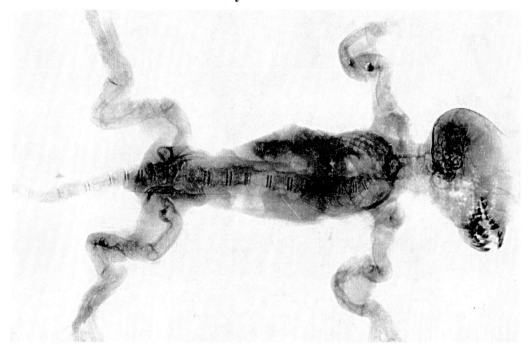

This problem of borrowing from the skeleton in times of stress may soften the bones so that they will be badly distorted. This is frequently seen as bow legs. An illustration of an extreme condition of bone softening by this process is shown, which is the skeleton of a monkey that was a house pet. It became very fond of sweets and was fed on white bread, sweetened jams, etc., as it ate at the same table with its mistress. Note that the bones became so soft that the pull of the muscles distorted them into all sorts of curves. Naturally its body and legs were seriously distorted.[97] An illustration of how the bones may be progressively softened by robbing them to make blood.[98]

In this x-ray photo, you see the badly pulled and twisted bones, softened by the monkey's diet of modern foods. This picture illustrates further evidence for the case against modern foods and provides a clue to why some children may have bow legs, or other misshapen features directly as a result of modern foods. A similar borrowing process is seen in the picture of the child's legs on the previous page, maldeveloped due to improper food intake. Dentist Melvin Page found that a key cause for the removal of minerals from the bones is an excess consumption of sugar. [99]

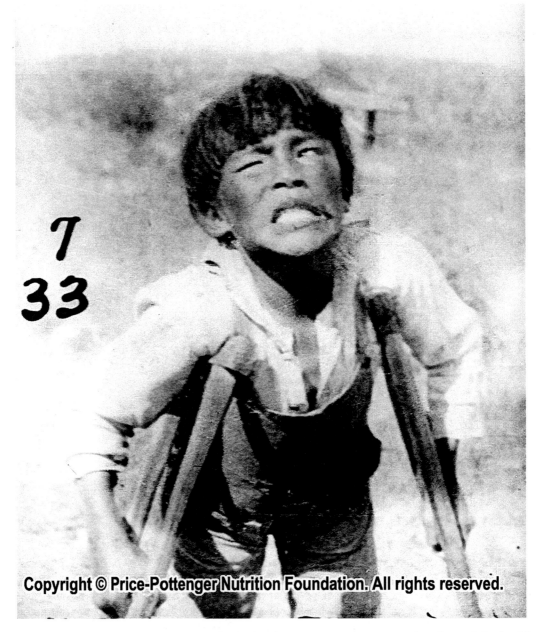

[O]ur bodies may be greatly injured by faulty food. Here we see a poor Indian boy of the far North living where the white man's foods were brought in to trade for furs of the trapping Indians. His bones were very badly injured and his teeth were decaying badly.[100] One can never forget the pathetic appeal for help of these boys and girls who are progressively becoming crippled and who seem to sense their doom like the young arthritic patient shown.[101]

You might think that these afflictions are a thing of the past. But children like this are just hidden away or their symptoms are treated temporarily with heavy doses of medications. A recent study by the Centers for Disease Control estimates the number of children in the U.S. with arthritis or similar conditions to be 294,000 under age 18 (or 1 in 250 children).[102]

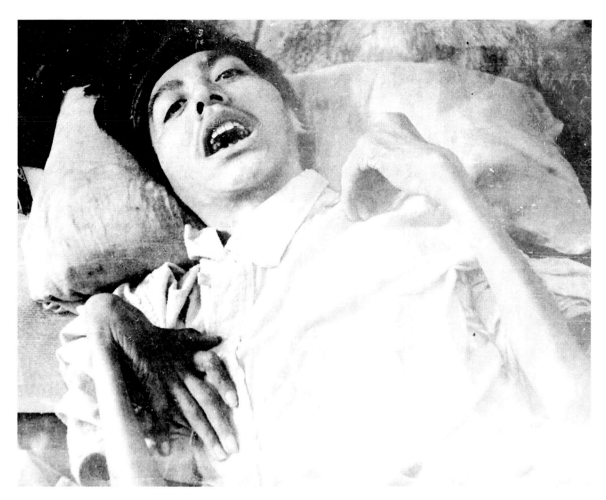

This Indian boy's dilemma is heartbreaking. He is physically helpless, is in terrible pain and cannot eat and was kept alive by an old Indian mother who fed and cared for him.[103]

*This young man's jaw is locked in the open position and note that his right hand has been distorted by the pull of the muscles so that the hand is folded back on the forearm. **The extremity of his suffering cannot readily be imagined.** [104] (Emphasis added.)*

I share with you Dr. Price's important images because this is the sort of suffering that we are inflicting upon our children. Perhaps the insidious effects of our lifestyle are not as grave and shocking as those seen in these pictures; yet nevertheless we are giving our children a diet and lifestyle that can cause grave diseases.

I once came upon a picture in a magazine of a modern girl in the United States suffering from a condition identical to the boy in the photo above. The magazine photo is now lost to me, but the girl was wasting away like this boy, with the same expression on her face and the same distorted joints. This disease is caused by an excess consumption of foods that wreak havoc on the body's blood chemistry, triggering a borrowing process that pulls minerals from the bones. At this point, the cause of this disease should be obvious to the reader, yet a majority of Western doctors remain oblivious to its cause.

A Sick Modern Child

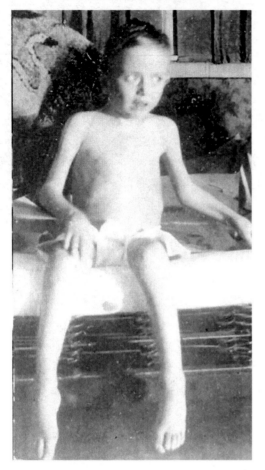

A mother asked my assistance in planning the nutritional program for her boy. She reported that he was five years of age and that he had been in bed in hospitals with rheumatic fever, arthritis and an acute heart involvement most of the time for the past two and a half years. She had been told that her boy would not recover, so severe were the complications. As is so generally the case with rheumatic fever and endocarditis, this boy was suffering from severe tooth decay... At this time the boy was so badly crippled with arthritis, in his swollen knees, wrists, and rigid spine, that he was bedfast and cried by the hour. His joints were still badly swollen and his spine so rigid that he could not rotate his head farther than shown in the picture. [105] *(This case is revisited in Chapter 14.)*

The Lesson to Be Learned

The lesson we should learn is that these primitive Indians living in that very inclement climate were able, before the advent of modern foods, to build superb bodies and that, in <u>even the first generation</u> after the arrival of modern foods, their children broke down with typical nutritional deficiency disease. [106] (Emphasis added.)

Every time you give your child commercial foods — ice cream, soda, cake, chocolate, fast foods, pizza, breakfast cereal, donuts — you are giving your child a dose of disease; a dose of suffering to come. This happens not just through the direct process of providing the wrong nutrition for our children; it happens before conception and during pregnancy, when mothers and fathers themselves unknowingly eat the wrong foods.

The Plague of Modernization

Our boasting civilization has failed to give our mothers and our children superb health. Even our advanced technology seems unable to replace living in harmony under Nature's exact laws. There seems to be not only a connection between physical health and vitality and the foods eaten, but also a sense of moral character in which the spirit of love, compassion and service to another takes priority over material values. When native people are introduced to "civilized" ways, diseases once unknown to them — tooth decay, tuberculosis, cancer and other diseases — become rampant.

Modern man, representing the collective consciousness and habits of the Western world, has imposed his ways and thus his suffering, on the many life forms of this planet. Modern man promotes a way of living that separates people from Life. The ego, that distorted consciousness, with its lust for power over everyone and everything, is given the highest priority. It is thus devoid of His and Her presence, which is filled with beauty and strength. The plague of the white man is not just a plague of the body; it is a plague of the spirit, where material values become primary to everything else. As Ch'I Po explained to the Yellow Emperor thousands of years ago, people have forgotten how to find contentment within themselves, and thus have to find fulfillment through the stimulating activities of the outer world. This disease, filled with destruction on all levels, is now destroying our planet.

In the United States, our "modern" civilization is founded on the massacre and exploitation of millions of native peoples, and the enslavement of millions more native people kidnapped from Africa. Isn't it blatantly obvious that there is something wrong with our society, with our culture, with our values, if we created our new world through murder and exploitation?

Yet, in the center of the heart of the steel pillars of our modern skyscrapers, and within the manufactured walls of the homes we live in; within the heart of the plastics, metals and composite materials that make our cars, computers, and weapons, lie the seeds of redemption. The divine, the formless consciousness that created life, is within everything. Many of us were born into this plague, this wrong way of living. Through honoring, accepting, and acknowledging the way we suffer internally, the suffering we now unconsciously impose on ourselves, on our children and on our planet, we can find our grace. We can rebuild the planet, and make it whole once again. The Garden of Eden is in the midst of us. We simply need to remove the weeds of the plague of modernization, and plant the seeds of love, redemption and grace. Let us begin this process of redemption in the place where we have both the most power, and the most responsibility: with ourselves and with our children.

Activity, Feel Your Feelings: If you've gotten to this point in the book — I cannot imagine that you are not feeling something now. This chapter has likely stirred something up in you. You may feel like the carpet has been pulled out from beneath your feet; maybe you've experienced the death of your old beliefs and assumptions, and so have a sense of disorientation. Whatever you are feeling right now, pause and pay attention to it. Don't change it, and if you have judgments towards it, notice the judgments

as well. Each time we acknowledge our feelings we are bringing ourselves closer to home. Through feeling your feelings you will again reach solid ground, where you can take effective action and find a safe way to be in the world.

The Fear of "The Plague"

One common fear that the popular media and entertainment industries like to perpetuate is the fear that a plague or some new superbug will come and wipe everyone off the face of the planet. Or at the very least, the plague will cause great suffering, great disease and numerous deaths. In the germ theory of disease, in which we are powerless to stop infection by diseases from the world around us, we have been taught that this plague will be a germ or a virus. News reports or stories about historic plagues randomly affecting the "powerless" disease victims are twisted and tainted with false knowledge that helps perpetuate the fear that you are powerless in the face of these viruses. Fear is never the ultimate truth. It is but a feeling that happens when a part of ourselves is blocked from the enlivening power moving through us. One way we experience the outer reflections of the feeling of separateness from life is fear.

But this scenario is far from the truth. The plague we fear is not a future event. It is the *white plague*, the plague of our modernized way of living. It causes war, creates disease and death as I have blatantly illustrated, and it scorches the beautiful earth. Everywhere, the modern medical man, the government, and almost everyone else is pointing his finger, blaming the world's problems on something or someone outside himself. Or, as our modern disease story goes, we cannot ever find the cause of _____ (insert disease name here). That is because the establishments searching — or *claiming* to be searching — for the cause of the disease are looking everywhere in the world, and somehow miss the real cause and source. Well, it is emanating from them and they are apart of it. We collectively and unconsciously choose as a society to be blind to the causes of our illnesses, because we don't want to feel the pain or see the decimation that we are causing. We are this plague; or at the least, we contribute in some ways to it.

The Failure of Modern Medicine

Modern medicine is the number one cause of death and disease in this country because it has become disconnected from its origins. Remember how the father of Western medicine, Hippocrates, said that our food is our remedy? Modern medicine ignores the causes of degenerative diseases because it is a part of the cause, it is a part of the plague of modernization in which we live. Most if not all degenerative diseases — commonly known as Alzheimer's disease, Lou Gehrig's disease, heart disease, cancer, atherosclerosis, diabetes, inflammatory bowel disease (IBD), Parkinson's disease, osteoarthritis, and osteoporosis — are both curable and preventable when we understand how we have created them through our ways of living.

A majority of infectious diseases are also not caused by viruses or bacteria, but rather take root in a weak and toxic body; they are created through the use of impoverished and toxic foods, and through exposures to other toxic elements. Some examples of modern infectious diseases that are created by our modern lifestyle include colds, influenza, tooth decay, respiratory infections, ear infections, AIDS, tuberculosis, polio, tetanus, meningitis, syphilis, and hepatitis B.

We have been locked into a disempowering belief system that encourages us to be victims to disease. And I say, "No more." Each mother and father, who stands up against disempowering beliefs by seeking real truths, helps end this disease-promoting system.

What Is The Root Cause Of the Plague?

If I merely told you about the plague that affects us — our modern lifestyle — that information would help you a bit. But I want you to know the root of this plague, so that you can uproot the entire weed. Without knowing the real source you are just hacking off the top, which will always grow back.

You have probably been touched in some way by seeing these pictures of suffering children. You are touched by this even though they are not directly connected to you, are not your own children. Because these children, like all children on the planet, truly are OUR children. When our children are mistreated it affects us deeply. That is why this book is called, "Healing OUR Children." When you find the similarities between your children and other children, you will see that their suffering, along with their happiness, is not just their own. It is a collective suffering. Likewise, by caring for and honoring your own children, you are caring for and honoring all children. This is the place of the unitive mind and consciousness, where there is no *mine* and no *yours*; there is only *ours*. By viewing other children's suffering with compassion, you help heal the real wound of the children suffering on this earth at the level that addresses the cause.

I touched upon the root of this suffering briefly by calling it the egoic mind. The root of this suffering is a false self or false personality that each one of us has. This false self is composed of our personal layers of thick and heavy clouds of distorted consciousness. You feel this part of yourself as anger, rage, pain, unhappiness, dissatisfaction and suffering. Nearly everyone on the planet has pieces of broken and trapped consciousness inside them. The best word to describe it would be pain or suffering. If you don't feel pain or suffering daily, in some way, then you probably feel the shell of it: numbness and indifference.

The pain within the human soul radiates and magnetizes with other people's pains, and in fact has literally created the world we live in — it even created birth and death. We can easily see the pain in the world, but usually have a difficult time acknowledging the pain within ourselves. This pain is caused by being separated from the source of life, the Creator. Separated consciousness can go by another name – evil.

Let's look at three evils which are a part of the plague of modernization. This evil is not just in the world around us; seek to identify it within yourself. What is within us not only defiles us, but defiles the world. It is our own separated and distorted consciousness that adds to the suffering on this planet. So if you wish to change the world, or make the world a better place for your child, then you will need to change yourself.

Michelle says: "There is a lot of beauty and a lot of ugliness in this world. Truths keep coming to us in waves. Yet we have walls around our hearts and armor insulating us. The waves of truths come, and we want to fight them off because we don't want to feel the pain of looking at the truth and seeing what is truly going on. But if you can endure the discomfort and feel the pain of others then it helps let your guard down. This is part of the process of becoming unified and not separate from others. The more we can look at our own negativity as individuals and work through it with help and guidance from sources of love the more we can influence the world. We can then create oases of beauty and tranquility. We can also choose to remain ignorant of the evil and darkness both outside and within. We can choose to remain as we are and nothing will change. The consequence of losing ourselves in this false contentment is that we do not experience true happiness. Our true nature is love and truth and it can look at darkness or evil with compassion and not feel harmed by it."

1. The Evil of Separation.

It takes a separated mind and separated feelings to do bad things to other people. One cannot do evil or destructive things to himself or others unless one feels this separation. Everything wrong in the world is earmarked by separation. Separation is a disconnection from the self; it is the feeling of being isolated from other living beings. Separation is like a child locked away in his room to be punished. In separation:

The perpetrator deludes himself to be unaffected from the further effects of his acts... The delusion of evil in the case of this first principle lies in the misperception that your brother's or sister's pain is not unavoidably also your own pain. On the contrary, the person filled with evil experiences excitement and pleasure when wringing havoc, destruction, suffering, and pain. [107]

In the many examples given, the modern and "civilized world" spreads its destruction to the world of primitive and isolated people. Since we are a part of the modern world, we may have inherited the tendency to experience excitement from watching others suffer. Perhaps this explains our addiction to tragic television stories and violent movies, as it helps the evil in us live.

Activity: Look at yourself and see if you feel compassion when you witness suffering, or if you feel excitement and pleasure? If there is excitement or pleasure, try not to judge it, but make a space for that root of darkness, the energy that feeds on negative excitement, to show itself.

2. The Evil of Materialism.

I am sure you are familiar with the phrase, "Money is the root of all evil." While that's not exactly the whole story, since right now most of us need money to exist and also to do good things in the world, it is close. A more accurate statement might be, "Materialism is a key root of evil."

Materialism is a lifeless realm absent of all vitality. As technology has improved, we have come to value the physical form in a way that is mechanical, such that we have lost touch with our inner vibrant being. We exist disconnected from the enlivening force of the Universe; and it is as if human beings have become machines living in an alienated reality, distant from life. In turn, we make the world lifeless by ripping out trees and pouring concrete on top of the soil. Then, because of the unbearable feeling of separation, we fill the world with objects of desire, with inventions and gadgets. And while those things are entertaining and interesting and even occasionally have some purpose, they cannot replace the true experience of living. We have become merged with our technology. People seeking fun through playing video games is a good example of this. The person playing the video game identifies with the hero in the game, and becomes merged with him or her — becoming more disconnected from their own true self in the process. Occasionally, video games or television watching can be an acceptable diversion, but as a lifestyle it is out of balance.

Activity: Look within yourself. Where do you feel lifeless? You might notice that you feel an inner emptiness that you might try to fill with material objects, food or entertainment. What is that emptiness? Why is it there? What is its purpose? Observe and notice.

3. The Evil of Half-Truth and Distorted Truth

This is perhaps my "favorite" evil, because I hope to squash this evil with my writing and sharing with others. A half-truth is a truth that has been layered with falsehoods for the purpose of creating confusion. The people in charge of disseminating information about our health or about the environment, people with sinister motives, are masters at the half-truth. They leave everybody confused or unsure about themselves. The half-truth:

> ...is the principle of confusion, distortion, half-truth, lie, and all the variations that may possibly exist in connection with it. It includes using truth where it does not belong, is not applicable, so that the truth subtly turns into a lie, yet cannot easily be traced as such because the divine truth is pronounced and seems unassailable per se. Thus confusion is wrought.[108]

A half-truth may be used to make a mere belief appear as real scientific knowledge, as incontrovertible fact. This is the concept of "balanced neutrality," and is one of the most insidious forms of the half-truth in our culture today. We are taught to believe that the Western medical paradigm represents a neutral and non-biased view of our health. We are taught to believe that newspapers and the news media present a neutral perspective, as if they were mere objective observers of the events. This is false neutrality that lulls us into submission. It is difficult to recognize outer world truth when we are given these white-washed "neutral" perspectives. It is important, however, to realize that half-truths and their variations also exist within us. A half or false truth occurs internally, for example, when we lie to ourselves or to another person in a subtle way for the purpose of deceiving ourselves about our real feelings, and thus hiding the real motives behind our behaviors. It may be fun to point fingers at all the half-truths and lies in the world, but how about looking for the ways we deceive ourselves? A half-truth can be those little lies we tell ourselves in order to keep things internally consistent. We make up stories to ourselves to justify our idiosyncrasies and contradictions.

Activity: Throughout your day, keep a watchful eye for when you tell yourself or someone else a story that is not exactly the full honest truth. Deception of self and others is an evil principle and keeps us from knowing ourselves, and from being in the world in a healthy way.

Modernization & Children's Health

We have examined the tragic manifestations of wrong nutrition — the diseases of childhood. While we tend to blame genetics for these problems, or believe the claim that the causes are unknown, I have shown evidence that these problems are indeed the ravages of modern civilized living, and primarily of the modern diet. Improper nutrition does not just cause disease; it makes our children less fit for life. At the very least, improper nutrition inhibits the natural formation of children's bones and muscles; it leads to narrow breathing passage ways, poor posture, crooked spines, swollen joints, weak organs, lowered intelligence, disturbed facial features and many other subtle and overt deficiencies. In the more severe cases, modern food and other modern habits cause severe suffering and disability, and an early and painful death in childhood.

No matter what your genetic heritage, no matter how fine your blood lines, your children's bodies will still break down under improper nutrition; it is merely a matter of time. Literally, we bear many of our children into a world that will be filled with their physical suffering. Unless we begin to seriously look at ourselves and the way we live, this will continue to happen; and the predicament will only get worse until we are forced to give up the insanity of our ways. Or like the Marquesans, who once lived in pristine health in a paradise on earth but who are now gone, we will die out.

4

The Origin of Many Birth Defects

The mainstream thought pattern claims to be ignorant of the cause of most birth defects. Without knowing their cause, we are powerless to prevent them.

Intention: To learn a real cause of birth defects so we can prevent them.

The cause of birth defects is not a mysterious secret and in fact is even understood by some perceptive doctors in other countries. For example, Foresight, the association for the promotion of preconceptual care in England, has worked with high risk couples over a period of ten years, and has been able to reduce the rate of birth defects in that group to 0.47%.[109] Compare this figure to the national average for birth defects in England of 6%. That is over a 1200% reduction in the rate of birth defects. If doctors can do it in England, shouldn't it be front page news here? The headline would shout "Birth Defects Are Preventable!" You can download free preconception resources at Foresight's website, **www.foresight-preconception.org.uk**.

It is now commonly accepted that pregnant women must have sufficient dietary folic acid in order to help prevent the birth defect of spina bifida in their babies. As with this straightforward example of cause and effect, so it is true with most other birth defects: **a lack of nutrients or the presence of toxic substances in the sperm, the egg, or the mother's body can produce a birth defect.**

A recently released report from the US Centers for Disease Control states that:

Major structural or genetic birth defects affect approximately 3% of births in the United States, are a major contributor to infant mortality, and result in billions of dollars in costs for care...<u>The causes of most major birth defects are unknown.</u>[110] (Emphasis added.)

With approximately 4 million babies born in the U.S. every year, about 120,000 of those children will suffer from serious birth defects. The infant mortality rate is the number of infants who die before the age of one; and in this country that number is 6.3 deaths per 1,000 live births,[111] or about 24,000 infants per year. Most infant deaths occur within the first four weeks of life. Think about those figures — they are staggering. When one child dies or is born with a serious problem, it causes great sorrow in the family. Now, multiply that single loss by thousands and you can see the tragic results of our modern lifestyle.

Birth Defects and "Modern" Civilization

If you reflect on Nature's plan for a moment you will see that she doesn't want any of her children to suffer from any type of physical disease. Disease is equated with failure to thrive and failure to survive. If Nature had designed humans or animals to suffer from disease, then we couldn't have survived as a species for so long. Nature naturally selected out genetic defects millions of years ago; that's why most people are born without noticeable defects. The modern theory of birth defects, including problems related to childbirth, places significant blame on genetics, which is something that is supposedly beyond our control. In light of that narrow assessment, let's reflect on these words of far-seeing warning from Dr. Price, recorded after he visited Australian Aborigines living in desperate conditions and confined to reservations:

The rapid degeneration of the Australian Aborigines after the adoption of the government's modern foods provides a demonstration that should be infinitely more convincing than animal experimentation. It should be a matter not only of concern but **deep alarm that human beings can degenerate physically so rapidly** *by the use of a certain type of nutrition, particularly the dietary products used so generally by modern civilization.* [112] *(Emphasis added.)*

If you are willing to accept the fact that our bodies can quickly degenerate from a poor diet, would you be willing to take one small step further and consider the effects this malnourishment would have on reproductive health? The symptoms of physical degeneration could easily include deteriorated sperm of the father and the egg of the mother. What can be reasonably expected when life begins from unsound building materials? After conception and as the fetus begins to grow, the mother's body lacks certain nutrients as a result of a poor diet, and this deficiency is passed onto the growing child; this could result in an improperly formed baby — in other words, a birth defect

The Indians of the Amazon

...share the belief of many peoples of the lower cultures that food eaten by the parents – to some degree of both parents - will have a definite influence upon the birth, appearance, or character of the child. [113] *(Emphasis added.)*

With the coming of the "white man" and his modern ways, came birth defects. Birth defects became prevalent in several healthy indigenous groups after the introduction of modern foods. [114]

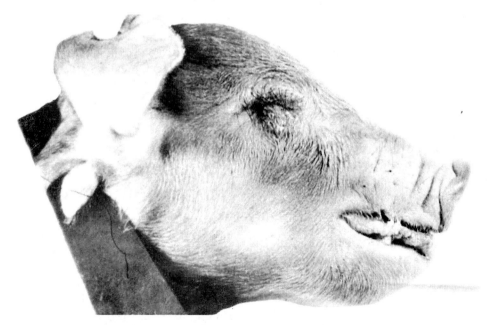

Above, this pig was one of fifty-nine born without eyeballs and with other serious deformities due to lack of vitamin A in the mother's diet. Offspring of these blind pigs when normally fed had perfect eyes and no deformities. [115]

Birth Defects from Nutrient Deficiencies

Let's first clarify what is meant by a birth defect. One of the most common is a cleft palate or cleft lip; this is when the lip or the surrounding tissue doesn't form properly or completely. Spina bifida is when the spinal bones do not fully grow around the spinal cord. Heart defects include problems like holes in the walls of the heart or malformed valves. There is a pattern to these defects. Almost every one is the result of tissue not forming fully. If improper nutrition during childhood causes malformations in the child's bone structure (and tendencies for diseases), then we might expect the same deficiencies to affect the environment of the womb and the health of the growing fetus. To put it simply, a majority of birth defects are the result of a lack of essential nutrients needed for proper development of the growing child.

I wish I didn't have to show these unpleasant images; but seeing is believing. The pig shown in the picture was born without eyes. This condition was not the result of a genetic aberration. It was induced artificially as part of an experiment by depriving this pig's mother of vitamin A. In the next chapter we'll explore how most modern mothers also lack sufficient vitamin A in their diet. When this pig and several others like it were given a diet that included adequate vitamin A, their subsequent offspring were born with healthy eyes. This demonstrates one example of a birth defect that is not hereditary in the sense of genetics, but hereditary in the sense of an inherited nutrient deficiency, in which the substance needed to build the eyes (vitamin A) was absent. This is where Nature's plan for success was *intercepted*. Again, Nature did not make the body of this pig imperfect. Rather, by being deprived of certain essential nutrients for fetal development, the pig developed imperfectly.

Fat-Soluble Vitamin A and Birth Defects

Deficiencies in vitamin A in these pig experiments led to defects in the snout, dental arches, eyes, feet (such as clubbed feet), and displaced kidneys, ovaries or testes. A lack of vitamin A produced extreme incoordination, spasms and paralysis. It also led to aborted and stillborn pigs.[116] In cattle, vitamin A deficiencies produced the birth of dead or weak calves and led to sterility in females.[117] Researchers were able to produce varying severities of birth defects based upon how much vitamin A they supplied in the mother's diet. The less vitamin A supplied, the more severe the birth defects. Again, in several experiments and variations, the pigs with defects had healthy offspring when vitamin A was restored to the diet.[118]

Modern science has now more accurately shown that a vitamin A deficiency in women can cause birth defects in the heart, central nervous system, the circulatory, urogenital and respiratory systems, and the improper development of the skull, skeleton and limbs.[119] Vitamin A is found in grass-fed liver, raw grass-fed butter, wild-caught seafood, farm-raised egg yolks, and raw grass-fed milk. This preformed and easily assimilated vitamin A is different from and yet complementary to the carotenes found in vegetables like carrots that the body can partially convert into vitamin A in some circumstances.

Birth Defects from the Father

Dr. Price was keen to point out that the father also plays a role in the child's susceptibility to birth defects. He gave an example of a male dog deprived of nutrients. This dog produced pups with birth defects with five different healthy female dogs. [120]

It is well known and accepted that birth defects can be caused by the father being exposed to certain chemicals. (We'll look at some of these chemicals in chapter 7.)

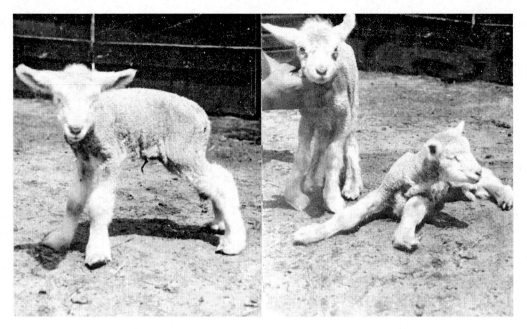

Many young of modern domestic animals are born with deformities...two blind lambs and one with club foot. [121] *The animals pictured above are not eating their native diet. Deformities in domestic animals are common, due to food substitutes.*

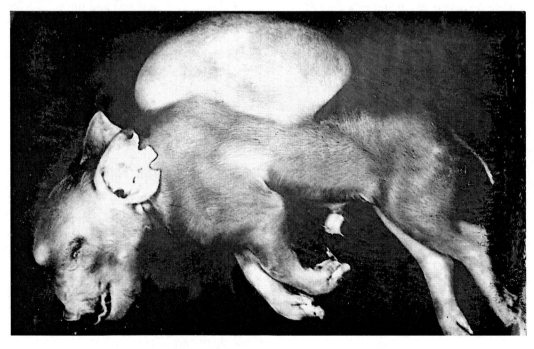

Pig has club feet, deformities of the ears, two tumors and no eyeballs due to lack of adequate vitamin A in the mother's diet. [122]

Miscarriage, Birth Defects and Our Modern Diet

A large percentage of naturally aborted fetuses are malformed.[123] Medical doctor Henry Bieler believed that miscarriages were caused by assaulting the body with toxic foods;[124] in other words, that miscarriage was caused by modern processed foods of commerce. A miscarriage is really a survival mechanism of the body. The fetus is no longer viable and becomes poisonous to the body, so the body expels it.

There is a significant correlation between deformed fetuses and miscarriages. Like the case of the pig in the (opposite page) image, the fetus may be deformed due to a lack of vitamins, in this case vitamin A. Lacking nutrients, the underdeveloped fetus dies, and the resulting miscarriage is the body's need to release it. A vitamin deficiency, therefore,

was most likely the cause of the miscarriage. Many sources indicate that the prevalence of miscarriage in the United States is around 25%. The number is difficult to track because many occur in the first few weeks of pregnancy.

Example of Preventing Miscarriage

Dr. Henry Bieler wrote of a patient who had seven miscarriages, each of which had occurred when she was seven months pregnant. [125] The patient looked pale, had swollen legs and frequent and intense headaches. He noticed that her hands showed a thick, red, scaly eczema. He associated the eczema with sugar poisoning, and thus the reason for her miscarriages was explained. Dr. Bieler put her on a sugar-free diet and she soon delivered a full term baby boy! [126]

Birth Defects in Humans from Modern Foods

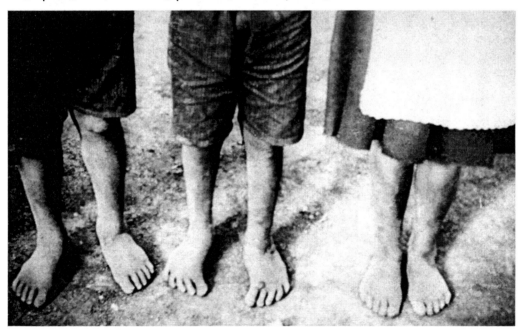

© Price-Pottenger Nutrition Foundation, www.ppnf.org

Three Maori children of New Zealand; the second child is smaller in stature than the third and gives more evidence of facial injury. While his older sister and younger brother have normal feet, his quite severe disturbance in facial growth is associated with club feet.[127] The same children are seen on the next page.

Same Three Maori Children, Full View

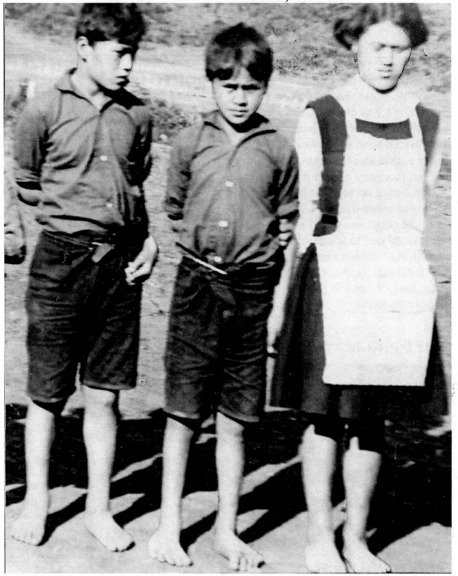

New Zealand Maori. Note the marked undersize of the second child and underdevelopment of the face associated with marked deformity of the feet.[128]

The children in this Maori family are lined up from eldest to youngest. The second oldest child is much smaller than his younger brother. Dr. Price explains:

> *The history of this family showed that the first and third children were produced when the parents lived near the sea in New Zealand. The second, the [club-footed] child, was developed when they moved inland and were living on the foods of commerce.*[129]

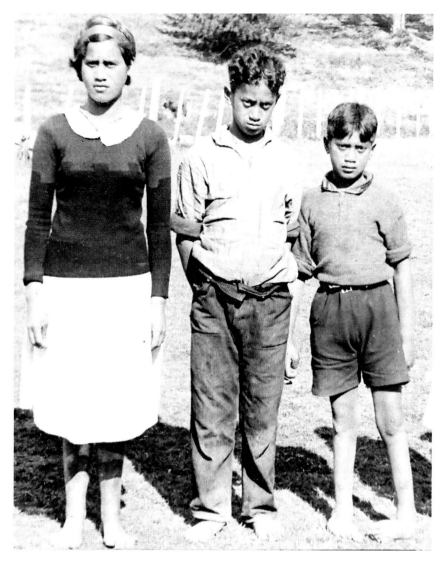

© Price-Pottenger Nutrition Foundation, www.ppnf.org
New Zealand Maori. Note the progressive change in facial form of the two younger boys as compared with their older sister. Then note the progressive change in their feet. Normal feet, flat feet, and club feet.[130] (Not Shown – When this family returned to their native diet, they had two healthy children without any defects.)

It would be remarkable if these disturbances in the physical pattern were limited to the face and dental arches. An illustration of other deficiency injuries is shown, which shows three children in a modernized Maori family. It will be seen that while the oldest girl has the typical Maori racial pattern of face, there is a marked lack of development of the middle third of the face, with

progressive severity of distortion in her two younger brothers. On observing the feet it will be seen that she has splendidly formed feet while the second child has flat feet, and the third child has clubbed feet.[131]

This image is an example of a progressive vitamin deficiency. Over time the mother's and father's bodies become depleted due to their use of modern foods. As a result, like the experiments with the pigs, the severity of the defects increases with the severity of the deficiency of essential vitamins.

Flat Feet

I always wondered why I had flat feet. I thought there was something wrong with me. In high school my feet would hurt often when other people's feet did not hurt. When I saw these pictures and several others like them in *Nutrition and Physical Degeneration* by Weston Price, the cause of flat feet became obvious to me: poor nutrition in the womb and during the growing years.

Birth Defects a Response to the Environment

I have given you several examples of the same birth defects (clubbed feet) being caused by essentially the same thing: deficiencies in the diet. Birth defects can also occur when the mother's or father's seeds for life are toxic, again due to toxic foods like white sugar and other processed sugars, and to exposure to other disharmonious substances like pesticides or heavy metals. It is widely accepted that a lack of folic acid in the mother's diet produces certain birth defects in her child. This understanding ought naturally to be expanded to conclude that vitamin deficiencies are a cause of most or all birth defects. I have demonstrated in previous chapters how the coming of the modern man to remote areas brought disease to native peoples, and how the modern diet brought physical imbalances such as poor formation of the teeth and facial structure. The case of the monkey and sick child illustrate how even our bones can become disjointed with modern foods. I have also shown that a lack of vitamin A produces birth defects. Vitamins and minerals are essential for good fetal development,[132] and an absence or imbalance of any one of a variety of vitamins or nutrients could lead to the same results we've seen in this chapter.

Let's reflect back on the important knowledge from Chapter 1. Nobel Prize-winning Alex Carrel stated, "The cell is immortal. It is merely the fluid in which it floats which degenerates." Throughout this first section of the book, I outlined the concept that Nature gives us a perfect design, perhaps even a design for immortality, yet something else causes this perfect design to fail. That something, as explained from several view points, is essentially how we live in the world. And how we live in the world is a reflection of how we feel about ourselves, about life, and our purpose on this planet. Let's also reflect again on the words of Dr. Price: "One immediately wonders if there is not something in the life-giving vitamins…" that builds a higher type of individual capable of putting moral values above material values. Healthy diets build healthy minds and bodies, and unhealthy diets, which are a result of human error and not Nature's error, create disease and in certain situations, birth defects. Let us cease pretending that there is a dark mystery shrouding the cause of birth defects. If we are made within the perfection of the creative force of the Universe, then we must be the ones responsible for any imperfections. If our fate is predestined, then we are not in control of our fate. But if we have free will and can make choices to affect ourselves and the world, then we can choose to heal and prevent disease. Disease does not just happen to us. It is a reaction to a set of knowable factors. These factors are primarily 1) toxic cellular waste and toxins from the environment: air, water, food and so forth; and 2) a lack of nutrients that our bodies are designed to have in order to grow healthy. When disease occurs in spite of all of those factors existing in an ideal balance, its cause can be found in toxic and/or split emotions or life force.

On the molecular level, the cells that build our bodies and our children's bodies are made up of substances that never disappear but that merely change form — they can be traced back to the creation of the Universe. In this divine order there can be only one thing that causes disease or creates health: ourselves.

Birth defects are a tragic result of our modern nutritional program, and our modern disharmonious lifestyle. If we are mistakenly contributing to the causes of birth defects, then we can also prevent them. Prevention comes when both the mother and father are in optimal health, with balanced body chemistries prior to conception. To reach this auspicious state the parents-to-be must be nourished by the proper nutrition, neutralize and then avoid toxins, and bring balance to their emotions.

With the advent of the plague of modernization and the inferior foods of commerce, as well as with the exploitation of nature and indigenous peoples comes a tragic end to our ideal state of health. To return to a state of grace, we must act consciously to heal ourselves from this plague.

Concluding Words on the Disease Of "Modernization"

Our modern lifestyle makes us prone to physical degenerative disease. It increases our children's risk for disease. Disease is not a cruel, incurable mistake made by Nature. Disease is a curable mistake made by humans, who violate their own nature.

One of the most tragic results of the errant ways in which we live is birth defects and the variety of diseases that affect our children. These diseases are not Nature's accidents, but are usually caused by humans who do not give the body the right fuel and level of internal cleanliness to produce fine children. Let us not waste any more time with complicated theories of the causes of disease. Let us now acknowledge that disease is inflicted upon us not by a wrathful god or deity, but by our own wrath: the separated evil and unconscious instincts within us. The plague that we are a part of and unconsciously and haphazardly participate in is a reflection of our collective dark and stagnant inert layers of consciousness. To heal the plague, we must take responsibility in the place where we have ultimate control and power: with ourselves.

By correcting lifestyle disharmonies in our children we can, fully eliminate birth defects, miscarriages, and most if not all childhood diseases — as well as the now common degenerative diseases such as cancer and heart disease — in our children's children. For thousands of years indigenous people lived in robust health, reaching the maximum potential in their lives. They lived fully, often peacefully, and to a ripe age with little physical pain or suffering caused by diseases common among us today. If we can simply mimic these practices, we will produce similar results today.

In light of this information, do you still want to practice and promote society's ill and misguided ways?

Our cultural pain exists as a seeping wound. It has been passed down from one generation to the next. It existed within the European colonialists, who sought contact with native groups in order to "civilize" and exploit them. The pain dwelling in the colonial settlers of the United States motivated the genocide of millions of Native American people, as well as the enslavement of African peoples, during the formation of our nation. This pain resulted in a disconnected way of existing in which the perpetrator could not feel or connect with his victim's pain. As a result, the colonialists lost an important spiritual truth: "that your **brother's and sister's pain is as unavoidable as your own pain.**" In the most severe state of numbness of the soul we derive pleasure from inflicting destruction and death upon others. Most of us, to some degree, still hold a piece of this inner numbness and unconsciously inflict subtle forms of suffering on ourselves and others.

This pain is passed from one generation to the next, from one culture to another, and most if not all of us carry or can tune into the residual violence that has been bestowed upon our native **brothers** and **sisters**. The pain comes not only from the violence that has taken place in this country, but from the destruction of native peoples around the planet, in Australia, Africa, South America, and beyond. I suggest you take a moment of silence to acknowledge and mourn this loss of life so that we can begin to heal both ourselves and others. The sins of the previous generations must be cleansed so that we can forge a path to the light and create a planet full of peace, harmony and brotherhood. We must acknowledge the tremendous tension field which exists across the globe, as hundreds of millions of humans, as well as animals and the Earth itself, are suffering as a result of our modernized ways.

Part II
Nutritional Wisdom For Preconception, Pregnancy, and Lactation

Indigenous Versus Modern Dietary Standards

Through proper nutrition, weakness and disease in children can be substantially reduced. The best time to start implementing superb nutrition in the diet is prior to conception. However, even if you begin your dietary improvements after you have become pregnant, it is important for you to understand that we have at each moment the possibility to put our best care, love and attention into our children and what nourishes them. Every little effort you make towards being healthier will substantially influence the life of your child to be.

Intention: To really understand what modern, devitalized foods are so that you can avoid them. To empower you to creatively take charge of your health through diet.

Nature gave us a blueprint. Nature gave us everything we need to be healthy and to heal: pure water and air, vibrant foods, and powerful plant medicines. Humans evolved over hundreds of millions of years always in symbiotic harmony with Mother Earth. Our bodies are therefore designed to react and respond when we do not follow Nature's blueprint — that reaction is a part of Nature's design, too. You won't hear a ringing voice warning you, "Don't eat that food; it is unhealthy!" Your body will simply tell you by giving you a bad feeling. Just as in mathematics or physics, our internal biochemistry obeys a set of known and unknown laws and rules. Our immaculately planned and constructed body cannot process or utilize foods that have been improperly altered by commercial industry, because the producers of these inferior foods did not take Nature's design to heart. Profit and greed are the motivating forces for the creation of these substitute foods.

Let me reinforce the central and crucial theme of Chapter 1: If the internal environment of our body is a primary determinant for our health, and thus for the health of our children, then what is the primary factor that determines our internal environment? It is the fundamental expression of our relationship to the world around us, the world of form and of Nature — food.

Many of us have not experienced the extent to which diet influences our health, because when we tried a new type of diet or a "health food" we did not really notice any results. That is not because diet does not influence our health or because the health food didn't work; but many times we are so numb and disconnected from our body's responses to what we are eating that we cannot feel what is happening any more. Many modern diets are based on the theory of deprivation, that in order to be healthy we have to minimize our intake of foods. While there are times for cleansing and minimizing food intake, in general I have learned that the opposite is true. If we are to nourish ourselves and as a result nourish our children, we must follow a diet that is based on abundance, fulfillment and nourishment. We need to give our bodies enough!

I had to practice yoga consistently almost every day for several years to retune my sensibilities to my own body. Eventually it dawned on me that the food I was eating was not satisfying or healthy for me, so I began to experiment with my diet. Even so, I became so fatigued and exhausted from my 1-2 hours of exercise per day that after a few years I had to stop. Finally, now that I am eating a healthy diet, my energy and enthusiasm are returning. The good news is that I and many others have spent several decades in total paying attention to what foods are healthy or not. In the next chapter, I will provide you with the shortcut route to health, with a clear outline of helpful and deleterious foods.

Activity - Feel your body. Feel your feet on the floor and notice the rhythmic vibrations of your breathing. Allow yourself to feel a calming wave of love and compassion coming from the abundant Universe. Direct your attention to your pelvis. Here is the root of your body, your organs of elimination, reproduction and pleasure. Feel how your body is resting upon the surface that is supporting you. Gently breathe in and out, and just notice any sensations within and without.

Why Native Peoples' Bodies Failed

Weston Price not only catalogued the physical disease and degeneration experienced by the indigenous groups who had abandoned their native diet, he also proved *why* these sad out-comes occurred. Dr. Price analyzed both the ancient and the displacing diets of the indigenous people he visited. He discovered that the modern displacing diet of the "white man," which is a diet that many of us largely partake of, did not provide the same amount of vitamins or minerals as the traditional diet. And everyone knows and acknowledges that we need vitamins and minerals to be healthy! On average, indigenous diets producing healthy people had 4 times more (400% more) water soluble vitamins and minerals such as calcium, phosphorus, and vitamin B, and 10 times more (1000% more) fat-soluble vitamins (vitamins A, D, E, and K).[133] Bound to the fat-soluble vitamins are hormones or hormone like factors that provide activating chemicals to trigger healthy growth. Many of these substances are not clearly identified. With these crucial vitamins and activating hormones missing or deficient in our modern diet, our bodies fail and break down. This breakdown has been illustrated in Chapters 2, 3, and 4. It is much like building a house out of stone, a solid substance, and building another house out of paper. When the winds blow, the stone house will keep you protected while the paper house will collapse. Eating modern food is like living in a paper house and expecting it to protect you from the elements; it simply doesn't work.

The Modern Deficient Diet

Modernized Diets	Calories	Fat-Soluble Vitamins	Calcium	Phosphorus
Averages of United States[134]	2,047	Low	0.76	1.3[136]
Eskimo and Canadian Indian[137]	3,000	Low	0.39	1.14
Swiss Alps[138]	2,000	Low	0.44	0.82
Outer Hebrides[139]	2,000	Low	0.84	1.30

Modernized, Low Nutrient Diets (all figures for calcium and phosphorus are given in grams)

What you see in the first chart are figures taken from several of Dr. Price's field studies, as well as some typical figures from the average diet in the U.S. Do you remember the photos of the unhealthy Eskimo adults and children? Note the low nutrient value of their diet. Do you recall the two brothers and the grandfather and granddaughter? Their diet is that of the Outer Hebri-des. Recall also the lost harmony of the high Alpine Swiss villagers. As you can see, the average,

U.S. diet (the figures are probably similar for Canada and England) is about the same as the diets that caused disease, death and suffering in native groups.

Indigenous Diets	Calories	Fat-Soluble Vitamins	Calcium	Phosphorus
Canadian Indians[140]	3,000	High	2.30	6.61
Eskimos[141]	3,000	High	2.14	5.70
Swiss Alps[142]	2,000	High	1.66	1.84
Outer Hebrides[143]	2,000	Very High	1.76	3.04
Averages	-	High	1.97	4.30

We have here the nutrient break down of a typical diet that produced robust health and freedom from disease. I am not presenting this information to impel you to follow them as guidelines, but to illustrate the striking and profound differences in the two diets. The health-building diet is extremely high in fat-soluble vitamins and offers an abundance of essential minerals like calcium and phosphorus.

The Synergy of Vitamins

As fate would have it, our ability to utilize water soluble vitamins and minerals such as calcium and phosphorus is dependent upon the presence of fat-soluble vitamins in our diet. Therefore, if you are eating a modern displacing diet, even if you have an adequate source of minerals, your body won't absorb or utilize them properly without the fat-soluble vitamins.[144] This is where the greatest breakdown occurs in our modern diet: the lack or near total absence of fat-soluble vitamins and related hormones.

(We'll soon learn where to get those!) The modern diet has very few vitamins and minerals and those that it has are not absorbed very well because of the absence of the fat-soluble vitamins. The indigenous diet is both high in fat-soluble vitamins and in minerals, so the body is nourished. Our white bread society produces children made out of white bread, whose bodies are going to be highly susceptible to disease.

A Recipe for Disease

It is quite easy to make people sick. If the body is deprived of essential nutrients for a prolonged period, and in exchange is given foods and drinks that cause havoc in the internal ecosystem, disease is the natural result. Let's review carefully these disease-causing diets.

The Modernized Diet of the people of the Swiss Alps[145]

Calories	Food	Fat-Soluble Vitamins	Calcium	Phosphorus
1000	White Bread	Low	0.11	0.35
400	Jam, Honey, Sugar, Syrup	Low	0.05	0.08
100	Chocolate and Coffee	Low	0.02	0.07
100	Milk	High	0.17	0.13
100	Canned Vegetables	Low	0.08	0.08
100	Meat	Medium	0.01	0.11
100	Vegetable Fat	Low	0.00	0.00
100	Butter (dairy)	High	0.00	0.00
2000		**Low**	**0.44**	**0.82**

Modernized Diet of the people of the Outer Hebrides[146]

Calories	Food	Fat-Soluble Vitamins	Calcium	Phosphorus
1000	White Bread	Low	0.11	0.35
400	Jam, Sugar, Syrup	Low	0.05	0.08
100	Chocolate and Coffee	Low	0.01	0.07
300	Fish Without Livers	High	0.57	0.60
100	Canned Vegetables	Low	0.06	0.08
100	Eggs	Medium	0.04	0.12
2000		**Low**	**0.84**	**1.30**

Modernized Diet of Canadian Indians and Eskimos[147]

Calories	Food	Fat-Soluble Vitamins	Calcium	Phosphorus
1200	Bannock Bread (white flour)	Low	0.13	0.42
1200	Jam, Sugar, Syrup	Low	0.05	0.08
100	Chocolate and Coffee	Low	0.02	0.07
300	Meat	Medium	0.03	0.33
100	Vegetables	Low	0.06	0.08
100	Vegetable Fats	Low	0.00	0.00
3000		**Low**	**0.39**	**1.14**

Dr. Price explains the effects of the modern Eskimo diet:

*Since their muscle meat, glands and other organs of animals of the land for the Indians and of the sea for the Eskimos, would be reduced approximately to one-tenth, this would decrease the total fat-soluble activators per day to **a quantity below the minimum bodily requirements of even an adult**. This will make it impossible for them to utilize properly even the small amount of minerals that are present in the foods ingested besides being insufficient to maintain the functioning of various organs and tissues of the body. It is at this point that their greatest injury occurs. Even if they could utilize all the minerals that are available the intake for those on modern foods is reduced to less than one fifth of that in the original diets for several of the minerals.[148] (Emphasis added.)*

Dr. Price continues and poignantly states:

This means tragedy especially for growing child life and motherhood because of their greater demands.[149] (Emphasis added.)

This sentence really sums up the essential lesson for the first half of the book. Our modern foods create a tragedy for our children and our mothers because it does not support the requirements for new growth and life. As a result, disease and a tendency for disease are induced, and at the worst end of the spectrum one finds poor facial development, poor bone growth, distorted body proportions, miscarriages, birth defects, and early infant deaths.

The Characteristics of a Modern Disease-Forming Diet

While we will explore a more specific food plan in the next chapter, here are some of the key ingredients of the modern diet. These foods are to be strictly avoided if you want to be healthy.

1. White Flour Is Everywhere

All of the modernized disease-promoting diets had their principal source of calories coming from white flour, which has been industrially processed with its vitamin content removed. Please note that whole wheat or foods containing organic flour are only marginally better than white flour, due to the unnatural way the flour is processed and stored. Many people eat white flour foods regularly; I know that I did in childhood.

Bread, crackers, pasta, noodle soups, muffins, cookies, bagels, doughnuts, biscuits, breakfast cereals, English muffins, pancakes, pizza, toaster tarts, cakes, waffles, croissants and snack foods.

2. Processed Sugar Is Everywhere

The second source of calories for energy in the modern displacing diet comes from sweets or sweetened foods. Let's review processed sugars a bit, as well as common foods that contain them.

Jam, commercial honey, soda, corn syrup, other syrups, sweetened drinks like iced tea, candy, candy bars, food bars, pastries, ice cream, cookies, toaster tarts, sweet rolls, cake, muffins, breakfast cereals, fruit juice, doughnuts, <u>chocolate and coffee</u>.

Many packaged foods contain added sugar. Sweetened foods with processed flour like pastries or muffins create a double-edged sword. Breakfast cereal is at the top of the list of worst foods (yes, even organic varieties). Many people mistakenly feed their infants breakfast cereals as one of their earliest foods. In an experiment with one name brand breakfast cereal, the cereal itself killed lab rats faster than when the rats ate only the cardboard box the cereal came in.[150]

3. Displaced Fats

The native groups of people obtained their fats from animal and plant sources, whole and healthy as nature intended. The modern displacing diet contained fats from vegetable sources. Think of something like margarine, canola oil, or just regular vegetable oil. Most indigenous cultures on their native diets did not obtain their fats from vegetable oils. Unfortunately, processed oils are what are most commonly used in restaurant cooking. Why? Because they are inexpensive. These days clever people convert these rancid oils into gasoline for their cars (biodiesel). Not exactly something that we should be eating regularly.

4. Low Quality Proteins and Vegetables

Native peoples generally consumed all parts of the animals they hunted or fished, including, and often preferentially, the organs such as liver, kidney, brain and heart. Vegetable foods were eaten in prime condition either freshly prepared, fermented to enhance nutrient content or preserved using time-tested methods of drying and fermenting. By contrast, foods prominent in the displacing diet were devitalized by the industrial processing to which they were subjected. Tinned meats and vegetables undergo high heat and pressure in the canning process, which damages protein quality and also destroys most vitamins and all enzymes naturally present in the fresh or fermented versions. These devitalized foods are drastically deficient in most of the health-giving factors of their unprocessed or traditionally processed versions.

A stereotypical example of a convenience food in our modern deficient diet might be a ready-prepared sandwich. Two large rolls of white bread, or the barely better whole wheat option, are smeared with a cheap, low-quality spread, containing rancid, MSG-flavored vegetable oils and labeled as mayonnaise. The sandwich might contain a mediocre assortment of limp, vitamin-deficient vegetables, and packaged meats that are highly chemically processed. This sandwich is usually accompanied by potato chips, which have been fried in poor quality, rancid vegetable oils, along with a sweet drink such as a soda or fruit juice, and a dessert. Here the calorie break down is similar to the displacing diet, with most of the calories coming from processed flours and sugars, and only a minor amount of calories coming from proteins and vegetables, which are usually of poor quality.

The Secret to Indigenous Health –
Liberal Use of Fat-Soluble Vitamins

Diet of Healthy Indigenous People in the Outer Hebrides[151]

Calories	Food	Fat-Soluble Vitamins	Calcium	Phosphorus
500	Oatmeal	Low	0.17	0.99
500	Oatcake			
100	Barley	Low	0.00	0.31
800	Fish with Livers	Very High	1.54	1.62
100	Eggs	Medium	0.05	0.12
2000		**Very High**	**1.76**	**3.04**

Their nutrition is provided by their oat products and fish, and by a very limited amount of vegetable foods. Lobsters and flat fish are a very important part of their foods. Fruits are practically unknown. Yet the physiques of these people are remarkably fine. [152]

For nutrition, the children of this community were dependent very largely on oatmeal porridge, oatcake and sea foods. [153]

The fishing about the Outer Hebrides is especially favorable, and small sea foods, including lobsters, crabs, oysters and clams, are abundant. An important and highly relished article of diet has been baked cod's head stuffed with chopped cod's liver and oatmeal. [154]

Keep in mind that to reproduce this diet, one would need to obtain fresh oats. Oats in stores, even health food stores, are heat treated and thus rancid and lacking important vitamins. The oats eaten by the people of the Outer Hebrides were also likely soured or fermented over a long period to enhance digestibility.

Diet of Healthy Indigenous People in the Swiss Alps[155]

Calories	Food	Fat-Soluble Vitamins	Calcium	Phosphorus
800	Rye Bread	Low	0.07	0.46
400	Milk	High	0.68	0.53
400	Cheese	Very High	0.84	0.62
100	Butter	Very High	0.00	0.00
100	Barely	Low	0.00	0.03
100	Vegetables	Low	0.06	0.08
100	Meat	Medium	0.00	0.12
2000		**Very High**	**1.76**	**1.84**[156]

The healthy diet of the remote Loetschental Valley villagers is probably the easiest to replicate today in modern America. But it takes great precision to do so. The 100% rye bread eaten by the Swiss valley inhabitants was sourdough and aged for 2-4 weeks before baking. The milk was of the highest quality imaginable. It is difficult today to obtain such high vitamin milk, although many states have some excellent grass-fed dairy farmers and locating such high quality milk, butter and cheese is possible. For a premium price, you can get Alpine summer cheese made in chateaux. One such cheese is called Beaufort d'Alpage. For several months my family and I would feast on Beaufort, which is a full-fat French cheese. Three ounces contains one gram of calcium. The cheese is so rich and creamy it tastes almost like chocolate. We are now on a break from our cheese habit, but when we were eating it regularly we got a bulk price of $18 per pound. That might seem expensive, but is equivalent to what you would pay for a good piece of fish or a high quality steak. Find your local gourmet cheese shop and if it is a good one you will be able to sample summer-made raw milk cheeses from Europe; there are many varieties. Cheese that is grassfed during the spring or summer time usually has a very pungent taste.

Diet of Healthy Indigenous Canadian Indians[157]

Calories	Food	Fat-Soluble Vitamins	Calcium	Phosphorus
2500	Flesh of Wild Game	Medium	0.58	4.16
400	Glands and Organs	Very High	0.10	1.49
100	Vegetables, Barks & Roots	Low	1.62	0.96
3000		**High**	**2.30**	**6.61**

The food of the [Indians] was found to consist almost entirely of wild game but this does not mean what we moderns would understand by a meat diet. [158] *It seems to be an inherent part of their conception of life that in order for man, woman or child to have a perfect body he **must eat some of every part of the moose**.*[159] *(Emphasis added.)*

This did not of course, include indigestible structures, such as hide, hair, hoofs, horns or bones, but did require that the marrow be taken from bones that even the walls of the intestine or stomach after having been thoroughly cleaned should be utilized for foods as well as the tissues of every organ and gland of the body of the animal. I was told by different Indians that even when plenty of moose were available the livers of small fur animals were utilized for food.[160]

This physical activity on the part of all required a daily intake of foods which consisted of various parts of the animal prepared in different ways generally cooked either on spits before the open fire or in kettles as stews. The average amount eaten as I would judge from the sample servings would be from 5 to 7 pounds per day per individual adult.[161]

*The Indian knows where these special life-giving substances are to be found and he like the wild carnivorous animal is wise in food selection. He accordingly selects the liver, brain, kidneys, and glands. Part of every day's food for the Indians includes eating some of these special tissues. **The parents provide these for the children and teach them their special values**.*[162] *(Emphasis added.)*

Diet of Healthy Indigenous Eskimos[163]

Calories	Food	Fat-Soluble Vitamins	Calcium	Phosphorus	Iron
1700	Salmon	High	1.24	2.68	0.05
200	Seal Oil	Very High	0.00	0.00	0.00
100	Plants, Roots	Low	0.49	1.40	0.04
500	Sea Animals	Medium	0.36	1.02	0.01
500	Caribou	Medium	0.05	0.60	0.00
3000		**High**	**2.14**	**5.70**	**0.10**

A ground nut that was gathered by the Tundra mice and stored in caches was used by the Eskimos as a vegetable. Stems of certain water grasses, water plants and bulbs were occasionally used. The bulk of their diet, however, was fish and large animal life of the sea from which they selected certain organs and tissues with great care and wisdom. These included the inner layer of skin of one of the whale species, which has recently been shown to be very rich in vitamin C.[164]

Like the Indians of the interior who live on the animal life of the land the Eskimos eat not only the muscle part of fish and other forms of aquatic life but the livers and hearts and in many cases the edible parts of the head; also the milt and roe when these are present as is the case when the fish are running toward their spawning grounds which is the time the principal harvesting is done.[165]

[Eskimos] also use at certain times of the year stems or roots of certain plants, particularly the growing parts.[166]

The severity of their weather requires that they provide their bodies with large quantities of fuel for production of heat... This would be provided largely by the stored smoked dried red salmon. This salmon is dipped in seal oil as it is eaten... Small quantities of parts of several plants are used when available... The flesh of walrus, seal, caribou, moose, sea cow, and occasionally whale should be a regular part of the menu according to season.[167]

Sea Cow Not To Your Liking?

In the Western part of the world it will be difficult to find caribou, sea cow or seal. However, there is a simple lesson to be learned from the diet of the robust Eskimos and Indians of Canada's north. Eat the entire animal.

Today, we have plenty of grassfed lamb, beef, chicken, turkey, bison, pork and wild sea

foods. Yet our modern culture still follows the displaced dietary standard of avoiding the organ meats in favor of the muscle meats, eating, for example, the thigh or the butt and not the liver. With their wisdom and superb health, Canadian Indians described how they used the excess lean muscle meats — they fed them to their dogs.[168] Take extra effort to obtain the organs of the animals that you are eating (organic only) and start eating them. The most readily available source of organs is fish. It is still easy to obtain whole fish and shellfish. Many times, fish merchants just throw away the fish or shellfish organs. This is a modern tragedy, as thousands of pounds of vitamins that could be used to make our children healthy, in the form of organs from healthy animals, are thrown into the trash or dumped into the ocean.

A Recipe for Good Health

Every successful indigenous group producing a high immunity to disease used fat-soluble vitamins liberally.[169]

Three principal sources for fat-soluble vitamins:

1. Dairy products from grassfed animals.
2. Organs and muscle meat from fish and shellfish.
3. Organs of land animals.

In a rarely reviewed 1936 article from the Journal of the American Dental Association, Dr. Price reveals this little known secret for 100% immunity to tooth decay and by inference other forms of physical degeneration.

On the basis of the fat-soluble activators or vitamin content of the foods used, I found that those groups using at least two of the three principal vitamin sources had the highest immunity to dental caries... All groups having a liberal supply of minerals particularly phosphorus, and a liberal supply of fat-soluble activators, had 100 per cent immunity to dental caries. [170]

It is important to note that vegetables do have fat-soluble vitamins (the same as fat-soluble activators); examples include the germ of wheat and other whole grains, coconuts, and avocados. I believe that vegetable food sources, with their vitamins intact, work synergistically with the principal sources of fat-soluble vitamins, producing a very high immunity to every sort of disease. [See mortality chart on page 280.] However an important distinction needs to be made. The hormone like activating substances that are related to fat-soluble vitamins in animal foods are not likely present in vegetable sources.

Other Interesting Indigenous Diets

I have briefly summarized some other healthy indigenous food habits.

New Zealand Maori: Some foods in their diet included: shellfish large and small, including sea clams, oysters and lobsters (including the organs) and scale fish, used with plants such as kelp, fruits and seeds of the land, including a fern root very similar to our potato.[171][172]

Masai of Africa: Raw and fermented milk was a staple of the diet.[173] The Masai treat their cattle with the highest respect. The diet also included blood, fat, and tree bark.[174] Vegetables were considered plant matter for cows.

Samplings from other African Tribal diets: Other superbly healthy groups in Africa ate dairy products from cattle and goats, together with sweet potatoes, cereals and bananas.[175] Also included were fresh water fish from the Nile River, and a fly that hatches in enormous quantities in Lake Victoria, which is gathered and used fresh and dried as a storage food. They also use ant eggs and ants.[176] Locusts are gathered in huge quantities and made into flour. (Locust or other insect flour could probably solve many modern food problems as insects are generally high in fat-soluble vitamins.) Also eaten were a variety of grains that were freshly ground and then roasted.[177]

South Pacific Islanders: Liberal amounts of sea foods (with most or all of the organs) including shellfish and scale fish eaten with a variety of plant roots and fruits, raw and cooked. Fermented taro root was eaten (poi). A sample dish is fish head soup, which includes the high nutrient fish eyes.[178]

Modern South Pacific Islanders: On today's South Pacific islands, the rates of diabetes and obesity are soaring. Modern foods include white flour, white sugar, canned meat and fish, margarine, mayonnaise, carbonated beverages, candies, cookies, and breakfast cereals.[179] Another source states that modern South Pacific Islanders are now the most obese people in the world, the sad result of trying to fulfill the body's nutrient needs with our modern foods.

	Calcium	Phosphorus	Vitamin A	Vitamin E
1. Averages of the previously listed Indigenous Diets	1.97	4.30	High	High
2. Dietary Reference Intake (DRI) – for Pregnancy, standards proposed by US Government, Ages 19-30[180]	1.00	0.70	2541 IU	15mg
3. Percentage of Adult <u>Women be-low</u> the RDA, averages[181] (RDA is not identical to the DRI, but the figures are similar)	65.1%	27.4%	56.2%	69.4%
4. Percentage of Adult Women <u>be-low 50%</u> of the RDA[182] (that is, per-cent of women who eat ½ or less of the RDA figures)	28.6%	4.7%	26.3%	22.8%
5. Percentage of Adult Men <u>Below</u> the RDA[183]	55.4%	13.0%	60.9%	64.4%

Here the guidelines for pregnancy intakes are compared with average intakes from indigenous diets mentioned. The recommended intakes are far below what the average healthy indigenous person ate in the native diets. Vitamins A and E are important fat-soluble vitamins. All figures for calcium and phosphorus are in grams.

1. Averages of the previously listed Indigenous Diets

The first row for comparison is the average figures of the four indigenous diets mentioned previously. The exact figures for fat-soluble vitamins (such as A and E) are missing, but due to their lack in our modern diet we know that the fat-soluble vitamin intake in a healthy indigenous person is several times higher than in the modern displacing diet. With Dr. Price's careful investigations, he found that the indigenous diet could contain as much as ten times more fat-soluble vitamins (A, D, E, and K) than the modern diet that replaced it. I know for certain that the tests Weston Price used for fat-soluble activators generally were related to tests for vitamin A.

2. Dietary Reference Intake (DRI)

The next row is a standard called the Dietary Reference Intakes by the National Academy of Sciences. This represents what our government agencies believe are healthy nutrient intakes for pregnant women. Keep in mind that the indigenous nutrient intakes presented were representative of what an average adult might consume, and they did not reflect the higher nutrient intake of food consumption during pregnancy; the true indigenous figures for pregnancy nutrient intake could have been even higher. The intake percentages for the modern diets are in reference to the figures in line 2, the DRI. If we were to compare nutrient intakes of the typical US citizen to that of healthy indigenous people across the globe, we would likely find that 5% or less of the US population is eating a healthy diet in terms of vitamin and nutrient intakes.

3. Percentage of Adult Women below the RDA

The RDA, Recommended Dietary Allowance, is now called the RDI, Reference Daily Intake (that is different from the DRI, but they are similar). Yes, these acronyms can be confusing. When the United States Department of Agriculture (USDA) did their 1994-1996 nutrition survey, they studied how many women on average were below the RDA standards. The DRI standards which I have listed are likely to be very similar to the RDA standards. In some cases, the figures may not be precisely the same but they are close enough to make the general comparison. Of particular note, the bone building nutrient phosphorus has a very low requirement. As a result of the abnormally low phosphorus standard, the food survey shows less of a phosphorus deficiency — 27.4% of 19-30 year old women are below the required level of phosphorus. The USDA survey found that only 5% of adult women ate the same or more than 1.4 - 1.6 grams of phosphorus a day.[184] A generous conclusion would be that about 5% of modern women get their daily intake of phosphorus. The reality is probably far more grim than that.

Even with the USDA's low designation for healthy mineral intakes (line one compared with line two) they conclude in their report that modern people may be lacking calcium.

> *Current calcium intakes by these groups may be insufficient to attain optimal peak bone mass and to prevent age-related loss of bone mass.*[185]

4. Percentage of Adult Women below 50% of the RDA

This is the number of women who are nutritionally starving. If they are pregnant, there is a significantly higher chance that they will have complications, birth difficulties and a child who is not in good health. A generous estimate would be that these women are eating approximately 25% of the nutrients required to be healthy. They represent approximately 20% of the US female population who are in their childbearing years.

5. Percentage of Adult Men below the RDA

At the onset of a new life, men contribute 50% of the genetic material necessary to make a baby. On average, 60% of adult men don't even meet the daily deficient DRI standards. At least half of our population is creating new life on very minimal amounts of nutrients, and so our children are not set up to thrive in the world.

Diseases of Pregnancy and Childhood Are No Longer a Mystery

Like those societies which have died out in the past or are on the brink of extinction, ours is in the midst of its collapse. Our modern diet is all too similar to the diet which led to the early death of thousands, if not millions, of native peoples across the planet. Perhaps this explains why the prevalence of many diseases continues to rise. In a large portion of modern pregnancies the diet does not even provide the minimum requirements for health.

We have a nutritional <u>health crisis</u> in our country today.

Let there be no more room left to wonder. With such a deficiency of nutrients, it is clear why so many women are infertile. Let us cease to fool ourselves — because we do know what causes so many miscarriages, birth defects, premature births, and infant deaths! I have laid out before you a case that I hope is now blatantly clear. It is a story that accounts, with anthropological evidence and the statistical analysis of our nutrient intakes, for the main cause of disease in our country. Our bodies are asphyxiated for nutrients; we starve ourselves with deficient foods, and the building material of our bodies is not fertile enough to create healthy children. The result is that our children may be born into a life of physical disease, and thus of suffering. As was so vividly illustrated in Chapter 4, the physical breakdown from a lack of vitamins and key nutrients is passed along from the parents to the child, when Nature's course is *intercepted by an improper diet.*

Let's examine our modern diet more closely, so that you can clearly understand which foods you must avoid, and which high-vitamin foods are available for you and your child, or child to be, to eat and grow healthy.

6

Dietary Guidelines For Preconception, Pregnancy, and Lactation

Good nutrition is the foundation of a more comfortable pregnancy, a safer birth, and the creation of a child with optimum physical health.

Intention: To learn about what is safe and healthy to eat, and what must be avoided.

Our bodies, after years of neglect and sometimes a lifetime of reliance on modern foods, cannot usually absorb all the nutrients of a whole foods diet based on indigenous practices. Our modern diet has damaged our digestive system, which is now literally clogged with gunk. Merely eating healthier won't necessarily clear up the residual toxic matter in your body. As a result, health improvements will be dramatic for some and less so for others. Most of us need to devote extensive time and energy to restoring our digestive function with special foods, diets, cleanses and alternative treatments. For many people, removing modernized foods from their diet will result in noticeable health improvements.

Now Is the Time to Create Optimum Health

It doesn't matter if you are in the phase of pre-conception planning, pregnancy, or lactation; each and every effort you take to improve your state of health makes a difference.

Preconception health matters a great deal. The truth is that our child's health has a lot to do with how healthy both the mother's and the father's bodies are at the time of conception. A healthy diet before conception insures optimal growth during the crucial first few weeks of pregnancy.

Pregnancy is an excellent time to significantly alter the health of your child to be. During this phase, nutrition is still a keystone of creating a robust baby.

During lactation, making dietary changes will still help you and your child in unseen ways. It will help you prepare for future children if that is in your plans, and ensure that your new baby is getting nourishing breastmilk.

Beyond these phases, you can apply these guidelines (and guidelines about children's health in Chapter 13) to give you and your child the fullest potential for health. Good food will give you a positive outlook on motherhood, and equip you with energy to enjoy the time with your new baby. If you have missed essential opportunities to prepare for a healthy pregnancy with nutrition, you might feel some remorse or regret. I have found that what makes this feeling linger is not past mistakes so much as it is not putting your full positive intention towards making the best out of your current life situation. Our only control over the past is to forgive ourselves for our mistakes, and to remind ourselves of our triumphs.

Marvelous High Vitamin Foods

Dr. Price wrote:

> *There is no good reason why we, with our modern system of transportation, cannot provide an adequate quantity of the special foods for preparing women for pregnancy quite as efficiently as the primitive races who often had to go long distances without other transportation than human carriers.*[186]

Foods high in fat-soluble vitamins and their related hormones are the secret to native health. These fat soluble vitamins A, D, E, and K are almost totally absent from our modern diet. High-nutrient foods contain essential nutrients and activating factors to help our body absorb other vitamins and minerals from the food we eat. Indigenous cultures knew that mothers and fathers needed to eat these special foods before conception because the continued survival of their people depended on their children, and their children's children, being in excellent health. They also knew that special foods produced children who were physically strong and highly intelligent. These foods can benefit mothers and fathers in all phases of parenting: during preconception, pregnancy, and lactation. Later, these special foods will benefit growing children.

Lobster and Crab

Lobster and crab from clean waters, that include the guts (mustard and tomalley).
In the picture (opposite) we see:

> *...a woman of one of the Fiji Islands who had gone several miles to the sea to get this particular type of lobster-crab which*

> *she believed, and which her tribal custom had demonstrated, was particularly efficient for producing a highly perfect infant.*[187]

> *These are known by the primitive tribes to be very efficient both in preparing the mother for reproduction and also for enabling her to produce a very healthy and robust child and preserve herself from the overload of child bearing.*[188]

Native people ate most or all of the internal viscera of the crab — the source of the life-giving fat-soluble vitamins. In Japanese cuisine, *kani miso* is a highly relished dish, and consists of a mixture of crab guts, sometimes eaten with a raw egg.

> *[At Suva, the Fijian museum director] provided me with a shell of a species of spider crab which the natives use for feeding the mothers so that the children will be **physically excellent and bright mentally**, clearly indicating that they were conscious that the **mother's food influenced both the physical and mental capacity of the child**.*[189] *(Emphasis added.)*

Fish Eggs

Specifically, the Eskimos, the people of the South Sea Islands, the residents of the islands north of Australia, the Gaelics in the Outer Hebrides, and the coastal Peruvian Indians have depended upon these products for their reinforcement. Fish eggs have been used as part of this program in all of these groups.[190] *Among the Eskimos I found fish eggs were eaten by the childbearing women... for the purpose of reinforcing reproductive efficiency.*[191]

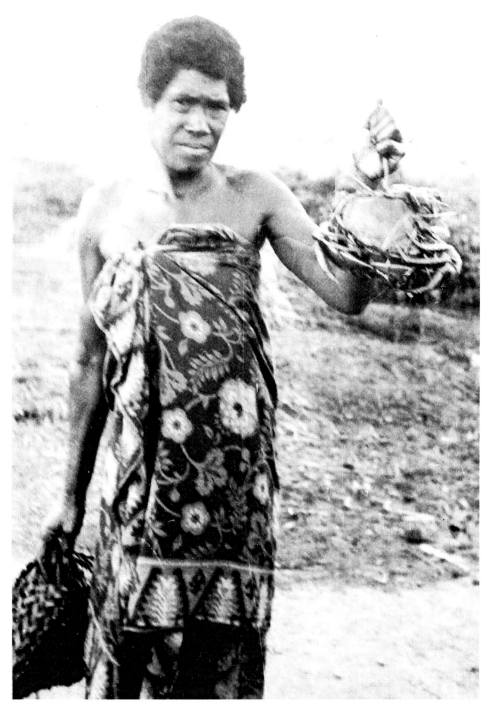

This Fiji woman has come a long distance to gather special foods needed for the production of a healthy child. These and many primitive people have understood the necessity for special foods before marriage, during gestation, during the nursing period and for rebuilding before the next pregnancy.[192]

Fish eggs are also special foods used by mothers-to-be.[193] Since fish eggs are not available year round, the Eskimos preserved their fish eggs through drying, so that they could be eaten year round.

Raw and Cultured Dairy Products:

milk, cream, butter, and cheese produced during the period of rapidly growing grass.

> *Among the primitive Masai in certain districts of Africa, the girls were required to wait for marriage until the time of the year when the cows were on the rapidly growing young grass and to use the milk from these cows for a certain number of months before they could be married.[194] It is their belief and practice that by the use of fresh grass milk for three moons, they will prepare their bodies for marriage and reproduction.[195]*

The rapid growth comes after a period of rain when there is good sunshine, usually in the spring and summertime. After three months of feeding on the special milk, the mother's body would be especially strong and fertile.

Octopus, including some or all of the organs.

> *We see a species of octopus which is used similarly as special nutrition for motherhood and for growing children.[196]*

Again this is not just the octopus flesh, but some or all of its organs.

Sea Foods with Organs

> *At this feast the chief appointed one or two young men to be responsible for going to the sea from day to day to secure the special sea foods that expectant mothers need to nourish the child. Recent studies on the vitamin content of crabs have shown that they are among the richest sources available. **We have then for modern mothers the message from these primitives to use the sea foods liberally**, both during the preparatory pe-*

> *riod in anticipation of pregnancy and during that entire period.[197]*

> *We were advised in different groups that the community life included providing the expectant mothers with something fresh from the sea every day. **Growing children living near the sea were taught to go at the time of low tide and feast upon the sea forms.**[198] (South Sea Islands) (Emphasis added.)*

Examples of the sea forms eaten are: sea cucumber, sea urchin, and a variety of oysters and clams, or anything else that is edible along the coast.

> *In this agricultural tribe, girls are required to eat special foods for six months before marriage, during which time they must not be required to do hard work.[199] Among the special foods used, fresh water fish play an important part. Here we see fish being carried off to great distances from the lakes and streams as special food.[200] (Kikuyu Tribe, Africa)*

In reference to the quote, "hard work," by tribal definition, was probably much different from our modern definition of hard work. I presume that the eggs of insects were also used as special foods in preparation for pregnancy in agricultural tribes in Africa. It is important to emphasize that when these fish were consumed, nearly every edible structure of the fish was eaten. In a photo found in the most recent edition of *Nutrition and Physical Degeneration*,[201] a man is seen carrying the head of a giant fish he has caught. He took nothing else, because the fish was so big. The fish head, when you eat the brains, the eyes, and other special meats, is extremely high in fat-soluble vitamins and related hormones.

> *For these people, the fish provide a very liberal source of the fat-soluble activators, since these native tribes eat practically all of the organs as well as the muscle meat.[202]*

This ancient wisdom provides recommendations quite different from the advice of modern conventional medicine and culture. Today, women are advised to avoid or minimize seafood consumption during pregnancy. But, provided you know that your seafood comes from clean waters and feel comfortable eating it, seafood is an excellent food for preconception, pregnancy and lactation.

Thyroid Gland & Other Glands of animals, after they have grazed for months on freshly growing green plants.

> *For the Indians of the far North this reinforcement was accomplished by supplying special feedings of organs of animals. Among the Indians in the moose country near the Arctic Circle a larger percentage of the children were born in June than in any other month. This was accomplished, I was told, by both parents eating liberally of the thyroid glands of the male moose as they came down from the high mountain areas for the mating season, at which time the large protuberances carrying the thyroids under the throat were greatly enlarged.*[203]

While it might be difficult to find the enlarged glands of a male moose, glands are available from other animals.

Hard Lining of the Large Intestine, the thicker part of the hard lining of the large intestine was a special food for some Native Americans. Eating it will give babies a nice round head. Pregnant mothers were not allowed to eat other parts of the intestine.[204]

Boiled tongue was served as part of a feast related to conception.[205] Tongue, then, is a special food particularly suited for preconception health.

Defibrinated blood that had been whipped in a gourd was a special food for growing children, pregnant and lactating women.[206] Many other cultures utilize blood as a special food.

Water Hyacinth was another special food. It was dried and burned, and its ashes placed into foods for mothers and growing children.[207] (Water hyacinth is a rapidly growing plant and may be high in vitamin E.)

Quinoa for Lactation

> *As an illustration of the remarkable wisdom of these primitive tribes, I found them using for the nursing period two cereals with unusual properties. One was a red millet which was not only high in carotin but had a calcium content of five to ten times that of most other cereals. They used also for nursing mothers in several tribes in Africa, a cereal called by them linga-linga. This proved to be the same cereal under the name of quinua that the Indians of Peru use liberally, particularly the nursing mothers. The botanical name is quinoa. This cereal has the remarkable property of being not only rich in minerals, but a powerful stimulant to the flow of milk.*[208]

Quinoa needs to be soaked for at least 12 hours to disable the anti-nutrients it contains.

Sources for Special Foods

Fish eggs from wild fish (farm raised won't do) are available from your local fish merchant, in whole fish during the correct time of year, and in preservative-free wild caviar. Dried salmon eggs, which you can put into capsules as a dietary supplement, are available at **www.alivesuperfoods.com** .

Sea foods are available from your local health food store, your local fish merchant or fish distributor, and farmers' markets. We found the location of the local fish warehouse; every business day they throw away thousands of pounds of fish carcasses, many times with the organs.

Organs and glands of land animals are sometimes available from local health food stores or farms. See **www.eatwild.com** for a farm near you. US Wellness Meats provides mail order grassfed meats including the organs and glands of many animals. They will provide a special offer for readers who place orders of less than 40 pounds. You can receive a 15% discount off your first order by using the code HEALTH15, **www.uswellnessmeats.com** .

Local ethnic food stores many times carry these special foods — just make sure they are preservative-free and from trusted suppliers.

Also be very mindful when buying seafoods from ethnic or conventional grocery stores. Ensure that the supply is trustworthy and comes from clean waters.

Raw milk products from the time of rapid grass growth are obtained through health food stores in some states, direct from farms (see www.realmilk.com for a list), and as pet food. Raw milk can even be purchased illegally, because in some locations it is illegal. For a related discussion on obtaining vitamin-rich butter, see the section in this chapter entitled "Activator X."

The Source of Indigenous Wisdom

The question has crossed my mind, as perhaps it has yours, of how these native groups knew what special foods to eat. What was the source of their wisdom? Dr. Price explains:

> In the studies of Indians of the far north of Canada, I asked an old Indian how they obtained their wonderful wisdom regarding foods and the art of living. He told me that **a great Power** taught the Indians to watch the animals to see what they ate.

> I found the native tribes in Africa using the same principle. When I inquired why they ate the organs of animals, particularly the liver, they reported that when a lion, the strongest of the beasts for its size, kills a zebra or another animal, it starts by eating at the flank and goes directly to the liver as the first of the organs to be eaten.[209] (Emphasis added.)

In Chapter 2, I described how the people of the Loetschental Valley "thank the kind Father for evidence of his Being in the life-giving qualities of butter and cheese." What could be more holy, sacred, or divine than a food capable of producing healthy children and safe births? All of these special foods are more imbued than most other foods with a quality of the creator of life, of humans, of the world of forms. Conversely, the foods most lacking this quality (special fat-soluble vitamins and hormones) are the modern foods devoid of nutrients and which produce disease and unhealthy children. No one consciously devised these rules of health and of Nature, yet if we choose to follow them we can be blessed with health, vitality, and in most cases healthy and disease-free children.

Guidelines for Preconception, Pregnancy and Lactation

The amount of food you eat will very greatly depend on what phase of child bearing you are in, as well as your body type and size. In indigenous cultures, each generation passed along the customs of health and vitality to the next. In our modern culture we have lost this tradition. If you are still connected to your ancestral roots, then a healthy diet can be maintained by following the old ways. Some people are fortunate to have a relative, or a grandparent who still eats or knows of the old way of eating, and thus they can be turned to as a resource and guide for continuing the way of living in a higher degree of harmony with Nature.

What follows is not intended to be a rigid protocol, except for the fact that you certainly need to avoid all modern foods. These guidelines will not heal all of your disharmonies (although they might), nor cure all of your health problems. They do, however, represent a good measuring stick for how to eat a healthy diet. Each person will need to modify the diet based on food preferences, availability of special foods, and personal level of health. If you cannot find raw milk then…buy a cow! I'm largely joking, but some people do consider raising livestock to get raw milk, although I understand it is quite a bit of work. Even if you cannot find raw milk locally you can still usually find good yellow butter, or raw pastured cheese instead. If you have trouble finding a local source, high quality raw butter and cheese is available online or through buyers clubs.

Dietary Program Outline

Use this as an outline for a daily diet to help you create your own dietary program.

A. Fat-soluble vitamins & hormones (vitamins A, D, E, K) twice daily from food-based sources. Choose two out of these three categories:

1. Organs of land animals
2. Organs or heads of fish or shellfish.
3. Raw dairy foods from pastured animals (milk, butter, cream, cheese)

B. Protein and fat foods such as: eggs, avocados, meat (beef, chicken, fish, turkey, lamb, etc.) butter, cream, coconut oil, suet, lard and so forth.

C. Vegetables. Consume vegetables cooked in soups, stews, or side dishes with plenty of fat, or make homemade vegetable juices, but don't frequently make excessively sweet juices using carrots or beets. Also limit the use of juices from vegetables that normally need to be cooked like kale, spinach or cabbage. Potatoes, though a starchy food, can be nutritious if not consumed to excess, and always with plenty of fat.

D. Assimilation enhancers. Probiotic supplements or foods like yogurt, kefir and sauerkraut help increase your digestive strength. Bone broths help you absorb proteins and fat when eaten together.

Daily Guidelines[210]

Food requirements are not exact. Don't force yourself to eat this much. This is an average guide to help you refine your diet or get started on your path towards better nutrition.

> ### Twice Daily
> ½ - 4 tablespoons organic/wild liver **or**
> $^1/_8$ - ½ teaspoon of fermented cod liver oil with meals
>
> *– together with –*
>
> 1 - 2 tablespoons of yellow butter **or**
> $^1/_8$ - ¼ teaspoon of high vitamin butter oil with meals

1 - 6 cups of raw grassfed milk such as cow, goat or sheep.[1]

1 - 2 cups of bone soup, made from slow cooking the bones and organs of fish. Beef, pork, chicken and turkey stocks are acceptable but usually lack the high amount of minerals in fish stocks. [211]

2 – 4 eggs from pastured birds.

1 – 4 ounces of your favorite organ or specialty food from the land or the sea. Examples: liver, tongue, heart, bone marrow, fish eggs, crab or lobster organs, oysters and clams.

Fermented condiments and beverages, such as yogurt, kefir, sauerkraut, and beet kvass. [212]

Eat substantial quantities of vegetables, such as carrots, beet greens, kale, chard, zucchini, broccoli, celery, and string beans. Dark leafy green vegetables should be cooked.

Weekly Guidelines

Eat several meals weekly of raw, seared, marinated, or stewed wild caught fish. [II]

Eat several meals weekly of raw, rare cooked, marinated, or stewed grassfed beef or lamb. [II]

Eat several meals weekly of raw, rare cooked, or marinated/fermented liver from grassfed beef, lamb, chicken, fish, turkey etc. (Liver is mentioned twice so you don't forget it!) [II]

Very high quality **raw, grassfed cheese**: cow, goat, or sheep. Cheese is best eaten with another fat like butter to help with digestion. (Can be omitted for a dairy-free option.)

1 - 3 tablespoons of bone marrow from grassfed animals frequently.

Replacement Foods

These foods can be added to your daily or your weekly plan or be used to replace other foods from the main list.

1/2 - 4 tablespoons of wild caught fish eggs can be used to replace a serving of high vitamin butter and liver.

[I] For a dairy-free diet, you will need to consume lots and lots of vegetables every day. Green vegetables that are very high in calcium come from the brassica family and include: broccoli, kale, bok choy, cabbage, mustard and turnip greens. Seaweed is another excellent source of calcium. Also include leafy green vegetables, a large variety of sea foods, and bone broths to provide the calcium requirements in a non-dairy diet.

2 – 4 cups daily of homemade vegetable juice between meals can be used to replace the vegetable requirement. Make sure to limit the use of sweet vegetables, such as carrots and beets. The juice can consist of a celery and cilantro mix. Use approximately one bunch of cilantro per one bunch of cel-

ery and add a small amount of clay to the juice (such as Azomite or TerraMin clay) that has been sitting in water for several days to neutralize toxins in the vegetable juice. Additional good juicing vegetables are zucchini, cucumber, and carrots (do not use carrot juice excessively).The Greenstar juicer (available at: **myultimatejuicer.com**) is an effective juicer for these purposes. Parsley juice limits breast milk flow. Both celery and parsley juice may promote miscarriage so replace it with cilantro or other vegetables for juicing. (This food replaces vegetables but not other special foods on the main list.)

Additional Variety and Diet Enhancements

Foods that can be added to your daily or weekly plan.

The cooked organs, mustard, and tomalley of crab and lobster can be eaten with the meat.

1 - 2 teaspoons of organic **extra virgin coconut oil** per day. [213]

Consider oily fish or lard daily, for vitamin D. [214]

Other organ meats and blood from grassfed animals and wild fish can be included.

Quinoa, for the time of lactation, (must undergo at least a 12 hour fermentation period, and be very well cooked.)

Seaweed can be a healthy source of much needed trace minerals.

Bread and grains made from freshly ground and fermented cereals.

[II] People with blood sugar problems or protein assimilation problems can resolve this by eating many meals frequently throughout the day. The meals should have small portions of proteins and fats, about 1-2 ounces, and be eaten with vegetables.

SUBSTANCES TO AVOID – Read This List Carefully. It Is Important Not To Cheat!

Avoid all modern, processed, genetically modified and denatured foods:

Sugar– white sugar, brown sugar, organic sugar, evaporated cane juice, corn syrup, commercial jams, jellies, jello, preserves, canned fruit, chewing gum, "health food" or energy-type bars, xylitol and agave syrup.

Flour & Grain Products– white flour, wheat flour, organic flour (unless freshly ground), and any unsoaked grain products. Examples: crackers, cookies, doughnuts, pies, **breakfast cereals**, granola, muffins, pastries, flour tortillas, bagels, noodles, pasta, pizza, bread that is organic but not made from freshly ground and fermented grains. Most store bought bread products, even from the health food store, need to be avoided along with store bought organic desserts.

Hydrogenated Oils – such as margarine or other butter substitutes.

Low quality vegetable oils – such as vegetable, soybean, canola, corn and safflower oils. Avoid potato chips, Crisco, and any food not fried in a natural fat. Unfortunately, most restaurants use these cheap cooking oils, which make their food unfit for regular consumption. Replace unhealthy fats with organic coconut oil, organic palm oil, organic olive oil, butter, lard, or tallow.

Pasteurized milk and homogenized milk are to be avoided — even if the milk is organic. Organic ice cream is usually made with pasteurized milk or cream with dry milk powder added for body, and contains high amounts of sugar. Limit the use of lower quality cheeses and yogurt, even if labeled organic. When animals are fed grain instead of their natural diet of grass, the quality of the dairy products are affected, despite the fact that pesticides, hormones and antibiotics were not used.

Table Salt– In general, foods with salt added to them, like salted butter and cheese, that have even the slightest bit of salty flavor, should be avoided. (Sea salt is acceptable, but use it mindfully.)

Any type of junk food, convenience food, or modern fast foods.

Coffee, Soft Drinks, NutraSweet, and anything with artificial flavors, artificial colors, or artificial ingredients.

Soymilk, protein powder, and excess tofu.

Most types of packaged or powdered green drinks (they contain excess sugar and usually are low in minerals), pasteurized fruit or vegetable juices, protein shakes and other supplement powders.

Excessive intake of fruit.

Non-grassfed, non-organic meat and eggs.

Farm raised fish.

Non-organic fruits and vegetables.

Foods that contain nitrates and nitrites.

Nut butters, except for homemade.

Alcohol and cigarettes.

Drugs, including most recreational and prescription drugs and vaccines (see Chapter 11 regarding vaccines).

Acceptable Sweeteners - Use In Moderation

The short list of acceptable sweeteners includes totally unheated honey, organic 100% pure maple syrup, rapadura (dried, organic 100% sugar cane juice). Unheated honey seems to be the safest sweeteners. Make sure the honey package says "unheated" otherwise it has been heated — even if it says "raw."

Trust your instincts. Your food habits and desires will fluctuate greatly from day to day and week to week. Relax, and give your body what it needs.

Food Intake Suggestions for Pregnancy and Lactation

	Calcium	Phosphorus	Vitamin A	Vitamin D	Vitamin E	Fat Calories
Pregnancy and Lactation	2.20+	3.40+	5,000 – 20,000+ IU	800 – 2,000+ IU	High[215]	40-60%

Caution: Under no circumstances should any synthetic supplementation for vitamins A or D ever be taken.

The figures for **Calcium and Phosphorus Intake for Pregnancy and Lactation** are based on averages of several figures including those mentioned in this book.[216] Fat calories are stored more densely than protein and carbohydrate calories. As a result, approximately ¼ of your food intake should be fat. Yum!

Summary of How to Obtain High Nutrient Foods

1. Shop at your local farmers' market or health food store.

2. Contact your local Weston A. Price Foundation chapter. Chapter members usually have gone through the work of locating excellent food sources in your area. **www.westonaprice.org/localchapters**

3. If these options aren't available, then order special foods online.

Special Foods in Other Countries– Many readers in other countries are closer to special foods because there are still people in their country following, to some degree, an indigenous diet. Contact local farms, health food stores, farmers' markets, and high quality restaurants to find out where you can obtain a good supply of nutrient-building foods. It does take a little work, but usually your efforts will produce results. Do not give up!

Living With a Whole Foods Diet

To live with this diet you'll need extra resources. One or both of these books can help with background, recipes and nutrition information.

Nourishing Traditions by Sally Fallon, includes whole foods and cooked and raw food recipes good for nourishing and sustaining the body.

Recipe for Living without Disease, by Aajonus Vonderplantiz, presents a 100% raw foods diet high in animal protein and fat and is especially good for regenerating the body and healing chronic illnesses. In general, the raw foods diet is more difficult to follow than cooked foods or semi-cooked foods. However, it provides significant healing for a body damaged by modern foods and drugs.

To help balance blood sugar and body chemistry, a simple program would consist of eating three or more meals daily, consisting of vegetables, animal protein, and animal or vegetable fat (olive or coconut oil, avocado, coconut, freshly ground grains). If your body tends toward an acidic condition (if you have indigestion or arthritis-type symptoms like joint soreness), then add more vegetables and have less protein, or add vegetable juice that isn't overly sweet between meals.

Michelle says: "It is not always easy to change our diet. However, if you take little steps to improve the food you are eating, it will gradually become easier and you'll feel a lot better. Regarding cooked and raw foods, most raw foods like vegetables, salads, juices, and raw fish are a good way to cleanse and cool down. Cooked foods like meat, soups, and vegetables are a good way to nourish and warm the body."

Animal Protein

Proteins are vital nutrient sources for our health and they must be used wisely. Protein is used to grow and repair the body. [217] The problem with proteins, which has caused many people to become vegetarians, is that heating animal proteins alters them in a way that increases the likelihood of their being improperly digested. And as a result of improper digestion, they putrefy in the intestine. [218] Urine tests have revealed that putrefactive acids are commonly left in the body after eating cooked proteins, which means the body is working hard to expel toxic material. And as a result, Dr. Bieler explains that "Many major and minor maladies arise from the toxemia that follows the ingestion of cooked proteins."[219]

When proteins are eaten raw they absorb water, and also easily absorb our digestive juices. Thus, raw proteins from raw fish, for example, are easier to digest than cooked fish. Cooked animal proteins repel water; that's why if you eat a piece of cooked protein like chicken, beef or fish, you usually find yourself very thirsty soon after you have eaten the protein. This effect is different with fruits and vegetables, and cooking is far less harmful to them than it is to proteins. [220]

This doesn't mean you must eat all of your proteins raw to be healthy. There is an exception here. When proteins are consumed with gelatin, the gelatin attracts water and digestive juices which make cooked protein easier to digest. [221] This means one of the best ways to eat cooked animal proteins is in a gelatin-rich bone broth made with the bones (and other parts) of chicken, beef, fish and so on. Recipes for proper preparation of broth are found at **www.westonaprice.org/foodfeatures/broth.html** and also can be found in *Nourishing Traditions*. Some examples are a rich clam chowder, or a rich beef stew.

Our western culinary culture also has a fine tradition of utilizing raw animal foods, such as steak tartar, oysters and clams, and raw milk, cheese and butter. Many people love sushi restaurants, where there are a variety of fish served raw. Many thousands of years ago, it is likely that most or all meat was eaten raw, and that bone marrow was a key part of indigenous diets. Eating a raw meat diet over time prevents constipation or indigestion [222] and can help heal illnesses.

Indigenous people ate their foods both cooked and raw, depending on the culture, the climate, and the particular food.

Generation after generation of indigenous people learned the special methods and purposes for preparing and utilizing every type of food in their environment. Understanding the usage of animals and plants was a key to the survival of indigenous groups. They knew what foods they needed to eat, how to prepare them, how to store them, and the best times to gather and collect them. Indigenous plant and animal foods are prepared and stored by drying in the sun, smoking, freezing, roasting on a fire, fermenting, stewing, slow cooking in underground pits, pounding and mincing.

Each food was likely prepared in a way to maximize its nutritional value, which was determined by which cooking method made food taste the best. Some examples of indigenous food preparation are: taro root eaten cooked or fermented,[223] liver eaten cooked and raw, blood eaten cooked and raw, sea snail eaten raw, [224] grains and meat roasted,[225] kidney fat eaten raw,[226] grubs raw or cooked,[227] lobster roasted,[228] and kangaroo seared.[229]

To make proteins easier to digest you can:

1. Rare Cook

Braising meat in butter or coconut oil for about one minute.

Sear meat on a grill for about 60 seconds.

Slow cook for pork, chicken and turkey, 140-150 degrees.

Boil meat by cutting it in chunks and boil for 45-90 seconds.

2. If you are concerned about parasites and raw meats:

Marinate raw fish in an acidic medium for approximately 7-24 hours. You can use lime, lemon juice, or whey. Cut the fish in small chunks or slices, fill a container to cover the fish with the juice, refrigerate and wait 7-24 hours. Recipes using marinating can be found in *Nourishing Traditions*. Marinating the fish chemically (acetic or lactic acid) "cooks" the fish while preserving the essential vitamins. Fish prepared this way is especially easy to digest.

Freezing Meat for 14 days will supposedly kill any parasites present in beef or lamb. Then you can consume it raw.

3. 100% Raw and Rare

Just eat whatever type of meat or fish you have fresh and raw. Raw animal foods rejuvenate the body.

My body had become too acidic and I was experiencing acid indigestion from eating too much cooked proteins (especially cooked eggs), so I was forced to eat most of my proteins in their raw or rare cooked form. Solutions to reduce acidity include:

- Bone broth consumed up to several times daily.

- Vegetable soup particularly rich in celery, zucchini and string beans.

- Fermented probiotic foods like yogurt and live sauerkraut help create a healthy internal environment.

- Raw fresh tomatoes, raw fresh figs, raw fresh pineapple, raw fresh lemons and raw fresh parsley are the most alkalizing foods.[230]

- Freshly made parsley juice with celery juice is effective at eliminating too much acid in the body. (Parsley can reduce breastmilk flow. Parsley juice or celery juice may promote miscarriage so replace with other vegetables if you are pregnant or breastfeeding.)

- Dipping food in a paste made with clay, or drinking clay water may neutralize acid.

Eating one protein at a time and not combining animal proteins may reduce acidity.[231] While I am not advocating this method of eating one protein at a time, if you are having problems with proteins it may be worth trying.

Poor use of oxygen also increases acidity in the body, so movement and exercise will help eliminate a high–acid condition.

Vegetables

- Raw vegetables contain cellulose, making them hard for us to digest. They can irritate the intestinal lining if the lining is already inflamed. Raw vegetables and fruits also have healing properties. It depends on your personal needs whether raw vegetables and fruits will be a benefit or a detriment.

- Cooked vegetables and fruits have their cellulose broken down so they are easier to digest. I recommend usually eating cooked vegetables or fruit with some type of fat like butter or cream.

- Fermented vegetables are sometimes made from raw vegetables, and sometimes made from cooked vegetables. Fermented vegetables are easier to digest because their cellulose has also been broken down.

- When vegetables are juiced, the cellulose is removed and the nutrients are free to be assimilated.

A Few Simple Food Ideas

Here are some basic ideas of what I consider good food (and that I eat personally).

Raw salmon ceviche (or any fish marinated with lemon, lime or whey) with a sauce consisting of plenty of raw butter, melted at a low temperature on the side. Raw tuna salad with an olive oil dressing.

Smoothies several times per day of 6-8 ounces of raw milk, 1-3 ounces of raw cream, 1-2 raw eggs, a drop of vanilla extract and sometimes a natural sweetener like unheated honey. (Caution: if you don't normally eat raw eggs it can <u>at first</u> cause intense intestinal cleansing/detoxifying in the form of nausea and even vomiting, diarrhea and flu like symptoms — be prepared. If the eggs are from a good farm then it's not food poisoning you are experiencing, but the gunk being cleaned out of your system.)

Miso soup, made with traditionally fermented miso. Place the miso in soup stock that is not overly hot, made from fish carcasses, including the heads. To this we sometimes add dried fish eggs and/or seaweed, and eat raw oysters and clams on the side.

Hamburgers. Rare cooked grassfed ground beef with shredded liver or kidney (or other organs) mixed in with it. Sauerkraut goes great on the side.

When we look towards indigenous people as role models for healthy eating, we need to consider that in their healthy lifestyles they did not have to heal their bodies from prescription drug poisoning, chemical exposures, heavy metals and food additives. For some, a totally raw diet will be the way to go. For others, nourishing stews will satisfy the body's needs without producing ill effects. If you have trouble assimilating proteins, eat them in small portions, 1-2 ounces throughout the day; this will also help balance your blood sugar levels.

Fat, Fat and More Fat

Just hearing the word "fat" might bring to mind all sorts of mostly negative images. In our culture we are taught to fear fat. It is rather odd that we are educated to avoid this food substance when it is actually the fat in our food that gives us a feeling of satisfaction from our meal. Healthy fats also aid in cleansing the body, as the fat lubricates the internal layers and promotes health. Many of us deny ourselves the basic pleasure and comfort of healthy fats. So, stop buying meat without the fat! Get full fat

products like whole milk, full fat cheese, and start eating fatty pieces of meat and fish.

Indigenous diets in general were much higher in fat than our modern diet contains, even consisting of as high as 80% calories from fat. For example, Canadian Indians sought the mature animals for the thick slabs of fat they had built up over a lifetime.[232] In addition, hunting older animals seems very ecological since the animal would have died soon anyway. Because fat nourishes the body, provides energy over the long run, and makes you feel good, I suggest a diet that provides between 40-60% of calories from fat. In our family, we don't measure how much fat we are eating or limit our intake. Rather, we eat as much fat as we can! When we first started eating extra fat, in the form of raw butter, all of us temporarily lost a little bit of weight, as the butter cleaned our bodies from the inside out.

Fat in our diet seems to be one of the key missing links regarding our health. Examples of healthy fats include organic nuts that have been soaked to remove phytates and enzyme inhibitors, organic coconut and coconut oil, organic avocados, cold pressed olive oil, butter, cream, lard, suet, tallow and any other animal fat from grass-fed animals. Margarine, cheap vegetable oils, most restaurant fried foods, fats from commercially farmed animals and non-organic fat sources are all to be strictly avoided, as they are debilitating to our bodies and lack vitamins.

Many people are afraid of eating fat. They believe the television, the newspaper, or the doctor who tells the public that fat is bad. It is important to differentiate between dangerous fats, which are man-made, and healthy fats that come from free-range, grass-fed, and wild animals, as well as the healthy fats from nuts, seeds, and certain fruit. Part of this fear-inducing story is the claim that eating too much fat raises blood cholesterol and thus increases the chance of heart disease. When examined more closely, you will see that cholesterol from healthy fats is not dangerous and that cholesterol levels do not bear any relation to the prevalence of heart disease.

Cholesterol and fat expert Uffe Ravnskov, MD, believes that guidelines from the National

Cholesterol Education Program will merely convert healthy people into patients. That is because there is no evidence — yes, you read that correctly—no evidence that animal fat or dietary cholesterol causes atherosclerosis or heart attacks.

> *For instance, more than twenty studies have shown that people who have had a heart attack haven't eaten more fat of any kind than other people, and degree of atherosclerosis at autopsy is unrelated with the diet.* [233]

> *People with high cholesterol live the longest... Consider the finding of Dr. Harlan Krumholz of the Department of Cardiovascular Medicine at Yale University, who reported in 1994 that old people with low cholesterol died twice as often from a heart attack as did old people with a high cholesterol.* [234]

A lean, low-fat diet can actually cause starvation. Indigenous people seemed to know this. For example, Native Americans would avoid eating female bison in certain seasons because they were too lean. [235] A famous Native American food, pemmican, is made from dried lean animal meat. But here's the catch: it is mixed with a very generous amount of animal fat. The Framingham heart study, most often cited as proof against saturated fat, actually says the opposite – that saturated fat decreases cholesterol. [236]

Modern fats, like the cheap oils used in restaurant cooking and the generic "vegetable oil" usually made with soy — all are poisonous to the body. It's a good idea to avoid anything fried or oily…unless it is made with "safe" fats like coconut oil, palm oil, olive oil, butter, ghee, or other animal fats. Indeed, eating foods fried in animal fats is a slice of heaven.

For more information about cholesterol myths, I recommend visiting the website of Dr. Ravnskov: **www.ravnskov.nu** .

Nourishing Ourselves by Eating Abundantly and With Care

We want to honor, cherish and deeply respect our bodies. From childhood, many of us have learned food habits based on the belief system of deprivation, or "not enough to go around." We stopped giving ourselves enough of what we really wanted, and as a result had to give ourselves other filler foods (usually processed) to make up for our hunger. Our food choices and standards have a lot to do with our hidden values. Let me explain.

On the superficial level we might think that certain dietary habits are health-promoting, and we just blindly follow them. The lowfat food habit is based on the belief that "I am not enough." If you believe that you are not enough (and by extension that life is not enough), then what do you think you are going to do with your food? Are you going to eat enough? No, you are not. It doesn't matter how hard you try, because the belief is what is controlling your behavior.

Feeling "not enough" comes generally from not getting enough when you were a child: not enough love, not enough attention, not enough positive care, not enough breastmilk, not enough good food, and not enough pleasure. As this experience is repeated throughout many years in childhood it becomes imprinted. As adults, we then unconsciously live out the "not enough" beliefs, and then deprive ourselves of what we need, like fat.

Activity: Are you feeling enough?
Do you feel satisfied the way you are, or are you always trying to strive and achieve to be **more**? Do you feel at ease with yourself and life, do you feel that what you need comes to you easily, or does life seem like a struggle and a burden? If you are always striving excessively or struggling, then you likely have an unconscious belief that there is "not enough." Look for it. Usually when we have this feeling, we feel weak and under-energized. This is not the ultimate truth. Rather, there is a welled up dam of energy inside of us that we need to open by opening to life.

I'd like to add a further observation: many westerners suffer from eating disorders, although not usually as severe as anorexia or bulimia. Many people have difficulty giving to themselves in a balanced way, so you are not alone on this one if you have this challenge.

I believe that one should not pay attention to the calories one is eating, but should eat until he has had enough and feels pleasantly satisfied.

A sample affirmation about self care: I want to take care of myself. I do not want to proceed haphazardly through life. I really want to feel that I have nourished myself and given myself what I have needed so that I may extend that fullness out to my family and community.

This is very similar to an affirmation I have been using from time to time, which in essence says, "I really want to live my life with purpose and meaning. I want to fulfill my purpose in being here to the fullest extent." Try it out yourself; you may find a sense of relief in having a clearer purpose.

Your dietary habits are also motivated by your emotions. Unconsciously or semi-consciously, it is likely that you use foods to try to control your feelings. You use food as a drug (in a negative sense) to help you leave this reality, to help you stay confused and distant from life. Food can be used to give the body temporary pleasure and to hide it from pain. Yes, we get pleasure from nourishing whole foods. But I am talking about that addictive satisfaction we get from foods that are made with stimulating ingredients like flour or sugar. Usually, a craving for junk food is really a craving for healthy protein or fat. Be aware of these habits when you make your food choices; stay present.

Other people use food as a method for self destruction. They eat food that weakens them. In this way, food becomes a drug in the sense that it supports underlying negative, self-destructive emotions, to which the individual is addicted. Many people are actually addicted to negativity and negative states of mind; they then eat accordingly.

Most important, listen to and trust the signals of your body. Make your time meaningful by paying attention to everything. Here are some other mindful food pointers.

Chew your food well; don't rush through the eating process. Make eating an opportunity to enjoy, take in, and receive nourishment that ultimately came from the earth. Don't eat sweet food all the time. Eating sweets too often (even natural ones like fruit), several times daily, can weaken your body. This is the act of getting your body's energy needs from sugar rather than from protein or fat. Also, don't be afraid to eat late at night, or have midnight snacks, especially if you are pregnant. Babies eat at night; it's natural. For example, warmed raw milk with ghee or raw butter and warming spices like cinnamon or cardamom with a touch of raw honey, or other easy-to-digest foods are good choices of foods to eat just before going to bed. It doesn't have to be a lot, but when we sleep our body rebuilds and repairs itself. Having nourishment before bedtime gives our bodies the building blocks it needs for this rebuilding process. If you are doing some sort of cleanse or are on a temporarily restricted diet then you would not want to eat before bed in order to aid the detoxifying and repair process.

Investigating the Roots of Vegetarianism

While we are on the subject of "not enough," we might as well talk about vegetarianism. First, if you are adamant about being a vegetarian, simply modify these dietary guidelines and remove all of the animal meats. You should still eat plenty of raw milk, raw cream, raw butter, raw cheese, and raw and cooked eggs. Many vegetarians can accept eating fish or taking fish oil supplements. You'll be much better off being a vegetarian if you take cod liver oil because it is really hard to get adequate amounts vitamins A and D otherwise. If you eat fish, then I don't consider you a vegetarian. You can be superbly healthy by eating only seafoods, especially when you eat some of the organs.

Even if you are not a vegetarian, you may still have unconscious patterns or habits that could be brought more into the light through reading this section.

Many people believe in non-violence. Some people take this belief far enough that they feel they should not eat animal foods because of the killing involved.

Some people have benefited from temporarily avoiding some animal foods or even from abstaining from all animal foods. This approach can be used as a part of fasting and cleansing: on a limited diet, liver functions and other bodily functions can be healed. Even though these limiting diets have created health and healing for many people, they are not body building diets. Many people erroneously see only the short term perspective of the healing and life enhancement they get from avoiding animal foods. Because of this rapid and great health freedom, they believe that their experience has proven to them that avoidance of animal foods is the optimal long-term diet. Yet, this is untrue if you plan on having children. Men also need to change their diet, as men deficient in fats and fat-soluble vitamins will be giving their partners deficient sperm and seminal fluids, and so the fertile ground for life will not be as rich as it could be.

For about two years, I was a vegetarian and then a vegan, and so I am sharing insights from my personal experience. Many years ago, I was fasting on a vision quest to help change the direction of my life. I hiked up to the top of a mountain (I did this with a group) and found my fasting spot. After two days without food my vision was clear: a turkey sandwich. From then on I began to eat meat again, but I did so conscientiously. Some people are upset with me for promoting the use of animal foods because they believe that eating animal foods depletes the earth of resources. To respond to this charge, I would point out that first, there is the law of conservation, in which every substance on earth stays on earth and simply transforms itself in the cycle of life. For example, the seed becomes a tree, and then a fruit, which is eaten, becomes waste, and then goes back to the earth. On the molecular level everything is made up of substances that are always here, and that never leave here. So nothing is ever lost. It is just changing form. The problem is that humans have seriously interfered with the natural cycles so that it appears as if there is a lack of resources.

If I could live off of a vegan diet and be healthy, I would do it. I surely would save hundreds of dollars a month on my food bills. Yet the spirit that created my body and yours gave our bodies certain requirements. While it may be possible to transcend these requirements, like the Himalayan yogis who can drink lead, or breatharians who don't eat at all, most of us are subject to the normal laws of hunger and nutrition, which means we need animal proteins and fat.

Weston Price specifically searched for healthy groups of indigenous people who were vegetarian. In the Fiji Island group Price encountered groups of people who had little access to land animals, and who lived far from the sea. Even among these people he observed, "No places were found where the native plant foods were not supplemented by sea foods."[237] The people who lived inland traded with groups who lived near the sea so that they would always have access to seafood. Fat-soluble vitamins and hormones in the organs and glands of land and sea animals are irreplaceable. Eat these special foods if you want superbly healthy children.

From the unitive perspective, all beings are equal; there is no "greater than" or "less than." Many of us have a secret part of ourselves that is not life affirming; it is life destroying. Under our conscious facade that says, "I give the best to myself," is an unconscious voice that says, "I won't give myself what I need." The reason for not giving ourselves what we need is that deep down we feel inadequate, undeserving, and we believe we are not "good enough."

I found a telling truth about vegetarianism in the life-sustaining work of Aajonus Vonderplanitz. He writes about a conversation he had with a Native American who came to visit him from the spirit world. Although now an omnivore, Mr. Vonderplantiz was once a vegetarian who was opposed to eating meat. He said to the Native American spirit,

I can't kill animals, I mean, even though I didn't actually kill them, eating meat is the same as killing,

The Native man replies,

To uproot vegetables, or bite into fruit is also killing. But when someone only kills to eat, it is according to the goodness of Nature. It is a natural agreement between all species. Death is quick in the hunt. Suffering is a lifetime in disease. You choose. [238]

So the choice is yours: the quick and brief suffering of an animal killed to sustain you, or a lifetime filled with disease and weakness from malnourishment.

If it were truly sinful or wrong to eat meat then the creator, or Nature, would not have made it necessary for animals to kill other animals to survive. We surely don't think lions, sharks, sea lions or bears are sinful, because it is their very nature to eat other animals to survive. So why not apply this logic to ourselves?

The trend towards non-violence, and hence non-killing, of animals has risen out of another extreme: the inhumane slaughter of animals. I do not have exact figures for each animal, but in the United States there are over 5 million commercially raised cattle slaughtered every year. Most of these animals are confined to crowded feedlots, poisoned with drugs to keep them alive in such conditions, and made to grow abnormally fast with chemicals, inappropriate feed, and selective breeding. These cows are fed toxic foods and live in horrid conditions, suffering daily. They are slaughtered by machines, in frightening, cruel and mechanistic ways. They have been objectified for the purpose of profit. The collective suffering we cause our animal friends is huge. It creates an enormous burden and negative energy field on the planet. We mistreat the animals that we need to sustain us. We are able to sense, although not usually consciously, this emanating field of pain caused by our objectification and mistreatment of animals. Many people understandably react to this repugnant extreme by resorting to the other extreme of avoiding all animal products. Very few people avoid animal products out of an inner conviction and commitment to a spiritual path which removes and isolates the seeker from the ways of the world. Most of us choose to remain

in and of the world, having children and families, and the attendant responsibilities to keep them robust and healthy.

For us, then, the solution to the deplorable treatment of animals used for food is not to simply avoid all animal products, but to avoid the animal products that are improperly produced. I try to buy all my meat from trusted vendors, and from the farmers themselves, where I know the animal was given the best care during life, and in death.

Outer cruelty only exits because of our collective inner cruelty. Each of us has that unloved part of ourselves that can at times act maliciously. By bringing love and compassion to those parts of ourselves, we can heal our inner cruelty, and thus stop it at its source. Love that does not deny feelings embraces them fully. This love feels, acknowledges and allows the feelings to be felt completely so that they can eventually be released.

Because of collective greed, violence, and other destructive forces of humanity, social movements have grown over time to counter these evils. Because of one distorted extreme, of only valuing life in the outer world, for example, the opposite extreme — denial of the outer world — was created. Many spiritual movements and schools throughout time have preached forms of asceticism, and use the denial of outer life to help point the seeker towards his inner spiritual reality.[239] Part of denying life can be a vegetarian diet. Again, this is fine for someone who does not intend to engender children; when you have children, however, your body requires vastly more nutrients. Where, for example, does all that breastmilk come from? Ultimately it comes from the nutrients you eat. So you must eat wisely if you want to remain strong and nourished while you nourish your child as well.

As a final note, I will mention Tibetan Buddhism. Many westerners regard Tibetan culture as one of the most spiritually oriented traditions on our planet. Their spiritual technology has evolved in parallel with the evolution of material technology in the West. Because animal foods — particularly pork — are available in certain locations where not much else is, many

Tibetan spiritual teachers (lamas) eat pork, at least occasionally. Even though they eat pork, the protocol is for someone else to kill it. So, there are spiritual role models and spiritual people who do eat meat and at the same time promote non-violence.

Fat-soluble Vitamins

The secret to superb indigenous health was a diet high in fat-soluble vitamins primarily obtained from three special food categories: raw grassfed dairy, organs of sea animals, and organs of land animals. Consuming high vitamin butter and a high quality wild or grassfed liver twice daily will help ensure that you are getting the needed fat-soluble vitamins. In addition to this, I suggest one special food per day, such as organ meats from land or sea animals. Fat-soluble vitamins are extremely critical for men to eat as well in the period of preconception. It makes their sperm vital.

Activator X

Activator X is the name Dr. Price gave to the special hormone like substance in the summer butter, the gift from the kind Father. When cows and other animals eat rapidly growing grass or similar substances (such as plankton in the ocean), their bodies synthesize via digestive fermentation plant hormones into Activator X, which "plays an essential role in the maximum utilization of body-building minerals and tissue components."[240] It is found in the butterfat of milk, the eggs of fish, and the organs and fat of animals who eat grass or plankton during the time of rapid growth. It plays an **important role in infant growth and also in reproduction**.

Activator X is largely missing from our modern diet, and modern parents and their children fail to benefit from this health building nutrient. Meanwhile, in most indigenous cultures studied across the globe, special foods containing activator X were a must for the times of preconception, pregnancy or lactation. Examples of this custom include: the Masai's special period of drinking milk after the rains, or the Canadian

Indians eating the thyroids of the moose after a summer of grazing on rapidly growing plants.

Follow indigenous wisdom by consuming foods containing activator X frequently before conception and during pregnancy and lactation, and you will exponentially increase the odds of having a healthy child.

High vitamin butter is naturally yellow or orange and contains activator X. Activator X is present in butterfat only when the cows eat rapidly growing green grass in the spring, summer or fall (depending on the climate).

Fish eggs contain fertility factors and activator X.

Other organs of animals eating rapidly growing grass will be high in activator X. (The intestine or stomach lining may contain concentrated amounts of activator X.) It is likely that the organs of the crab and lobster and certain other fish are also very high in activator X.

Obtaining Yellow High-Vitamin Butter

1. Sources for local butter from grassfed animals are available at: **www.realmilk.com**. The yellow butter is available from local sources during the spring and summertime. You can save high vitamin butter for the wintertime by freezing it.

2. Pure Indian Foods ghee is a very high quality ghee made from spring, summer and fall high vitamin butter. This particular brand of ghee is also excellent for baby food and cooking and can be shipped to you, **www.pureindianfoods.com** .

3. Anchor Butter is a New Zealand butter that has a nice orange hue. Call 1-888-869-6455 to find a local Anchor supplier. You can also contact your local organic grocery store and request that they carry Anchor Butter. Anchor butter is pasteurized, as required by U.S. import laws. Get the unsalted variety.

4. Kerrygold Butter is a high quality grassfed butter available in many natural food

and even conventional stores. It usually has a nice yellow color. Kerrygold butter is pasteurized, as required by U.S. import laws. Get the unsalted variety.

High Vitamin Butter Oil is produced by Green Pasture's™. Butter oil is a food-based supplement of concentrated spring or summer yellow butter. If you want to buy a real "multivitamin" for pregnancy, get this product. Buy it at: **www.codliveroilshop.com**

Obtaining Fish Eggs

Fish eggs should be wild caught and not from farm raised fish, otherwise they may be lacking in many vitamins.

1. Obtain fish eggs from your local fish merchant.

2. When you buy a whole fish you may find the eggs, as well as many high quality organ meats. Various types of fish produce fish eggs at different times of the year. Usually fish merchants throw the eggs away because it is too much work to harvest them and the demand is low.

3. Caviar is cost prohibitive for most people. Only use caviar from wild fish. Many high priced caviars are farm raised and probably lacking essential vitamins. Make sure the caviar does not have coloring or food preservatives added (most of them do).

Fat-soluble Vitamin A

True vitamin A is only found in animal foods. Provitamin A is what is found in yellow, red, orange and dark green fruits and vegetables and must be converted into true vitamin A in the upper intestines. This happens when fat is present. [241] High levels of true vitamin A, from safe food sources, do not have toxic effects despite the widespread fear of consuming excess amounts of this life-giving vitamin. [242] The claim that over 10,000 IU of vitamin A can cause birth defects came from just one scientific study. Other studies show in general that vitamin A either decreases or does not increase the

risk of birth defects in doses less than 40,000 IU daily. [243] The dietary suggestions of 1 teaspoon of fermented or high vitamin cod liver oil daily provide about 10,000 IU of vitamin A, and 4 tablespoons (or about two ounces of liver) provides anywhere from 6,000-20,000 IU of vitamin A, depending on what type of liver you use. This is well within the safety guidelines. If you are at all concerned of excess vitamin A just take a break from vitamin A food sources for one or two days a week. By the way, a lack of vitamin A is what caused the birth defects in the pigs in Chapter 4.

Fat-soluble Vitamin D

"Vitamin D is not found in plants, but must be sought in an animal food." [244] Dr. Price found four key sources of this necessary vitamin, which is closely tied in its functions to vitamin A and activator X.

Milk, butter, cream, cheese from cow, camel, sheep and musk ox.

Organs of animals, and eggs of wild and domesticated birds.

Sea foods, including oily fish and shellfish, containing most or all of the organs.

Small animals and insects.

Studies show that growing fetuses need vitamin D. [245] While all of the roles of vitamin D are not yet known, it seems to play an important part in organ and bone development. In addition to the foods mentioned, vitamin D is found in very high amounts in liver, and in smaller amounts in lard.

Fat-soluble Vitamin E for Reproductive health

Researchers called vitamin E *tocopherol,* which in Greek means "to bring forth a child," in recognition of the vitamin's role as a fertility factor.

In the modernized methods of food processing, the germ of the wheat kernel, which contains the delicate vitamin E, is removed when producing commercial flour. This process increases the flour's shelf life, making it a profitable product, but a devitalized and valueless food item. In studies with rats, partial vitamin E deficiencies have caused prolonged gestation and abnormal offspring.[246] I believe these essential vitamins help our hormonal glands (such as the master pituitary gland, which controls all the aspects of pregnancy and fertility) to control and regulate our hormonal system.

Modern mothers are most likely deficient in vitamin E because this vitamin is oxidized during wheat processing. Thus, we have a partial explanation for reproductive health failures in the modern world — a lack of fat-soluble vitamin E.[247] Vitamin E can be obtained from freshly ground wheat, wheat germ oil, and other grains freshly ground. One of its most absorbable forms is found in butter.[248]

Whole grains also contain phytates, which prevent the body's ability to absorb certain minerals in the grain. That means that in addition to being freshly ground, grains need to be sprouted, or fermented in some manner, before we eat them. This ensures that the nutrients in the grains are accessible as well as digestible.

Nature's Ultimate Life Giving Food

High vitamin butter contains essential health promoting factors such as activator X, and a highly utilizable form of vitamin E. This works in excellent combination with Nature's number one health food, liver. Dr. Price writes:

Some of the tribes [in Africa] are very tall, particularly the Neurs. The women are often six feet or over, and the men seven feet, some of them reaching seven and a half feet in height I was particularly interested in their food habits both because of their high immunity to dental caries which approximated one hundred per cent, and because of their physical development. I learned that they have a belief which to them is their religion, namely, that every man and woman has a soul which resides in the liver and that a man's character and physical growth depend upon how well he feeds that soul by eating the livers of ani-

mals. The liver is so sacred that it may not be touched by human hands. It is accordingly always handled with their spear or saber, or with specially prepared forked sticks. It is eaten both raw and cooked.[249]

Again, take note of how the indigenous cultures considered the life-giving liver to be sacred, much like golden summer butter was to the isolated Swiss. Take this advice to heart, and add high quality liver to your diet.

Getting your RDA of Organs and Glands

The Canadian Indians believed that eating every part of the animal was necessary to create health. For this reason, organs and glands are highly recommended. Liver is the best and most easily obtained gland. Liver is high in fat-soluble vitamins A and D, as well as in many minerals. In Chapter 4 we examined birth defects caused by a lack of fat-soluble vitamin A. The solution to this problem is eating liver. Eating many different types of glands regularly is a sure way to build your health. This is what makes mollusks like oysters and clams an exceptional food. They are usually eaten whole and include all the organs.

Some people might have difficulty finding organ meats. When you make soup with fish carcasses that include the organs, the resulting stock will be rich in many of the nutrients that were stored in the organs. Also, one decent substitute for liver is freeze-dried glands from grass fed lamb, available at **www.drrons.com**

Organs should be from wild or grassfed animals, with no hormones or antibiotics of any sort added.

Organs also contain vitamin C and other vitamins. Indigenous people ate vitamin C in the form of green succulent "shoots" from the spruce trees, raw adrenal glands, and the fat layers from a species of whale.

A precaution with organ meats: avoid organs from commercially raised animals, which contain high amounts of unnatural hormones or antibiotics.

To obtain organ meats:
Some health food stores have good quality organs. Whole wild fish has all of the organs.

www.eatwild.com will help you locate a local pasture based farm.

Order online from retailers like www.uswellnessmeats.com (coupon code HEALTH15 gives you 15% off.)

Get Your Cod Liver Oil Fix

Using a high quality cod liver oil is a simple method for ingesting vitamins A and D. Dr. Weston Price always administered cod liver oil mixed with high quality butter oil. Dr. Price observed that the two exert a synergistic effect and produce better effects when taken together than either provides alone. Liver or cod liver oil is a must for men and women preparing for conception, because of its important vitamins and activators.[250] If taken regularly over a long period, such as many months or years, regular commercially produced cod liver oil can be mildly toxic because of the harsh processing methods used. To minimize any of this concern, take cod liver oil with butter or butter oil. In addition, I recommend fermented cod liver and skate liver oils as the best choice, as these have either little or no toxicity, due to a more natural process of extraction. The following sources of cod liver oil are ranked in order of preference:
Fermented Cod or Skate Liver Oil is produced by Green Pasture's™. I recommend and use this brand. You can buy it at: www.codliveroilshop.com
Store Cod Liver Oil. Not all cod liver oils are alike. Cod liver oils purchased at health food stores do not have any of their natural vitamin D intact. Commercial cod liver oil production includes alkali refining, bleaching, winterization which removes saturated fats, and deodorization which removes pesticides but also vitamins A and D. In this process fat-soluble vitamin D is completely destroyed, and fat-soluble vitamin A is mostly destroyed.

The best available cod liver oil in health food stores seems to be Nordic Naturals® Arctic™ Cod Liver Oil without vitamin D added. This product contains no natural fat-soluble vitamin D. If a brand of store-bought cod liver oil has vitamin D on the label, it is highly likely to be artificial vitamin D3 added to the cod liver oil.

Calcium

We need calcium to grow our bones. In my estimate of dietary recommendations, I have given a rough figure of 2.2 grams of calcium per day for pregnancy and lactation. Dr. Weston Price suggested 1.5 grams of calcium per day for pre-conception (a normal adult). Here is how much calcium may be found in certain foods.

- 1 cup of milk contains about 0.3 grams of calcium, 3.5 cups of milk contain 1 gram

- 1 cup of yogurt contains about 0.3 grams of calcium

- 3.5 ounces of hard cheese contain about 1 gram of calcium. Softer cheeses contain less, but they still contain significant amounts of calcium

For people who cannot drink milk or do not like drinking milk, I will mention some alternatives. First, there is the option of goat milk, goat milk yogurt, sheep's milk, sheep's milk yogurt, and goat and sheep's milk cheeses. There is also fermented milk in the form of kefir. Lactose is mostly or totally consumed in the fermentation process, so the resulting cultured product should be easier to digest. Many people have a milk sensitivity because their digestive organs where damaged during childhood from eating low quality cheese, and low quality pasteurized milk. However, many of these alternative dairy products will not produce an allergic response in the body.

There were many groups of indigenous people that Dr. Price studied that consumed a high amount of calcium in their diets, and yet they ate little or no dairy. In the case of the Canadian

Indians, calcium came mainly in the form of tree bark and special plants. In the case of the Eskimos, calcium primarily came from salmon, which must have contained some bones that had been prepared in such a way that they could be eaten. Eskimos also ate fermented fish heads, which would contain high amounts of calcium from bones. Other calcium sources include: the burnt ashes of certain plants, stems and other special parts of plants, grains that have a high calcium content, taro root, the blood of the animals and perhaps certain tissues containing high calcium, animals with shells soft enough to be eaten like a soft shelled crab, and insects (their crunchy parts contain calcium). Calcium may also have been obtained through grinding oyster shells, crab shells, bones, egg shells or antlers. One half teaspoon of calcium in a powdered form would contain at least two grams of calcium.

Other calcium sources include sea-food, broccoli, beet greens, nuts, beans, seeds (sesame, sunflower, and pumpkin), cauliflower, figs and olives.[251] Bone broths, made with beef, chicken, or fish bones that have a bit of vinegar added when simmered, may also contain appreciable amounts of calcium. Sea vegetables and different types of algae are also high in calcium.

Phosphorus helps bones to grow

Phosphorus is the second most abundant mineral in the body. Phosphorus is needed for bone growth, organ function and cell growth.[252] Dr. Price also found that phosphorus is a key element in the diet of native groups highly immune to physical degeneration.

Since I have given you specific data for phosphorus of at least 3.4 grams per day during pregnancy, it is important to understand the amount of phosphorus found in foods. Phosphorus is obtained from meats and fish, and from grains and nuts. Many foods have some amounts of phosphorus.

3.5 ounces of a hard type of cheese provides approximately .7 grams of phosphorus.

4 cups of milk provides about 1 gram of phosphorus.

1 cup of wheat .6 grams of phosphorus.

8 ounces of beef contains about .5 grams phosphorus.

8 ounces of salmon contains about .8 grams phosphorus.

8 ounces of cooked lentils, .4 grams of phosphorus.

You can obtain more information about foods high in phosphorus by visiting **www.nutritiondata.com** .

Raw Dairy - Raw Milk, Butter, Cream, Cheese, Kefir and Yogurt

Many indigenous people created superb health using milk and milk products. These indigenous groups include: isolated Swiss, the Masai in Africa, the Anchola in Uganda, the Bahema and Balendu tribes in the Congo, many tribes along the Nile near Ethiopia, the Neurs in Sudan. Indigenous Arabs used camel milk, and Pathans in northern India ate soured curd. Due to their high calcium content, raw dairy products are essential to building bones.

It is essential that the dairy food be raw. However, if raw dairy products are illegal in your state, try a top quality yogurt and take action to get your local laws changed. Unpasteurized cheese is almost universally available. In many states, many raw dairy products are illegal and this encourages a black market for raw milk. It is a sad state of affairs when one of the most nutritious foods on the planet is illegal to buy for human consumption.

Some people are concerned about becoming ill from consuming raw dairy foods. Initially, you may have some minor symptoms of detoxification from drinking certified raw milk. A few people will need to take the time to allow their bodies to adjust to the milk and its live cultures. You may have heard of dietary guidelines that say to avoid drinking raw milk. But consider that healthy indigenous people drank their milk raw or in a raw fermented form, and also preserved their milk through a slow fermentation process in the form of cheese. Butter and cream were also never pasteurized, as there was not an irrational fear of bacterial contamination. Some people believe that casein (a protein) in the milk is toxic, but I believe this refers to damaged and indigestible proteins from pasteurized milk.

Due to the propagation of faulty information, I need to respond to the anti-raw milk propaganda. Raw grassfed milk is safe to drink. This type of milk is far different from the typical grain-fed pasteurized milk from confined animals that you buy in stores. For example, 1.9 cases of food-borne illness were reported per 100,000 people from raw milk[253], whereas, 4.7 cases of food food-borne illness per 100,000 people were reported for pasteurized milk.[254] That makes raw milk about 2.5 times safer than pasteurized milk.

The presence of enzymes and probiotics in raw milk help to disable the growth of any pathogens.[255] It should be clear that high quality raw milk is much less likely to cause food-borne illness. In fact, unpasteurized high-quality raw milk has a better safety record than even vegetables and fruits.

The reports we hear about the "dangers" of raw milk comes from test results on milk from commercial dairies, which is held in bulk tanks prior to pasteurization. This milk comes from cows that are kept in horrible conditions, given hormones, fed genetically modified grains, and crammed into small stalls. No one would recommend that you consume this milk raw! That milk averages 5% contamination with listeria.[256]

Speaking of raw milk safety let me remind you of something I said back in Chapter 1. Disease is not usually, if ever, caused by bacteria. It is caused, rather, by the environment in which the bacteria live. This explains why dirty milk will have higher counts of the bacteria associated with the cause of disease.

Dirty environments produce certain bacteria; but it is the environment, not the bacteria, that is the disease (or cause of disease). The advice to avoid raw milk because of potential listeria poisoning and other bacteria is unfounded. The information propagated by the Centers for Disease Control says, "*Listeria monocytogenes* is found in soil and water."[257] In other words, listeria can be everywhere; so why fear it? Listeria is non-existent in high quality raw milk. Pasteurized milk is far more dangerous than raw milk because enzymes and bacteria that help prevent the growth of harmful microorganisms are destroyed in pasteurization.[258] The real advice that should be given to pregnant women is to avoid pasteurized milk, since this once healthy product is now diseased material.

When the director of the FDA's dairy and egg safety division was asked if there have been any documented cases of illness directly caused by raw milk, his response was that he didn't know of any cases in the United States *in the last 20 years*.[259] A question to reflect upon is why should a food scientifically shown to be safe and healthy be legally restricted?

I have shown in Chapter 5 that a majority of women are deficient in calcium and vitamin A, among other nutrients, because of our deficient and modernized diet. Unpastuerized grassfed milk is an abundant source of usable vitamin A, as well as calcium.

Any policy that advises pregnant women to avoid raw grassfed milk is a policy aimed at thwarting Nature's laws for health. These policies and guidelines must have been designed with one purpose — to propagate weakness and deficiency in pregnancy and early childhood.

Learn more about raw milk at **www.realmilk.org**, which also has a resource for finding local raw milk suppliers. Also, see the "Report in Favor of Raw Milk" at **www.rawmilk.org** .

Lacto-Fermented Foods and Enzymes

Enzymes act as catalysts in most of the bio-chemical processes in our bodies. Enzymes help us digest our food. When we cook our food, the enzyme content of the food is lost. So, it is vital to consume both raw and/or fermented foods along with a meal of cooked food, as these additions will provide needed enzymes. Recipes for fermented foods are found in *Nourishing Traditions*.

Many indigenous groups ate certain foods, such as soured and fermented foods, to promote a healthy intestine. A healthy gut with a balanced bacterial ecosystem is crucial for the absorption of nutrients, and for the maintenance of overall health. Many people in our modern culture have minor illnesses, and most of these begin in the gut. The gut can be healed through a variety of programs, such as Aajonus Vonderplanitz's raw food diet, or the specific carbohydrate diet as described in *Gut and Psychology Syndrome* by Natasha Campbell-McBride, MD. Probiotic supplements and probiotic foods also help balance the gut ecology.

Vegetables and Fruit

Eat lots and lots of vegetables, and eat them with fat. Some vegetables need to be cooked; others are best raw or lightly cooked. Do not eat fruit excessively, or as your main source of energy throughout the day, as this will cause excess blood sugar fluctuations. In general, eat fat along with the fruit, such as a smoothie made with cream to slow the rate of digestion and enhance nutrient assimilation. Each meal of sweet foods can cause blood sugar fluctuations of three to five hours. Eating natural sweets like fruit is fine when not done to excess as the blood sugar then has a chance to return to normal. But if sweet foods are eaten consistently throughout the day, then the blood sugar never returns to normal. This can cause key minerals to be pulled from bones as well as promote glandular imbalances.

Muscle Meats – Lamb, Beef, Chicken, Fish and others

A nourishing supply of fat and nutrients comes from eating animal flesh. Many of the successful indigenous groups that Dr. Price studied consumed large amounts of animal flesh. Depending on the needs of the individual, some of these flesh products can be consumed raw; others can be prepared through marinating and slow cooking. It depends on what type of flesh you are eating and what your personal desires are. Eat the meat with plenty of fat. Since muscle meats are a common food in our culture, one needs to make sure to balance these with eating enough fat and vegetables. Good quality muscle meat contains phosphorus, amino acids, and other minerals that can build healthy bones and teeth.

Grains and their Problems

In Weston Price's field studies, a diet centered on white flour, refined sugar and vegetable fats was devastating to the health, teeth and gums of native peoples worldwide. From this evidence even Dr. Price himself concluded that consuming grain products in their whole form would resolve a part of the problem of tooth decay. The natural health community, and now even the US Government and food manufacturing giants, have embraced and promoted the view that whole grains are better for our health. But this perspective is incorrect.

The famous professor and doctor Edward Mellanby wrote that "oatmeal and grain embryo interfere most strongly" with the building of healthy teeth and bones. He called the effect of the germ of grains on teeth "baneful." He also found that a diet high in grain germ or embryo led to nervous system problems in his dogs such as leg weakness and uncoordinated movements. Dr. Mellanby concluded that most cereals contain a toxic substance that can affect the nervous system.

Phytic acid has a strong inhibitory effect on mineral absorption in adults, particularly on the absorption of iron. Grains also contain tannins which can depress growth, decrease iron absorption, and damage the mucosal lining of the gastrointestinal tract. **Grain bran is high in insoluble fiber that your body cannot digest.**

To make grain, nut, legume, and seed consumption healthy we need to remove as much phytic acid and other grain toxins as possible. Lectins are another form of grain toxin that can be poisonous. Agglutinin is a lectin in wheat germ that passes through digestion and into the body and produces intestinal inflammation.

Each indigenous culture that used grains, had specific procedures to make their grains safe to eat. Without following their careful example, of storage, sifting, and fermenting, modern grains, even whole grains can be toxic to eat.

Grain advice: barley, kamut, spelt, rye, wheat, corn and probably oats must have their bran and germ removed before consumption. Rice is best when the bran is partially removed and then soaked with a starter. In addition to removing the bran, grains should usually be fermented before consumption, one example is sourdough bread. Do not eat store bought sprouted grain bread products. For more information about grains please go to: **www.healingourchildren.net/wholegrains**

Folic Acid

Folic acid is also known as vitamin B-9, or folate. It is preferable, as with all nutrients, to consume it in a form that is whole and unrefined, which means either from a whole food or a whole food supplement. Whole foods high in folic acid are liver and leafy green vegetables. Some examples of green leafy vegetables are spinach, turnip greens, cabbage, asparagus, collards and seaweed.

Other Nutrients are also important

If I have left out anything else, omega-3 or omega-6 fatty acids for example, it does not mean that these other nutrients and trace minerals are less important. Some of these other nutrients I will discuss here. Many trace minerals are likely obtainable from all the different parts of certain plants and herbs (the roots, leaves, flowers, and bark). However, a complete guide to

indigenous uses of herbs and plant foods for nutrients is beyond the scope of this book. Many of the food sources are listed, to some degree, with the most potent source first and progressively less potent sources listed afterward. Other sources of these minerals exist that <u>are not listed</u>.

Vitamin B-12 is discussed in more detail in the chapter about preconception health (chapter seven). A lack of vitamin B-12 can lead to infertility and other health problems.

Sources: mollusks (clams, oysters, mussels, etc) liver and fish eggs, trout, salmon, beef sirloin, yogurt and milk.

Zinc — A deficiency of zinc can lead to birth difficulties and lack of care for offspring.[260]

Sources: oysters, pumpkin seeds, sesame seeds, beef, lamb, crab, chicken liver, wheat.

Magnesium — A deficiency of magnesium can cause abnormalities, calcium deposits, and kidney damage.

Sources: clams, chard, spinach, buckwheat, rye, quinoa, fish sauce, sunflower seeds, pumpkin seeds, almonds, peanuts, and black beans.

Iron — A deficiency of iron can cause eye, bone and brain defects and neonatal mortality.

Sources: goose and duck liver, beef, lamb and pork spleen, clams, oysters, turnip greens, spirulina.

Chromium — A deficiency of chromium can cause eye abnormalities.

Sources: nutritional yeast, broccoli, turkey thigh (not many foods have been analyzed for their chromium content).

Copper — A deficiency of copper can lead to anemia, fragile bones and depigmentation.

Sources: beef and lamb liver, oysters, crab, clams, cashews, sunflower seeds, pumpkin seeds, nutritional yeast, and spirulina.

Cobalt — Part of the structure of vitamin B-12, cobalt helps reduce iron deficiency (see B-12 section for cobalt sources).

Iodine – A deficiency of iodine leads to poor mental development in babies.

Sources: seaweed, cod, shrimp, haddock, perch, salmon, tuna and milk.

Manganese – A deficiency of manganese (different from magnesium) can lead to still-birth.

Sources: pine nuts, mussels, pecans, macadamia nuts, pumpkin seeds, rye, and sweet potatoes.

Potassium – A deficiency of potassium can lead to fatigue, listlessness, insomnia and weakness in adults.

Sources: quinoa, rye, prunes, bamboo shoots, dates, beet greens, sunflower seeds, cabbage, peanuts, acorns, Swiss chard, yam, octopus, cuttlefish, taro, salmon, clams, potatoes, spinach, mustard greens, and squash.

Selenium – A deficiency of selenium has been linked to Down syndrome. Fluoride in water depletes selenium stores in the body.

Sources: oysters, turkey giblets, Brazil nuts, whole chicken or turkey, beef, pork and lamb kidneys, tuna, anchovy, fish eggs, chicken, turkey and duck liver, pancreas, kidney and spleen of several animals, and cremini mushrooms.

Silicon – Silicon helps form connective tissues, bones, and the placenta.

Sources: barley, partially milled rice, root vegetables, lettuce, tomatoes, onions, cucumbers, beets.

Vanadium – A deficiency of vanadium decreases reproductive abilities and impairs growth.

Sources: buckwheat, rice, green beans, carrots, cabbage, mushrooms, dill seed, black pepper, shellfish, radishes, olive oil, oysters and lobster.

Nickel – A deficiency of nickel can cause liver cirrhosis and kidney failure in adults.

Sources: green leafy vegetables, lentils, peas, and nuts, especially almonds, cherries, bananas, pears, asparagus.

Clay. Clay can be used as a dietary supplement to provide trace minerals, as well as to provide balance of the body's ecosystem. Dr. Price writes:

> *It is also of interest that among this group in the Andes, among those in central Africa, and among the Aborigines of Australia, each knapsack contained a ball of clay, a little of which was dissolved in water. Into this they dipped their morsels of food while eating. Their explanation was to prevent "sick stomach."* [261]

Clay, to be safe, must not contain lead from its sources. Two suggested sources are Teramin clay, www.terramin.com and Azomite (trade name for montmorillonite clay), www.azomite.com. These clays can be consumed in small amounts.

Dr. Price's Food Suggestions

This is a diet that Weston Price gave to growing children to help prevent tooth decay. It is either identical or very similar to a diet he used to support health during pregnancy.

> *About four ounces of tomato juice and a teaspoonful of a mixture of equal parts of a very high vitamin natural cod liver oil and an especially high vitamin butter was given at the beginning of the meal. They then received a bowl containing approximately a pint of a very rich vegetable and meat stew, made largely from* **bone marrow** *and fine cuts of tender meat: the meat was usually broiled separately to retain its juice and then chopped very fine and added to the bone marrow meat soup which always contained finely chopped vegetables and plenty of very yellow carrots; for the next course they had cooked fruit, with very little sweetening, and rolls made from freshly ground whole wheat, which were spread with the high-vitamin butter. The wheat for the rolls was ground fresh every day in a motor driven coffee mill. Each child was also given* **two glasses of fresh whole milk.** *The*

*menu was varied from day to day by substi-
tuting for the meat stew, **fish chowder or
organs** of animals.[262] (Emphasis added.)*

*This reinforcement of the fat-soluble vi-
tamins to a menu that is low in starches and
sugars .., and with milk for growing children and for many adults, and the liberal
use of sea foods and organs of animals,
produced the result described.[263]*

For pregnancy, Dr. Price suggests:

*The use of milk, green vegetables, sea
foods, organs of animals and the reinforcement of the fat-soluble vitamins by very high
vitamin butter and high vitamin natural cod
liver oil. [264]*

You'll notice that all of Dr. Price's dietary
recommendations have been incorporated into
the dietary guidelines presented in this book. Dr.
Price's regularly included organ meats and sea
foods in his recommendations.

**Whole Food Supplements to Enhance Nutri-
ent Levels — may be helpful for some.**

Natural vitamin C from food sources such as
in the form of acerola berry or amalaki fruit.

Evening primrose oil, black currant oil, or
borage oil. Consider taking one of these oils
as they contain an omega-6 fatty acid called
gamma-linolenic acid, or GLA. When our
bodies are not totally healthy, or if we have
a certain genetic background, we may not be
able to produce enough GLA because of a
lack of the enzyme delta-6 desaturase
(D6D). [265]

Spirulina contains high mineral and protein
content and may be a good supplement to
take.

Bee pollen.

Probiotics to support healthy intestinal flora.

Red Raspberry Leaf Tea is one of the
most famous female tonic herbs, especially for
pregnancy. It is rich in calcium, iron, phosphorus, potassium and vitamins B, C, and E.[266] To

make, pour boiling water over 2-6 tablespoons
of the herb in a quart size mason jar and let
steep for 15-20 minutes, covered. Drink three or
more cups per day during pregnancy or prior to
pregnancy. It does wonders for the body.

I encourage the use of herbs prior to preg-
nancy, during pregnancy, and during lactation.
They provide missing trace elements and other
activating substances that help enhance health.
For more about herbs I suggest: *Wise Woman
Herbal for the Childbearing Year* by Susun
Weed, *Rosemary Gladstar's Family Herbal* by
Rosemary Gladstar, and *The Natural Pregnancy
Book* by Aviva Jill Romm.

Be Aware: Herbs can interact with prescription drugs, and sometimes with other herbs,
and produce negative effects. In general, herbs
do not interact with each other or with other
drugs; however, it is important to know that
sometimes they do.

The Safety of Fish Containing Naturally Occurring Mercury

Mercury occurs in several forms; inorganic mercury is contributed to the environment via such
natural sources as volcanoes, forest fires and the
erosion of mercury-containing rocks. Inorganic
mercury is also a trace constituent of fossil fu-
els, yet their large-scale burning for energy creates many tons of elemental mercury that are
released into the atmosphere each year, which is
eventually rained down upon the world's wa-
terways. Organic mercury is a carbon-containing
compound, which is formed when inorganic
mercury is acted upon by microorganisms living
in the sediments of lakes, rivers, wetlands and
the open ocean. Methyl mercury is a common
example of an organic mercury, which is the
product of anaerobic organisms acting on both
natural and manmade sources of inorganic mercury. In the past it was also produced as an industrial waste product of the manufacture of
chemicals such as vinyl chloride. Methyl mercury, then, can be seen to be both a natural constituent of ocean water as well as being contributed to by the fallout of human industry. The
issue of mercury contamination in fish is a complicated and confusing story, but compelling

evidence suggests that fish can continue to be part of a nutritious diet as long as the consumer chooses wisely.

The natural red color in plankton (food for fish) comes from methyl mercury. Methyl mercury has been a part of humans' diet for thousands of years through the consumption of sea food; some conjecture it might even be a necessary nutrient for health.[267] Furthermore, fears that mercury levels in fish are rising may be unfounded. In California's landmark mercury-in-tuna case (2006), in which Superior Court Judge Robert Dondero, University of Connecticut marine scientist Dr. William Fitzgerald reported that there are no peer-reviewed studies that show any increase in methyl mercury in fish over the last 100 years.[268]

Industrial mercury pollution is the true culprit of mercury poisoning. It is present in all of our lakes, rivers and oceans, and the use of mercury as an additive in food and as a component of vaccinations and other medications poisons us and our children still further. While you are vehemently told to eat limited amounts of fish because it contains mercury, you are told at the same time that vaccinations, which contain synthetic and highly toxic mercury in much higher amounts, are necessary for both you and your children. Even today's vaccines, labeled as mercury free, have been independently tested and found still to contain some mercury. The flu vaccine's key component is mercury. The mainstream medical establishment and government have done little to stop or change the real sources of mercury poisoning. If they really wanted to prevent mercury poisoning in pregnant women and children, they would focus on eliminating the true and most obvious sources first: vaccinations, food additives, mercury fillings, prescription drugs and industrial pollution. Instead, they suggest that we avoid naturally occurring mercury in fish.

Fears about mercury poisoning from fish arose in the 1950s, when large amounts of organic mercury (methyl mercury produced as an industrial waste byproduct) were released by a chemical company into the Minamata Bay in Kyushu, Japan.[269] The enormous concentration of methyl mercury in Minamata Bay caused horrific health effects for decades for pregnant women and other villagers who consumed fish and shellfish caught from the bay. But it is interesting to note that there has never been any other recorded case of harm caused by mercury poisoning from fish consumption, except for the cases in Japan that were due to massive industrial pollution.[270] The evidence in favor of fish safety does not stop here.

A study done in the Seychelles Islands, where women routinely consume large amounts of fish (12 times per week), and have higher than normal levels of mercury in their blood, found that there was no negative effect on their children from the fish consumption.[271] The same Seychelles Island studies concluded that mercury exposure from eating fish produced no negative effects at all.[272] In a landmark scientific study appearing in The Lancet, researchers found "no evidence to lend support to the warnings ... that pregnant women should limit their seafood consumption."[273]

What surprised scientists most was that of the 11,875 women included in the Lancet study, the children of the mothers who ate less than twelve ounces of fish per week had, in general, lower I.Qs.[274] The study concludes that the benefits from a diet rich in seafood and fish outweigh any potential risks of their mercury content.[275]

As previously mentioned in Chapter 5, many women are deficient in a variety of nutrients — the result of eating a modernized diet. Many indigenous people had special protocols that pregnant women and children should eat foods from the sea (both regular fish and shellfish). Seafoods are extremely high in minerals and, when eaten with the organs, are very high in fat-soluble vitamins and activating substances, which help facilitate new growth. The Lancet study found that lower fish intake is associated with less intelligent children.

Therefore, one can conclude that the forces trying to limit our use of sea-foods, through scare tactics not based on any valid scientific evidence, promote a system that increases our chances of illness and increases our chance of having mentally inferior children.

Detoxification

If you've been mostly eating foods from the "to avoid" list and then switch to the healthy foods, you may experience a detoxification response. There is a learning curve for adjusting to a healthier diet, because for the first time your body will be ingesting the foods it needs (and we hope is absorbing them). Take care when you switch your diet, and if you should become ill, it is likely that your body is releasing trapped goo from years of an unhealthy diet. My family has experienced several detoxifications, the most severe being caused by raw eggs. Each time, I know I have experienced a detoxification because I am healthier afterwards.

Small Head or Big Head

You might have a hidden fear or belief that eating better foods will produce a bigger head for the baby, and thus create a more difficult birth. While it is possible that the baby's head will be bigger, this isn't necessarily what will happen. In fact, the opposite occurs. When our diet is full of unhealthy foods, it creates a glandular imbalance and the baby's body can become swollen and out of proportion, making the birth more difficult. What happens when the diet is more densely packed with nutrients, on the other hand, is that the baby's body becomes more densely packed with nutrients. So your nutrient-dense baby might be heavier. But very experienced midwives can tell you that the size of the baby's head is rarely the cause of a birth complication; rather, it is the positioning of the baby that causes problems. An unhealthy diet can also create children with wide shoulders, because the unhealthy diet causes children to grow out of proportion, which will definitely add to birth difficulties.

Shopping and Eating with Integrity

Indigenous people who began eating store bought food rapidly succumbed to disease, and their children became weak and frail. Many indigenous cultures have eventually become extinct, or come close to extinction, from adopting modern dietary habits.

Yet, most of us must face the fact that we need to buy our food from the store. So we must choose our food wisely, and choose it with integrity.

Buying organic, biodynamic and grassfed foods, and supporting farmers who care more for the type of foods that they produce, is a good place to start. These organic foods are generally richer in vitamins, so they will support a higher level of health.

But remember, just because a food label says "organic" does not mean it is healthy for you. Certainly the organic variant has fewer additives and chemicals, but that does not mean it is a whole food that is life sustaining. Because of the processing needed to preserve shelf life and enhance flavor, convenience foods cannot sustain life. Additionally, in order for packaged food companies to remain in business, many of them try to find ways to cut costs by using inferior ingredients; and it is not uncommon for them to enhance flavor so that you continue to buy their products. Sugar and sweeteners are usually added, even to organic packaged food, to stimulate this desire for the product.

Eating whole foods does not mean you need to forsake pizza, cookies, or ice cream. However, it is important to acknowledge that there are almost never healthy versions of these foods available premade in stores or restaurants. You need to make these foods at home using more traditional methods.

A common food-choice pitfall that people trying to be healthy blunder into is to buy the following foods labeled "organic" when they should be avoided altogether: breakfast cereals, pasta, bread, crackers, cookies, frozen foods, pizza, potato chips, premade sauces and salad dressings, granola, chocolate, any drink that is unnaturally sweetened, or fruit and vegetable juices from bottles (which have been pasteurized).

The Life Force in the Foods

Our food is alive; it has *beingness*. Many indigenous people considered it unthinkable to plant, harvest, transport or eat food without acknowledging the life force within the food. They recognized and respected the mysterious confluence of forces that created the possibility for growth and life. One metaphor for the force that gives life to a particular object is the concept of a guardian spirit, or deva. Before we plant our foods we should acknowledge and welcome the guardian spirit in the seeds. Ideally, honoring the spirit of the seed would continue throughout the plant's life, through harvesting, transportation, storage, and finally, at the time of eating. When I eat, I remember to acknowledge the powers, both human and spiritual, that gave me the food.

In an ideal situation, all the foods we eat, both plant and animal, would be foods whose spirits were honored during their lives. This honoring of the spirit is manifest when the land is carefully cultivated and the livestock cared for humanely. Foods that have been tended in this way have not only physical vitamins and nutrients, but ethereal vitamins as well, which nourish our soul and strengthen our connection to the earth and to life. Native peoples knew that their survival and sustenance ultimately came from this ethereal source, and they honored it. In modern times food is rarely, if ever, produced through honoring the aliveness within it.

The Life Force in a Seed

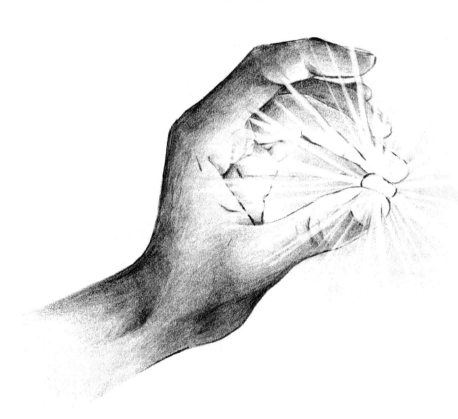

Everything contains within it a spiritual force that permeates everything else. It is important to welcome and acknowledge this force in our food, beginning at the time of planting the seed, up through the time of eating.

Deadly Food

When food is not mindfully and carefully grown and prepared, it contains very little of its life giving qualities. Because foods that have been processed pose a serious risk to our health, they were outlawed in 1906 by the Pure Food and Drug Act.[276] The purpose of the Pure Food Act was to protect the consumer from foods and drugs that might be harmful because of improper processing. The act was eventually repealed, after it wasn't enforced due to corruption in the Food and Drug Administrations (FDA). The FDA no longer legitimately protects us from most harmful foods or drugs. According to the Journal of the American Medical Association, there is a conservative estimate of 106,000 non-error (approved drugs properly prescribed according to established standards) drug deaths per year.[277] The wisdom of the pure food law is clear. Foods that are processed and adulterated in a manner that makes them poisonous — the vast majority of foods sold today — need to be outlawed. We cannot continue to poison ourselves, our land, or our children with these life-devoid and toxic foods. It is wrong that there are no laws to protect us from these harmful foods and drugs. However, that is no excuse for the ignorance of the consumer who buys them.

The only reason one might buy impure or overly processed foods is cost. Yet the few cents saved in the short term are exchanged for long term physical depletion and degeneration of health—with very expensive repercussions. At the same time, we need to acknowledge the malicious forces that advertise, promote and sell unhealthy foods, as they hide their true disease-promoting nature. Modernized foods that caused debility and disease in the indigenous populations around the planet in the early part of the 20th century probably contained few if any additives. Today's commercial foods are far more toxic than the foods of the past with the possibility of containing several of over 10,000[278] different additives (including pesticides, hormones, stimulants, artificial colors, chlorine, fumigants, gas residues, solvent residues, polymers from plastic, and much more). Today's soils are also far more depleted of nutrients than the soils of the 1930s.

In parting, just remember this prophetic statement which brings us an important truth. "It is store food that has given us store teeth." [279] And, we might add, store bodies….Now, imagine how this applies to your child developing in your womb.

To Keep Us Sick and Numb

Knowledge has been hidden from us to keep us sick. Many medical authorities might still recommend and suggest using the harmful modernized foods that I have shown to cause disease. Even many health-related organizations promote harmful foods indirectly, because they do not tell us about the dangers of modernized foods. To advocate for, or to do nothing against, modernized food and drugs in the face of overwhelming evidence of the harm they cause is wrong, and a sinister form of evil. Let us cease denying that modern foods are a source of tremendous physical — and as a result, emotional — suffering. I have already spoken about the connection between emotions and eating in the earlier section on abundance. But I will mention it again.

Many people are unaware that they use modernized foods as drugs. Many foods contain MSG, which is often labeled under different names. White sugar numbs our body and our feelings by increasing our pain tolerance; it encourages us to withdraw and not be present. As Dr. Bieler put it, the typical person

> is not aware that nearly all bad food habits are stimulation habits: that is, the body has almost automatically found out what makes it feel better for a half hour or so and what will mask the depression and fatigue symptoms momentarily.[280]

Modern food diets are based on stimulation habits and not on nourishment. They operate as methods to mask and hide our pain and as a result, we suffer.

Foods to Avoid

Knowing what not to eat is almost as important as knowing what to eat. The following foods poison our bodies and make us unfit for life. Our government agencies fail to protect us from dangerous foods. Food corporations cannot let go of their motives of profit and greed, so we wind up with a food system that is highly detrimental to our health, as well as to the health of our environment.

Avoid Non-Organic Food

A recent study, published in Environmental Health Perspectives,[281] documents how pesticides from fruits and vegetables rapidly appear in children's saliva and blood stream after being eaten. And it is now a proven fact that the poison sprayed on food will enter your body. These chemicals cannot just be washed off the food, because the use of systemic pesticides incorporates the pesticide into the very cells of the plants, making the entire plant a pesticide. Foods that are not organic also contain intentional chemical food additives, many of which have never been carefully tested for safety. Something every new mother should know is that pesticides present in foods can pass through her breastmilk to her child.[282]

Do not eat commercially processed foods such as cookies, cakes, crackers, TV dinners, soft drinks, packaged sauce mixes, etc. Avoid white flour, white flour products and white rice.

White flour that is not fermented may not be properly digested. Refined flour lacks vitamin E. Many of these packaged foods are loaded with MSG and other food additives, whose danger levels may not even be known. Packaged foods may also contain ingredients that are not listed on the label.

Avoid all refined sweeteners: sugar, dextrose, glucose and high fructose corn syrup.

Excess sugar consumption causes an imbalance in blood sugar, which can cause an imbalance in the ratio of calcium to phosphorus in the blood stream. In general, the more refined the sugar, the more dangerous it is. These refined sugars will cause a prolonged and more extreme fluctuation in blood sugar. If you want to be healthy you must avoid these sweeteners.

Special note: avoid on the polyol sweeteners (these are not natural) such as erythritol, sorbitol, and xylitol. Avoid agave "nectar," as all brands have more fructose than corn syrup and agave is contraindicated for pregnancy because its saponin content may cause miscarriage.

Avoid all hydrogenated or partially hydrogenated fats and oils. Avoid all vegetable oils made from soy, corn, safflower, canola, or cottonseed. Do not use polyunsaturated oils for cooking, sautéing or baking. Avoid commercially fried foods.

The high temperature heating common with commercial vegetable oils causes linoleic acid to break apart, creating dangerous free radicals. Industrially manufactured fats are toxic to the body and can enter the cell walls and wreak havoc on our internal body chemistry.[283]

Hydrogenated oils are probably one of the most dangerous of the processed foods. Many restaurants and natural food stores cook their food in canola oil. Restaurants save money by using these oils in place of healthier ones like olive or coconut oil. Saving money, while polluting our bodies, seems to be considered sound business sense. It is shameful that hydrogenated butter replacements are marketed as health foods. This oil makes me sick and causes coughing and congestion. These denatured products must be avoided.

Avoid pasteurized milk. Avoid homogenized milk and do not consume lowfat milk, skim milk, powdered milk, or imitation milk products such as soy or rice milk.

Commercial milk — the type that most people drink — contains fecal matter, blood, and pus. Pasteurization cooks this material, creating a toxic soup. What's more, significant portions of vitamins are lost in the pasteurization process. Homogenized milk renders milk unusable because it breaks apart the milk fat's cellular structure. Powdered milk has been exposed to high heat, damaging protein structure and rendering its fat rancid. Low fat milk is not satisfying, but can be used to create some good cheese (provided it comes from organic, grassfed cows). Soy milk contains enzyme inhibitors and excess estrogen. I have read of a fermented soy drink that can cure cancer, but this is not the same as the cheap, denatured and overly processed soy products sold in the grocery stores. Store bought rice milk is not a healthy drink. It is excessively sweet, and the manufacturing process doesn't seem to maintain the nutrients. If you are a rice milk lover, make it at home yourself. Don't settle for cheap imitations.

Most milk, and even milk labeled organic, comes from cows that are poorly treated and deprived of their natural diet of grass or carefully dried grasses. Instead, they are fed genetically modified grains and other inexpensive waste material that is certainly not what anyone would consider appropriate for cattle, such as bakery waste, orange peel cake and stale candy bars. As a result, the milk from these animals lacks vitamins. Modern, commercially-raised cows are bred for certain traits so they will produce more milk, which can make their milk out of balance and unsuitable for human consumption. Finally, the animals are also injected with rBGH (recombinant bovine growth hormone), a synthetic hormone that can cause negative health effects in humans when consumed through the milk.

Avoid battery-produced eggs and factory-farmed meats. Avoid highly processed luncheon meats and sausage containing MSG and other additives.

Packaged lunch meats contain many harmful food additives. It seems that many organic products (such as salami and hotdogs) containing natural nitrates (sea salt and celery juice) and nitrites, promote glandular imbalances but are less disruptive than the chemically-laden alternatives. Factory-farmed meats and eggs promote a profit-driven system of disease in which animals are misused and mistreated. The cesspools in these factory farms pollute the air and the environment. The animals are barely allowed to move, are loaded with drugs and chemicals to keep them alive, and are not fed their natural diet. It is unwise to eat the unhealthy meat from these animals.

Avoid the rancid and improperly prepared seeds, nuts and grains found in granolas, quick rise breads and extruded breakfast cereals. They block mineral absorption and cause intestinal distress. Avoid nut butters unless made at home.

Breakfast cereals, even when labeled organic, are not healthy and have little or no nutrients. Breakfast cereals are manufactured at high temperatures and pressures. A study found that rats that ate only puffed wheat died before rats that were given no food at all. Remember that at least one breakfast cereal has killed lab rats faster than when the rats ate only cardboard.[284] Also, phosphorus in the bran of whole grains — including organically produced grain — is tied up in a substance called phytic acid. Phytic acid combines with iron, calcium, magnesium, copper, and zinc in the intestinal tract, blocking their absorption. Many people unwisely continue to eat breakfast cereals because of the sweet-induced high it provides, and ignore the digestive distress that follows. But these high-inducing products also cause a rapid rise in blood sugar, and thus promote tooth decay.

The same policy goes for the store-bought granola that many people eat, which is almost always unhealthy. You can make delicious granola at home that is not stale and rancid, and preserves the vitamins of the grains. Avoid all nut butters unless they are homemade. When you grind nuts at home, you'll find that they become a powder, not a gob of goo. I have found nut butters in general to be a waste of money that provide little nutrients. Nuts should always be soaked first to disable the phytates and to make them more digestible. I do not know of any companies that have gone through the trouble of soaking nuts first. That being said however, if you eat packaged nut butter once in a while, it won't hurt you.

Note: Recently, I've come across some expensive granola in stores that is made with sprouted grains (such as buckwheat), and it is usually labeled as a raw food. Because the grains are sprouted, these cereals are an acceptable food, although usually the cereals are over sweetened. Rather than buying them at the store, you can make them at home for a fraction of the cost.

Avoid soy milk, soy meat, soy protein, soy formula, and tofu, including those that are organic.

Phytic acid in soy impinges upon the absorption of calcium, magnesium, copper, iron and zinc. Diets high in soy can cause growth problems in children. [285]

A friend of mine thought eating tofu was a good idea. In a short time after she began eating lots of tofu, her hair began falling out and her skin turned pale. Soy contains plant hormones that need to be disabled through a careful fermentation process, which tofu does not undergo. Fermented soy products, such as special fermented soy drinks, natural soy sauce, miso and tempeh can be acceptable. However, use fermented soy with care and awareness.

Avoid caffeine-containing beverages such as coffee, tea, and soft drinks. Avoid chocolate.

Many of these substances put an undue strain on the liver. Soda contains phosphoric acid, which inhibits the absorption of trace minerals and impairs the immune system. Caffeine overstimulates the adrenal glands, causing them to release a chemical which in turn causes sugar to be released into the blood. [286]

Wine and unpasteurized beers appear to be acceptable when used in moderation. In excess, wine and beer are overtaxing to the liver. Pasteurized beer should be strictly avoided. Soft drinks contain excess sugar and acid, robbing the body of calcium and filling it with empty calories.

Avoid canned, sprayed, waxed, bioengineered, or irradiated fruits and vegetables.

As discussed earlier, Dr. Price studied the decline in health experienced by indigenous groups who came in contact with modern food sources. Canned vegetables and meat were some of the foods that contributed to this rise in illness.

Avoid products containing protein powders.

The high-temperature processing of most protein powders renders the protein hazardous. Some high-quality protein powders made from high-quality whey or goat's milk may be of benefit to people, but this is not known for sure. What is the point of consuming protein powder when you can have *real,* healthy protein?

Avoid artificial food additives, especially MSG, hydrolyzed vegetable protein, and aspartame. These are all neurotoxins.

Most store-bought soups, sauces, broth mixes and commercial condiments contain the neurotoxin MSG, even if not so labeled. Vaccines also contain MSG. [287]

Avoid aluminum-containing foods, including commercial salt, commercial baking powder, and commercial antacids. Do not use aluminum cookware or aluminum-containing deodorants.

Avoid synthetic vitamins and any foods containing them.

Synthetic vitamins, and foods with synthetic vitamins added, offer little real benefit for our bodies. Synthetic vitamins are made with cheap substances and are not in a biochemical form that is easily absorbable by our bodies. Most actually put quite a bit of internal stress on our organs because our bodies view the vitamins as toxic substances that need to be rapidly eliminated (hence the unusual odor or color of urine after consuming many types of vitamins). A stalk of celery or a serving of fresh salad greens has more vitamins and minerals than a bottle of synthetic vitamin tablets.[288]

Do not drink distilled liquors.

These can easily cause glandular imbalances, and they weaken your primary organ of energy utilization and detoxification, the liver.

Do not use a microwave oven.

Microwaved foods do not taste good and there is a logical reason for this. Using radiation to cook one's food is unnatural, and the food molecules are damaged. Microwave ovens are the only cooking source that needs a shield to protect those nearby. If we have to be protected from microwaves, wouldn't it follow that our food needs the same protection? Studies have shown that microwaved food can pose a greater health risk than foods cooked by other conventional means.[289]

Do not use cigarettes or drugs — not even prescription drugs.[290]

Remember in Chapter 1, Dr. Bieler's second conclusion about creating health was, "*in almost all cases the use of drugs in treating patients is harmful.*" If disease is caused by a toxic or deficient internal environment, then a drug will **add** to the toxicity or deficiency, and thus contribute to the problem. That's why prescription and over the counter drugs are very dangerous to health and should only be used in urgent cases (if you want to be healthy). Western drugs are a primary cause of disease; they usually poison the body, and their residues get stuck in our tissues and weaken the efficiency of the body. Antibiotics are especially harmful to our digestive health. And our digestion is our first line of defense against disease, and the best opportunity to create health.

Now that you have some guidelines to follow for what is healthy and what is not, you can create your own diet. You can eat foods you enjoy, and that nourish your body. Keeping in mind the mental framework of healthy and unhealthy foods learned here, you can eat according to your tastes, inspiration and desires. Align with Nature's plan for health and success, again and again! At least once per day, just feel or visualize (or both) the vibration of health, aliveness, and wellness in your body.

7

Preconception, Fertility and Pregnancy Vitality

In order for us to start creating peaceful, healthy, strong and vibrant children, we need to start improving our own health before conception.

Intention: To give you the fundamentals to create a healthy and vibrant child, as well as a more comfortable pregnancy. To focus attention on the importance of preconception health.

It is time we start taking care of our children, by creating a fertile soil for them to grow in. If you're a gardener, you know that if you want plants to grow and thrive, you cannot just toss some seeds on the ground and expect wonderful results. If you want to plan for success, the soil needs to be fertile and healthy, alive with symbiotic organisms. You must carefully prepare the seedbed to accept the seeds, and provide enough moisture so that the seeds will sprout and take root. Yet when we create children, we rarely put any thought or effort towards the foundations of our own health. Attention to preconception health, by the way, is not just for prospective mothers; it is a requirement **and absolute necessity** for fathers as well.

Preconception is a part of Nature's symphony. This symphony guides the rhythms of all life forms. Animals migrate in response to the changes in sunshine and the nutrient content of the foods they eat. And they mate when they have the highest stores of nutrients in their bodies and are therefore most fertile. Indigenous groups producing physically excellent and emotionally stable children followed these cycles as well. Dr. Price explains:

This they have achieved by a system of carefully planned nutritional programs for mothers-to-be. It is important to note that they begin this process of special feeding long before conception takes place, not leaving it, as is so generally done until after the mother-to-be knows she is pregnant.[291]

To deeply honor and care for our child-to-be we need to take time before conception to heal our bodies and to nourish our bodies with special life-giving foods.

A Time for Preconception Health

It takes time for certain vitamins and nutrients to saturate deeply into the body. The time needed for this saturation depends on the foods utilized, and the health of the individual. The nutrients are used to build the foundations of new life. The spermatozoa of men are produced in the testes using nutrients in the man's body. The spermatozoa are immersed in a nutrient-rich plasma created from the seminal vesicles, prostate, and bulbourethral glands. The ova are created in the ovaries and go through a cyclical process of maturation. The health and vitality of the ova in women, and spermatozoa and seminal fluids in men, will be a direct reflection of their bodies' internal balance, which in turn is significantly influenced by their nutritional habits.

The production of sperm takes approximately 72 days.[292] Ova may take approximately

100 days to mature.[293] This scientific fact finds expression in the cultural habits of indigenous groups. The Masai, whom I have mentioned earlier, required that young women preparing for marriage spend a period of three months prior to conception consuming special foods in order to create a healthy child. This wise practice is based on the time it takes for the ovum to develop. If the women's fertile time is in the middle of the month, then you'll have 3 months plus 10-15 days, which is nearly the exact amount of time (100 days) the ovum needs to become ready for conception. For men, three months is also a safe bet as a minimum time for preconception health. The food consumed, and the health of the individual during the 100 days prior to conception, will significantly influence the creation of the ovum and spermatozoa. Therefore:

Every little health effort you make before conception, during this 3 month period of maturation and growth, will influence the health for your child-to-be.

In some of the tribes whose diets were dependent largely on grains, the special preparation time before conception was several months to one year. [294] Since many of us use grains in our diet, or are not in ideal health, the ideal length of preconception preparations is one year or more. This doesn't mean that you should or need to wait one year to have your baby. We do emphasize that one year is ideal, three months is a good idea, and anything you can do will help quite a bit.

Why We Need Preconception Health

Weston Price found that "heredity has been blamed wrongly for much of our modern deformity" [295] because the imbalances, birth defects and degenerative diseases only developed at the point of contact with modern civilization.

Heredity is our cultural excuse for imperfect physical development. We blame imperfect genetic combinations and mixed blood lines for causing problems in physical development. But the following pictures will illustrate what is really happening — our true heredity cannot properly come into manifestation because it is *intercepted* (blocked). Interception refers to something that is obstructed, or directed toward a new path by some type of force. Our children's heredity is, in a way, stolen from them. This *interception* is not caused by faulty genetics; but by nutritional deficiency (sometimes heredity is *intercepted* by toxic substances such as drugs, chemical exposure, and vaccines as well). And if you'll remember Chapter Five, I clearly illustrated how a majority of modern people lack essential vitamins, especially the fat-soluble vitamins and their related hormones, which are known to be important for reproduction. The diet and internal ecosystem of the mother and father during maturation of the germ seeds before conception is **the most important determinant** of how healthy their child will be. The deficient diet leads to deficient germ seeds, which then prevent out children from obtaining their full genetic heritage

On the next page you will see a picture of four young men. Even though they look as though they are related, they are not brothers; actually, they are from *different islands*. Note how well formed their faces are. The middle sections of their faces are wide, and have an even proportion to them with a mostly equal width from the top of the head down through the jaw. Since they all ate similar healthy native diets, and since their parents all regularly consumed special foods prior to conception, their similar genetic heritage was brought to full expression by the full development of their physical bodies. From this perspective then, they appear to be brothers even though they are not related.

Similar Facial Features in Unrelated Polynesian Girls

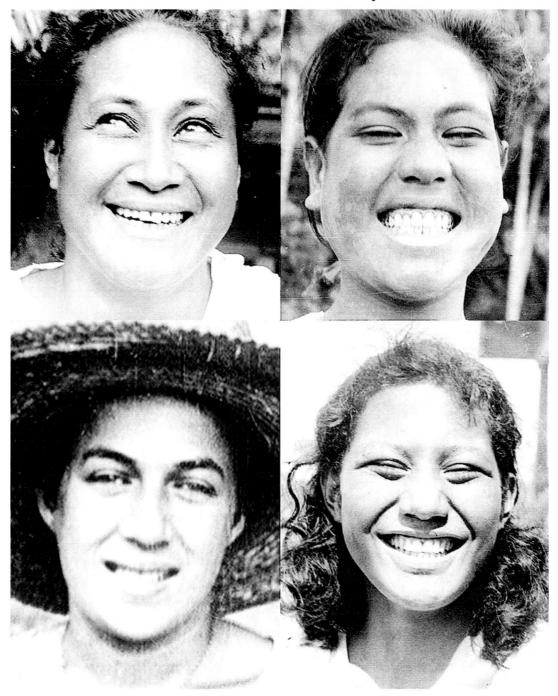

These four Polynesian girls live on different islands and are not related though they look like sisters. They record their racial type by undisturbed heredity.[296]

Similar Facial Features in Unrelated Melanesian Boys

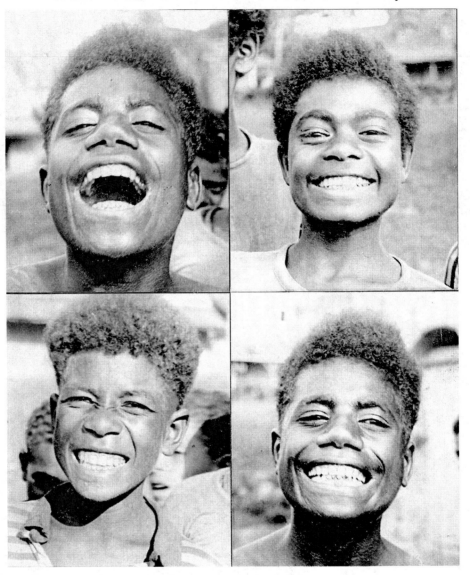

© Price-Pottenger Nutrition Foundation, www.ppnf.org

These four Melanesian boys born on different islands look like brothers but are not blood relations. They illustrate the role of heredity in reproducing racial type. Heredity, however, can only operate normally when the germ cells have not been injured.[297]

When nutrition is excellent, even unrelated people with similar genetic heritage look as if they belong in the same family, because their full genetic potential has been reached. Now let's consider a different phenomenon. In the following pictures we will see sisters and brothers who, even though they *are* related, have dramatically different facial features from one another. These differences are not caused by genetics, but by the *interception* of genetics as a result of a modernized nutritional program. The older sibling is a product of the native diet, while the younger, a modern diet.

Different Facial Features in Brothers and Sisters

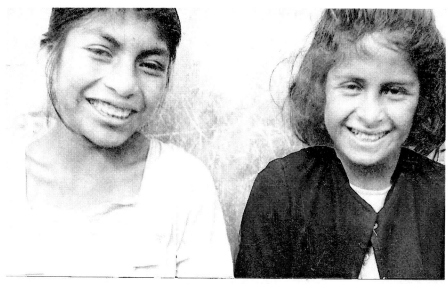

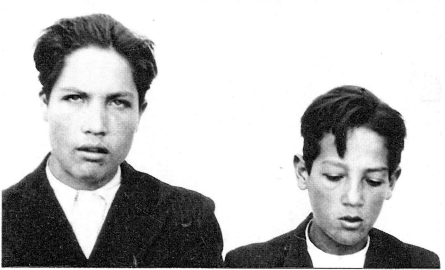

Disturbed heredity. Quichua Indians. Note the marked change in shape of the face and dental arches of the younger sister at the right. Also of the younger brother at the right. These families demonstrate a lowering of reproductive capacity of the parents with the later born children. [298]

In the above pictures, notice how the shapes of the faces of the two sisters are dramatically different. The sister on the left has fully developed features and a beautiful countenance. Even though her sister on the right is younger, her face is less defined and has a pushed in appearance. She looks so different because her genetic tendencies cannot blossom due to improper nutrition from modern foods. Now consider the brothers. On the bottom right, the brother's face is much more narrow, less square and defined than his brother's. This is due to impaired nutrition that began at preconception and continued through pregnancy, and is not the result of poor genetics.

Different Facial Features Observed in Brothers and Sisters

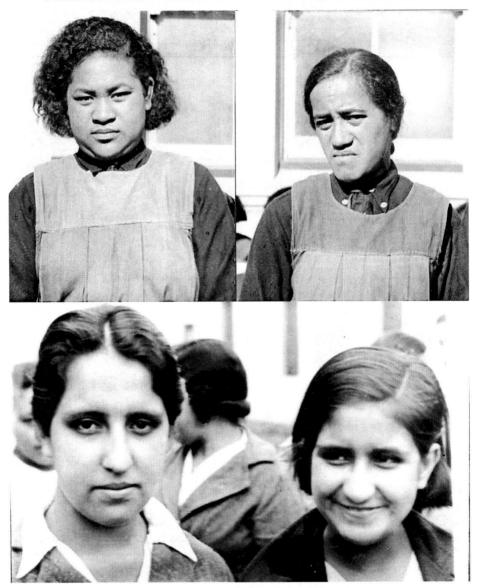

© Price-Pottenger Nutrition Foundation, www.ppnf.org

Above, two Maori girls in New Zealand and below, two white girls in Peru. Note the facial change in the girls at the right compared with their older sisters.

Here again, notice the significant change in the overall shape and structure of the faces of the sisters in the top photos. The girl on the (top) right has a narrow face, which is far different from the wide and square face of her sister. Of the sisters in the lower picture, the one on the right has a smaller face. Now, turn back a few pages and again look over the first two sets of pictures of unrelated young people raised with healthy nutrition. And then look over the second two sets of pictures of actual brothers and sisters, and see how much the faces changed as the result of the parents having eaten devitalized foods.

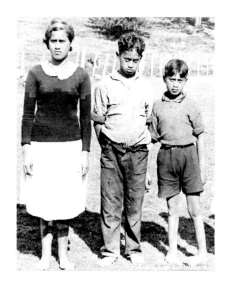

© Price-Pottenger Nutrition Foundation,
www.ppnf.org

Revisiting this picture from page 57, we see a progressive decline in the health of these offspring. Again, this is not a genetic defect, but a result of impaired heredity that began with the seeds of the mother and father.

When Nature's laws of proper nutrition are followed, our physical form develops to perfection. When these laws are not obeyed, the physical beauty and health of our children suffer greatly. After examining the disturbed hereditary features of the people shown on these pages, you might begin to notice these disturbed features and bodies in the people you see in your day-to-day life. And you may come to a profound and startling realization. Almost all of us modern folk, because of our impaired nutrition, suffer from physically abnormal development.

Disturbed Heredity Happens with Improper Nutrition

The physical growth of our bodies, and the growth of the prenatal infant, is controlled primarily by the hormones secreted through our glandular system. Our ability to develop fully, physically and emotionally, is greatly affected by the health of our glands. Each gland corresponds to the physical development of a different part of our body; therefore a weak or un-

healthy gland will manifest ailments in a particular part of the body.

Lab studies on rats have shown that when the pituitary gland (the master gland located in the base of the brain) did not function properly, it created a narrowing of dental arches and a mal-development of the face. But in the cases where pituitary extracts were used to correct the pituitary gland deficiency, the rats grew normally.[299] What can be concluded is that proper physical development is a result of the proper development of the gland (pituitary, thyroid, adrenal, sex glands, etc.) related to the particular area of the body. And it is fat-soluble vitamins and related hormones, which are almost totally absent in our modern foods, which promote the proper functioning of these glands.[300] Glands are also essential to the process of birth, so healthy glands will significantly increase your chances of a healthy and natural birth.

Child Spacing

When children are spaced too closely together, the mother's physical body as well as her emotional health is strained. Her nutrient stores have been depleted, and the mother needs time to recover and rebuild. The first child will have a more difficult time completing the phase of attachment and bonding with his mother, and this will put an emotional strain on both of them. Attachment and bonding are discussed in the next two chapters, but I will mention here that it takes approximately 6 years for girls and 7 years for boys to complete the bonding stage. (Boys take a little bit longer to mature probably because of the difference in physical size.)

Indigenous people took time to regenerate their bodies after having one child.

> *[In some tribes]...they considered that in order to develop the most perfect babies, the mothers must have a rest period after each baby. It was also for the purpose of permitting her to nurse her baby for three years in order to tide the baby over the stress period from infancy to childhood.*[301]

In researcher George Brown's study of the Melanesians and Polynesians, he observes that if a child is ever weak or sickly people would blame the parents for poor habits (not poor genetics).[302]

With the Ibos in Nigeria it is not only a disgrace but an abomination to have children closer together than three years. If a child is born sooner than this they fear that its health will be compromised.[303]

The Indians of Peru, Ecuador and Columbia abstain from intercourse throughout lactation to avoid children born too close together. At least two and a half years of space is achieved through this method.[304]

Cattle tribes in Africa use a system of multiple wives to create a child interval of two and a half to four years.[305]

In the Fiji Islands among "one of the tribes the minimum spacing was four years."[306]

To maintain child spacing, a healthy and safe version of birth control is needed. Later in this chapter I will discuss a method of birth control, Fertility Awareness Method (FAM), which can be used to support child spacing and is reliable when used carefully.

Infertility — Causes and Solutions

Infertility is an aspect of our karma, as it has to do with our present and past actions and unresolved life patterns. Infertility usually does not just happen to us; we are not victims of it. Infertility will result in a cycle of life lessons and thus fulfills a spiritual purpose: we must become more present and deal with the difficulties it may bring up. Many of us have the potential to transform our infertility into fertility. The Foresight preconception program, without using artificial methods such as drugs or implantations, has achieved a 78.4% success rate of reversing infertility.[307]

When coming into contact with modern civilizations, many native tribes, like the Marquesans, once numbering in the hundreds of thousands, quickly became extinct. Along with other health detriments resulting from this contact was the inability to produce healthy offspring. And the cause of this failure? Yes, the deficiencies of the modern diet. By simply correcting imbalances caused by our industrialized diet, many modern couples can restore their fertility.

When people are in sub-optimal health, their reproductive systems fail to function properly. This is the body's clever survival mechanism. It turns off the least important part first. The fact that reproduction ranks less than your health and survival as an individual is determined by Nature rather than by you.

Even though indigenous peoples were generally fertile and enjoying high levels of health, many groups nevertheless expended extraordinary efforts to provide their young adults of childbearing age special foods to enhance their fertility and reproductive ability. Fish eggs are one such special food which enhances fertility.[308] (Other fertility-enhancing foods were mentioned in the beginning of Chapter 6). Again, foods which enhance fertility are high in activator X. These foods include: butter made when the animals consume rapidly growing grass in the late spring, summer or fall; animal organs, especially after those animals eat rapidly growing grass; fish, as well as shellfish, including the organs.

It is important to know that infertility usually concerns both the man and the woman intending to have children. I came to this conclusion after reading that in one Native American group, if a couple couldn't have children the man was to eat bear meat (probably certain organs), and then it would be guaranteed that there would be children. Usually, both the prospective parents have similar lifestyle habits, which can result in infertility. Infertility is rarely an issue of a birth defect (such as a crucial organ not forming properly) and is commonly an issue of our bodies failing under our modern dietary program.

It was discovered that birth rates in European countries declined when refined grains became prevalent in the diet, and essential B and E vitamins were lost.[309] A lack of vitamin B6 can cause infertility and deficiencies of this vitamin can be caused by the use of birth control pills.[310]

Vitamin B6 is found in the highest abundance in raw liver, and then in raw milk, raw meat, raw cheese and raw fish. Cooking can also destroy vitamin B6.

Infertility can be caused by any damage to women's internal chemistry that makes their reproductive system too acidic. Spermicides, lubricants, birth control pills and other chemicals can be absorbed into the uterus and damage ova as well. Consuming blended drinks made with raw milk and raw eggs, taken 4 days weekly for 6 months and up to two years, along with other raw animal foods, can help heal infertility.[311]

Toxic excretions in the body can also create malformed spermatozoa or ova. Other sources of such toxins (in addition to modern processed foods such as sugar and flour products) are discussed later in this chapter.

Sometimes, we may actually be fertile and the barrier preventing a successful pregnancy is the sexual act itself. In *Dr. Bieler's Natural Way to Sexual Health,* Dr. Henry Bieler describes how a lack of sexual response can be a result of toxic accumulations in the body. This is a problem involving both men and women — that's why there is now a billion dollar industry for male enhancement drugs like Viagra.™ Impotence in men and lack of sexual desire in women are many times the result of their bodies breaking down from the effects of modern foods. Usually this is connected to emotional imbalances, such as unhappiness with life. Good sexual response requires that your glands are healthy and that your body has enough fat-soluble vitamins. For men and women many foods can be aphrodisiacs. Eating egg yolks (preferably raw) replenishes the adrenal glands, and eating avocados can help build vitamin E stores.[312] Eating foods that help replenish minerals, especially raw animal foods that are highly dense in nutrients and absorbable, helps with sexual vitality. Eat foods like raw oysters and clams, raw beef, raw fish, and raw eggs. (If you cannot tolerate these foods raw, cook them in any way that you prefer, but be sure to include them in your diet often.)

In addition to the aids discussed in this book, natural medicine can provide additional support for infertility. Homeopathy, Chinese herbal medicine and acupuncture are examples of several systems that can offer potent and effective natural solutions for infertility. Dr. John Christopher, an American herbalist, has created a herbal formula to promote conception and women's health called Female Reproductive Formula (NuFem). This and other similar herbal formulas can be purchased on the Internet or at some natural pharmacies.

Menstruation and Toxins

Proper internal cleansing along with adjustments in diet can lead to a great alleviation of symptoms that women commonly face in their lives. An accumulation of toxins can exist in the body and in the womb prior to conception, and thus result in an ecosystem not conducive to creating a healthy baby. If your body swells during the menstrual cycle, this is a sign that you are toxic. PMS is not necessarily normal or an inherent part of women's cycles, but the result of the elimination of toxic blood through menstruation. The cleansing menstrual flow could be one reason why women tend to live longer than men.[313]

Revitalizing the Body — A Program for Preconception Health

The principle of preparing the prospective mother for childbearing well in advance of the opportunity for conception has been the practice of primitive tribes in quite remote parts of the earth.[314]

If you observe the following symptoms in yourself, you may be seeing indicators of sub-optimal health: allergies, constipation, skin blemishes or disorders, headaches, muscle or joint pain including back pain, irritability and anger, mood swings, unclear thinking, fatigue, hair loss, tooth decay, vision loss or poor vision, and lack of sexual energy. All of these, in addition to other similar conditions, are signs that your body is physically degenerating.

A successful preconception health program contains the following:

Creating Physical Health

Absorbable Nutrients– Building up a reserve of minerals and fat-soluble vitamins and activators.

Recovering from drug and contraceptive use (birth control pills and IUD). The nutrients especially important to restore in this case will be zinc, manganese, vitamin A and the B-complex vitamins.

Cleansing and Healing– Removing toxic residues in the body.

Identifying and healing any minor types of ailments such as allergies, lingering or hidden infections, physical aches and pains, and low energy.

Maintaining Health– Avoiding future toxic accumulations and energizing the body.

Avoiding electro-magnetic and microwave fields, western drugs, and environmental pollutants in food, air and water.

Regular exercise such as yoga, tai chi, swimming or walking to build physical health.

Emotional Health

Taking time to feel your feelings.

Building and cleansing emotions through searching for and integrating lost emotions. Use healing techniques and/or journaling, while engaging in positive and supportive relationships.

Mental Health

Clarify thoughts and feelings through meditation, journaling, talking, and reading spiritual or harmonious texts.

Clarifying your intentions around parenting, family, your intimate relationship and your community.

Spiritual Health

Align with your life's purpose as a parent.

Engage in spiritual practices such as prayer, meditation, reading religious or spiritual texts, yoga, and selfless service.

Most of us subscribe to the common belief that rather than take care of ourselves, and heal the root of our problems, we should let someone else, such as a doctor or midwife, take charge of our health — all the while staying in our unrealistic, unsatisfied and unhealthy lifestyles. A visit to the doctor typically involves certain exams and tests which are often totally meaningless and useless. These tests don't resolve problems and they don't create a better potential for health. With few exceptions even most midwives try to provide services and tests identical to what conventional doctors would provide. At best, the many tests identify a potential for a problem but offer little to no real solutions. That is why I say they are meaningless; if a potential problem is found, there usually isn't much to do about it. In fact, I just got a psychic hit — many of these tests are performed solely to generate income. If a potential problem is found, it's a good way to justify more procedures and thus more profit. It's like when you go to get the oil changed in your car; the garage offers you all these other services to try to make more money off of your visit. As sick as this is, it is all a part of the "business of disease" that manipulates health problems to make obscene amounts of money. Doctors with such motivations will order many tests to see if they can offer you more profitable services.

Many tests are invasive and carry a significant risk for harm. The test for pregnancy diabetes, for example, requires the pregnant mother to ingest large amounts of very unhealthy sugar. Many disease conditions of pregnancy have obvious indicators that don't require tests; they can be noticed by intelligent and attentive practitioners. Unfortunately, most midwives and doctors spend their energy protecting themselves from potential lawsuits by performing only tests and procedures that are sanctified by conventional medical protocols. There are effective ways to help prepare yourself for birth and to have a healthy pregnancy, but it is rare that you'll get even 25% of that information from even the most alternative birth care provider. Hence, the need for this book.

Preconception is not just for Women — It is Essential for Men, Too

Men are not excused from participating in pre-conception health preparations. The seeds of the man exert a strong influence on the health of his child, as the evidence I provided in Chapter 4 suggests. Since you now know this, you cannot consciously deny that your lifestyle can affect your unborn child. Habits like drinking alcohol (even small amounts), or smoking cigarettes could make your seed deficient. Abstaining from these health-depleting substances for at least four and a half months prior to conception is necessary.

On the emotional, mental and spiritual level, women need men to be there with them. Women have a difficult time succeeding as mothers without the loving and supportive presence of the father. On one hand, men can find fulfill-ment and an improved quality of life from being fathers; but on the other hand, they can create more suffering for everyone involved if they don't take care of themselves.

Creating Physical Health — 3.5 months to one year prior to conception

Build up a reserve of minerals and fat-soluble vitamins and activators.

	Calcium	Phosphorus	Iron	Vitamin A	Vitamin D	Vitamin E	Fat Calories
Preconception	1.50	2.0	0.05	5,000 – 20,000 IU	500 – 2,000 IU	High[315]	40-60%

General Dietary Guidelines for Preconception Health

Avoid the foods of modernization (see Chapter 6).

Avoid smoking, alcohol and unnecessary drugs.

Eat two of these three foods regularly (daily or almost daily).*

Raw grassfed dairy foods

Seafoods, including all edible organs

Organs of land animals

Animal foods should usually be eaten raw, or seared, marinated/fermented, or cooked in stews.

Eat an abundance of vegetables.

Regularly consume fermented foods or other probiotic foods like yogurt, kefir, sauer-kraut, kombucha or other raw, cultured ani-mal foods.

Bone broths can be used regularly to restore, cleanse and nourish the body.

Eat the special preconception foods (as de-scribed in Chapter 6 and in the preconcep-tion timeline which follows).

*As an alternative or as a supplement for one of the categories, you may use mixture of fermented cod liver oil with high vitamin butter oil daily.

Adjust the dietary guidelines in Chapter 6 for pregnancy and lactation according to your particular needs. I have already discussed healthy nutrition in depth, as well as the foods that comprise a healthy diet. The most important impact will be made with a diet high in fat-soluble vitamins.

Preconception Health Timeline

Your preconception program includes:
Beginning the preconception health diet
Consider stopping the use of birth control pills or IUDs in favor of FAM

5 years B.C. (**Be**fore **C**onception)	Begin preconception health program.
	Safe to fast if necessary. Heal the body utilizing raw foods and/or fermented foods, and special cleanses.
2 years B.C.	Eat building and nourishing foods like oysters, raw or fermented milk, raw butter, raw cream, *fish eggs,* eggs and liver.[316]
	Wild seafoods with organs included, or organs of land animals.
6 months B.C.	Eat at least one special food regularly. Crab and lobster including "mustard" and "tomalley" (from clean waters). Milk, butter, and cream when the cows graze on rapidly growing grass. The *glands* of land animals when the animal is grazing on rapidly growing grass. Octopus. Fish eggs.
3.5 months B.C.	Men, eat soft roe (milt) and/or other foods high in Activator X, such as the special foods listed above (frequently-daily).
	Women, eat fish eggs and/or other foods high in activator X, such as the special foods listed above (frequently-daily). Or as an alternative to, or a supplement of special foods, take a mixture of yellow butter and liver, or high vitamin butter oil with high vitamin cod liver oil.
Day of Conception	Boiled tongue conception feast, and make sure to consume one of the special foods once or several times that day/s.

Conception!

The preconception health timeline can be adjusted to fit your needs. Anyone in optimal health who has been eating mostly native foods their entire life (including foods high in whole fats and activator X) can simply follow the preconception program that begins 3 or 6 months prior to conception. In indigenous groups, preconception nutrition had been practiced for countless generations. The parents traditionally consumed the proper nutrient-dense foods and their child-to-be was thus nurtured to its full potential of health. Through this child's entire life, he was provided with special foods to grow into a healthy adult. Then as an adult preparing for marriage, even within this ideal setting, the prospective parent will consume the special foods in preparation of conception.

Realistically, most people reading this book will need 1-5 years of preparation time prior to the conception of their child. If most of this material in the book is new to you, a longer preconception period might be better for your situation. Then again, babies happen when they happen, so try not to be too rigid about these things. The 1-5 year figure may be an ideal guideline for some, but certainly won't be suited for everyone. Don't wait too long for conception and then blame me if something doesn't work out because you were blindly committed to my 5 year plan! The time of your child's conception is your choice. My advice is to take as much time as you realistically can to improve your health. Even if you are on a limited time frame, every little bit of improvement before conception will make a big difference.

Preconception for Men

It is of the utmost importance that men practice eating whole foods rich in fat and fat-soluble vitamins. This should begin at least 3.5 months before conception, and ideally for 6 months to 5 years or more before conception. It is also important for men to be aware of the toxin levels in their bodies — the accumulated result of toxic lifestyle habits. Men also need to take time to meditate and go within themselves and search inwardly for ways to increase their level of health and vitality.

Fish Milt and Male Fish Organs for Men "Among the Eskimos I found…the milt (sperm) of the male salmon [was eaten] by the fathers for the purpose of reinforcing reproductive efficiency…The coastal Indians in Peru ate the so-called angelote egg, an organ of the male fish of an ovoviviparous species. These organs were used by the **fathers-to-be.**"[317]

The angelote egg is likely the testes of the angel fish (angel fish is similar or the same as an angel shark).[318]

Vitamin B-12

Vitamin B-12 deficiency can cause a low sperm count.[319] B-12 deficiency can also lead to infertility and miscarriages. Restoring B-12 levels by eating foods high in B-12 will help resolve or prevent these problems.[320]

Food sources of B-12 — Potent sources: Mollusks (clams, oysters, mussels, etc) and liver (turkey, duck, goose, beef).

Less potent sources still high in B-12: trout, salmon, beef sirloin, yogurt and milk.

Obtaining the special preconception foods for men. Sperm sacs, such as from salmon or cod, should be obtainable. To do this, you would need access to the whole fish, from which the sacs or glands could simply be removed. Some traditional Japanese restaurants serve shirako, which are cod sperm sacs. Perhaps your local sushi chef could help you identify which organs are the sperm sacs. A good fish merchant may also be able to help. A good Japanese restaurant offers many opportunities to support preconception health. In addition to shirako, there is the previously mentioned kani-miso (crab guts), along with uni, sea urchin, ikura, salmon roe, tobiko, flying fish roe, and also many other dishes with fish eggs. (Unfortunately, some of these foods also have preservatives when they come from restaurants, so be aware of your choices.)

The angelote, or angel fish, has a one-pound special gland, but will be more difficult to obtain. Other substitutes may be skate testicles or special glands, oysters (from the sea), rocky mountain oysters (bull testicles) or testicles from other animals. If these are unobtainable (or the thought of eating these is unfathomable to you), then consuming octopus with organs, crab with the mustard, sea foods including the organs, and/or milk products after the cows have eaten from rapidly growing grass, is an acceptable alternative. Again, if you can take the opportunity to get the special glands or soft roe, you will surely increase the vitality of your child-to-be. A little work now can change an entire life. In this case, in which you invest in the effort to consume special foods for the sake of your future child's health, people will remark years later about how fortunate you and the mother are to have such a vibrant, delightful child. You'll just smile to yourself, knowing that fortune had little to do with it.

The ideal time for conception is after three months of rapid grass growth. Depending on your location, this would range from June through September. (Again, don't go crazy trying to be perfect here; have your baby when you want to.)

Vitamins Lost from Contraceptive Use

Birth control pills and the IUD, along with alcohol and smoking, deplete the body of vitamin B6. When planning a healthy pregnancy it is a good idea to discontinue use of birth control pills and other synthetic drugs. Stop taking these well in advance of pregnancy. Later in this chapter I will discuss natural family planning (FAM), which is an effective method of natural birth control when practiced carefully and mindfully. When not practiced extremely carefully, babies will soon follow. This comment comes from personal experience.

Oral contraceptive pills contain hormones (steroids) that are usually synthetic. These hormones are estrogen and progesterone. The birth control pill alters one's internal copper and zinc levels and interferes with other mineral balances (magnesium, iron, iodine, chromium and manganese). [321]

If you have used birth control pills at any time in your life, the levels of vitamin A, C, B1, B2, B3 and B6[322] (and magnesium, iron, iodine, chromium and manganese) in your body need to be restored. To recover these nutrients, eat foods containing them more frequently, along with foods containing fat-soluble activators (butter, cream, etc.) to help in the absorption of the nutrients. See Chapter 6 for recommended foods and additional trace mineral suggestions.

Food sources high in B1 (Thiamin): nutritional yeast, pork (especially the loin), spirulina, oats, barley, macadamia nuts, sesame seeds. Sugar depletes B1, so avoid it.

Food sources high in B2 (Riboflavin): beef, pork, lamb, turkey, chicken, liver and kidney, spirulina, cuttle fish, fish eggs, almonds, raw eggs.

Food sources high in B3 (Niacin): beef, lamb, pork, chicken, turkey liver, anchovy, peanuts, chicken, tuna, salmon, spirulina.

Food sources for vitamin B6: raw liver, raw milk, raw meat, raw cheese and raw fish.

If you look carefully through the list, you will see that liver, especially eaten raw or seared, contains significant vitamins and minerals needed to restore the body to health after the depletion caused by birth control pills or the IUD.

Nourishing Raw Liver Shake/Smoothie

Makes 2 cups (courtesy of Michelle Smith)

2-8 ounces of raw milk
2 ounces of raw cream
1 - 2 raw eggs
1/2 - 1 tablespoon liver grated or chopped
1/2 - 1 cup frozen strawberries (or raspberries and other fruit)
Optional: 1/2 to 3/4 teaspoon of unheated honey

Blend.

Notes: You can replace the raw cream and raw eggs with 4 ounces of milk, so the recipe can be made using eight ounces of raw milk. If you cannot obtain raw milk, use the best quality yogurt as a milk replacement. When you use more than one full tablespoon of liver you can taste the liver. Kids will drink this smoothie! If you are prone to cavities or have sensitive teeth, eating strawberry smoothies all day may not be the best course for you, also omit the honey.

Cleansing and Healing

A healthy gut (digestive tract) is the basis for creating physical health. Our health begins with the delicate internal balance of flora and other inhabitants of our digestive tract. When the integrity of the digestive tract is compromised, healthy foods become toxic and can leak into the bloodstream unprocessed. So to create health, your gut balance must be restored. There are many routes to achieving this, and it usually takes a long time to come back to health. If your body is really clean and healthy then you have the possibility of having a healthy pregnancy. At the beginning of pregnancy the body will cleanse itself normally, and this is what we call morning sickness. Morning sickness occurs when the organs responsible for cleansing blood (like the liver and kidneys) become overloaded.

If you are taking any medications, these types of cleanses will likely alter the dosage requirement.

If you want to try cleansing your body, food-based cleanses are the most well rounded approach. **A word of caution**: any health changes are done at your own risk, if you feel unsure of how to proceed, please consult a natural health care provider.

The raw milk cure, written and described by Dr. J.R. Crewe in 1929 from the Mayo Foundation (requires good raw milk).

> *The therapy is simple. The patients are put at rest in bed and are given at half hour intervals small quantities of milk, totaling from five to ten quarts of milk a day. Most patients are started on three or four quarts of milk a day and this is usually increased by a pint a day. Diaphoresis [copious perspiration] is stimulated by hot baths and hot packs and heat in other forms. A daily enema is given.[323]*

Each quart is 4 cups, so that is 20-40 cups of milk in a day. Results may also improve by adding raw eggs and some raw cream to the milk. The milk should be at room temperature. This program can be used anywhere from 2-10 or more days. Adrenal exhaustion and fatigue respond well to the milk cure.

Raw foods cure and heal diseases. Hippocrates prescribed raw milk for tuberculosis and later physicians used fresh raw blood as a beneficial treatment of this disease.

Raw liver and raw fish for health benefits. Dr. Bieler explains:

> *Raw liver was commonly used by the Plains Indians to rehabilitate exhausted and diseased people... Even today raw fish is used by the Eskimos as well as by the South Sea Islanders for the cure of disease.[324]*

Raw fresh vegetable juice and raw eggs. Drinking vegetable juice helps heal the body. A good vegetable juice can be based on celery with additional vegetables like parsley, zucchini, cucumber, cilantro and/or carrots. (Using a Greenstar or other low speed juicer is best if you juice frequently.) I have already mentioned Aajonus Vonderplanitz, who healed himself of blood and bone cancer.[325] Mr. Vonderplanitz's protocol is called the *Primal Diet* and can be found in *Recipe for Living without Disease*. The diet includes all raw avocado, coconut, cream, butter, fish, meat, chicken, milk and vegetable juices. Of course, you can modify the diet to your liking within reasonable guidelines. Vegetable juices are part of many different healing protocols including Max Gerson's cancer curing method (**www.gerson.org**). I was forced to follow a raw foods diet (which included animal foods) when my toes started to swell and became red and painful. Over time, a mostly raw foods diet has significantly improved my health, and this particular condition went away.

Raw food protocols work because they restore lost nutrients to the liver and fatigued glands; at the same time, raw foods help the body to heal because they're easy to digest.

There is another class of cleanses, which places more burden on the body because they involve almost complete fasting, which in turn causes deficiencies that can last months or longer. I am sharing them with you because they have been highly effective for some people. Their effectiveness will depend on your body type and overall health. Use these cleanses with mindfulness.

Tissue cleansing through bowel management helps clear out toxic accumulations from the bowels. As described in detail in *Dr. Jensen's Guide to Better Bowel Care* by Dr. Bernard Jensen, the cleanse program involves fasting and high colon enemas, and believe it or not, just as in the pictures in the book, most people have ropes of black goo in their intestines. This program gets these out in 3-7 days! Other cleanses similar to Dr. Jensen's program, including options that don't require enemas, are the Blessed Herbs® cleanse, www.blessedherbs.com, Health Force Herbal Colon Cleanse, Arise and Shine cleanse, www.ariseandshine.com **and** *The Master*

Cleanser by Stanley Burroughs (a slightly different cleanse program that has been helpful for some people, but can promote tooth decay or other deficiency conditions).

Total fasting (no food, but lots of water) can be a liberating and spiritual experience, and it can help the body cleanse. It is recommended that you not do this within two years of conception (it must be done 2 or more years prior to conception).

When you follow any one of these programs you will likely experience disease symptoms such as a cold or flu. Many times people experience nausea, fever or headaches. During a cleanse, these symptoms arise from the body burning up old debris such as left over waste products or other unhealthy contaminants. Many people have eaten toxic foods and absorbed toxic medicines for years. So it is going to take months or even years to get back into perfect health.

Healing With Vegetable Soup

Maverick physician Henry Bieler used to help his patients cleanse their bodies using a careful selection of special foods, and particularly through the use of a broth containing mineral-rich vegetables. The minerals feed and strengthen the glands, nourishing them with needed elements like sodium and potassium. During pregnancy, Bieler's broth may be effective in helping to restore balance to a sick body. Its alkalizing effect can help bring balance to a diet that is high in animal fats and proteins.

Bieler's Soup

1 pound of string beans, ends removed

2 pounds zucchini, chopped

1 handful of curly parsley [1]

Enough water to cover the vegetables

Add all ingredients to rapidly boiling water and boil for 10-15 minutes, until a fork will pierce the rind of the zucchini. Purée using the cooking water (it is important to use this water as it contains vitamins and minerals) and thin the soup to the consistency you desire.

[1] Lactating women should limit their parsley intake as it dries up breast milk.

This specific recipe is designed for healing when the body is ill. Feel free to modify this recipe by adding all kinds of different vegetables to suit your personal needs.

You can also modify this recipe to make other types of nourishing broths by adding one or any of the following: chicken or beef stock, celery, carrots, bone marrow, unpasteurized miso, raw butter or cream, herbs, spices, leafy greens, seaweed.

Hippocrates' Soup

There are many variations of vegetable broths, and they're all very easy to create. Another soup that may be helpful is based on a recipe supposedly recommended by Hippocrates. Of course the addition of New World vegetables (tomatoes and potatoes) is a more recent amendment!

For one person, use a 2-quart pot, add the following vegetables, and cover with water:

1 medium celery knob (if not in season, use 3-4 stalks of regular celery)

1 medium parsley root (use carrots or another type of whitish root vegetable if you cannot find parsley root)

2 small leeks (substitute 2 small onions if leek is unavailable)

2 medium onions

A little parsley (avoid while lactating)

1½ pounds of tomatoes or more

1 pound of potatoes

Do not peel any of these vegetables, but wash and scrub them well, chop coarsely, cook slowly for 3 hours, and then put through a food mill in small portions; scarcely any fibers should be left.

Healing and Cleansing Practices

A castor oil pack placed on the skin will increase circulation and promote elimination of toxins and healing of the tissues and organs beneath the skin. Castor oil packs are made by soaking a piece of wool or cotton flannel or cloth in castor oil and placing it on the skin. The flannel is covered with a sheet of plastic or other material, and then a hot water bottle is placed over the plastic to heat the pack (the plastic is used to prevent the castor oil from getting on other things, as it does stain, but you don't have to use it). Place the castor oil pack on various parts of the body, over various organs, and leave it there for 5-30 minutes. Repeat as often as necessary, several times per day or per week.

I have found that the brand Home Health, available in some local drug and health stores, is a far more effective castor oil than another commonly available brand. Castor oil packs can work miracles for some seasonal types of allergies.

During Pregnancy. I have read that castor oil may not be safe for use during pregnancy or lactation, but I do not know for certain if this is true. Consult your healthcare practitioner and your inner guidance for this.

Absorb nutrients through your skin. Some of the natives whom Weston Price studied in the South Sea Islands rubbed coconut oil all over their bodies (they lived mostly or totally naked). The natives believed the coconut oil was an important source of nutrition. [326]

Consider rubbing or massaging part or all of your body with the following oils frequently, and even sunbathing with these oils. Shea butter can work as an effective "sun block" but it is not as strong as the commercial sun blocks you may be used to. Coconut oil helps lessen the harmful effects of the sun and has some sun blocking properties.

Organic Olive Oil – The olive oil is a complete food itself and will penetrate into the body to feed and rebuild muscles, flesh, and the entire system. [327]

Organic Coconut Oil – High in vitamins and minerals, it is anti-bacterial, and can help protect the skin against harmful effects of the sun.

Unrefined Organic Shea Butter – Shea butter is one of the most potent healing substances I have used. It nourishes the body with vitamins, and helps you feel more vitally alive. It can heal damaged skin and offer protection from the sun. Be cautious in your selection, though — some varieties have too many synthetic substances added, and any variety may be harmful if you have allergies to nuts. There are some varieties that are hand made, organic, and totally unrefined. These are the most effective. It is a bit greasy, and can have a distinct and fairly strong smell.

A Note about Massage during Pregnancy. If you get a professional massage, be aware that there are certain types of massage techniques that are harmful for use during pregnancy — deep pressure, for example, or massaging near the belly. Provided you are not allergic to the oils listed above, there should be no ill effects from topical rubbing.

The sun is the all-giving light in the sky and is considered by some to be the world's greatest doctor. [328] The sun exemplifies selfless service—being constantly present to give unconditionally to all life on earth. The sun can strengthen us, as it induces positive chemical reactions throughout the whole body (provided you do not burn yourself). Sun bathing on most or all of your body as often as possible is health promoting. The sun does not cause cancer, as has been wrongly reported. [329] You need to be extremely careful in using sun blocks, as a majority of them contain toxic chemicals, which then absorb directly through your skin and into your blood. Many sun blocks also block or decrease the sun's healing power. Eating more fat helps the body protect itself against the sun.

Walking barefoot is a great health promoting practice, especially when you walk on uneven surfaces. When barefoot and touching the ground, energy is exchanged between you and the earth, and the stimulation of pressure points on your feet can also help soothe and relax your entire body. Shoes are in general bad for us. They promote unnatural walking habits and cause stress and tension to build up in the body. Sandals, slippers, clogs, moccasins or anything else that allows your feet to breathe and stretch are an acceptable variation (of course, some are much better than others). One solution is flip-flop like shoes like the Tarahumara Huarache running sandals worn by the Tarahumara, the running tribe in Mexico. These shoes have an extremely thin sole and there is a wrap around the ankle so they stay secure. (**barefootted.com/shop/**). Of course if you live in a cold climate you'll want something different, such as a moccasin. In any case, pay attention to how your feet feel. I myself have mostly given up wearing shoes and now usually wear very thin flip-flops made of leather.

Taking a very hot bath in filtered water can help cleanse the body. You can also take a hot bath using a few teaspoons and up to ½ cup of clay. There are various clays available in health food stores (some may be healthier than others). Just be mindful because clay can cause a mess in your bathtub and your drains; so try a small amount first. You can also add up to 8 cups of Epsom salts (available at drug stores) into the bath water to create a super concentrated solution that will help pull toxins out of the body. Do not use the salts at the same time as the clay. You can also add many types of minerals to your salt bath, as well as tea, essential oils and/or aluminum free baking soda to help relax and soothe your body. Before, during, or after you bathe, consider brushing your skin using a natural bristle brush or slightly rough washcloth/dead skin scraper. This removes dry skin and toxic accumulations on the skin.

During Pregnancy: Do not take excessively hot baths, and start with very small amounts of bath additives to see if they affect you negatively or not.

The sweat lodge is a native tradition found in several cultures across the globe. A sweat can be used for more than just purification of the body; it can purify your mind, body, and spirit. The purpose might be to enter the spirit world and connect with your deeper and most intimate self. The sweat lodge is a powerful tool for cleansing negative energies from your body. The prolonged and excessive sweating allows deeper layers of tissues to release their contents. Infrared and other types of saunas can be used to replace a sweat lodge. And remember: not all saunas are created equal; you don't want to use ones that have any chemical smells.

Preconception: Do not participate in sweat lodges or visit saunas within 6-8 months of conception. When your body sweats vigorously, it also can become depleted of many essential nutrients. Once you are in the 6 month time frame before the time of conception, avoid this purification technique. (Times may vary according to your clear intuition.)

Pregnancy: Saunas and sweat lodges must be avoided as they are dangerous during pregnancy.

Maintaining Health by Avoiding Toxins

A crucial part of creating health in the preconception phase and during pregnancy and lactation is to avoid the countless environmental toxins that are typically part of our daily life. It is of the utmost importance that men also avoid these toxins.

The existence of toxins in our environment and in our lives is a tragic reflection of how we live — of how our lives are far out of balance. But we do not have to live these toxic lifestyles anymore, or continue to mistakenly maintain a realm that is filled with suffering buffered by fleeting sensory pleasures. If humanity's consciousness and awareness as a whole were to change, we could easily eliminate all of the toxins in our lives and in the planet. We have the power to create a heavenly realm on earth. But before earth becomes a heavenly realm we need to take the first step to avoid and stop using toxic chemicals.

Environmental poisons can cause the germ cells of the man or woman to be altered. Environmental toxins can lower our vitality, as they create a burden that our body has to eliminate, and they weaken our immune system. It is also very difficult to avoid all toxins, unless you live in some very remote area of the planet. Even if we cannot rid our lifestyle entirely of toxins, we can significantly reduce them.

The Influence of Toxins on the Developing Child

The content of the child's bowels before birth is known as meconium. Meconium does not exist in animals in nature. It is the collection of toxic elements that have been filtered by the infant's body, particularly the liver, while in the womb. The product of the filtration via the liver is dumped into the intestines as the child grows, waiting for an opportunity for release (usually within one day after birth).[330] Excess mucus may also build up in the nose or mouth of your child. This excess mucus is also a response in the infant's body to toxins; it's rather like an infantile cold, and can make it difficult for the child to breathe when emerging from the birth canal.

Our second daughter, Yeshe, had meconium even after many health building and cleansing practices. There seemed to be much less than with her older sister, Sparkle, however, and it was very soft and came out quickly. She also was born with a slight bit of congestion, and we never identified the cause. Michelle removed the congestion not with one of those infant nose sucker devices, but gently, using her own mouth.

The child in the womb is affected by the mother's internal chemistry. I bring back a reminder here of Chapter 1, where we learned that disease is a response to some sort of stimulus. If a child is born ill, the illness is his or her body responding to a set of conditions. Dr. Bieler explained that the baby's body is at first protected by the mother's liver, and then the placenta. After that, the fetus' liver can filter toxic blood, although it takes great effort to do this. The next line of defense is the kidneys, which also filter the fetus' blood. If the fetus is toxic, urine can enter into the amniotic fluid. The final line of defense is the unborn child's glands — the thyroid, for example. The thyroid is responsible for putting mucus into the throat and lungs. Again, this mucus deposition is a cleansing mechanism of the body in response to toxins in order to keep the fetus' blood clean. [331]

Finding Love and Acceptance even of Pollution

Toxic substances seem to be everywhere in our modern world — the result of the modern plague. We create things with very little reverence for the life force in the Earth, in Nature, and in the humans who live here. Few if any of us are in the position to eliminate single-handedly all the toxins we encounter in our outer world. I am reminded of a story by Yogi Sri Yukteswar.

There was a town in India where the bodies of the dead were cremated throughout the day. There was a large and intense cloud of smoke that hovered above the town because of the activities of the crematory. Now, there was a great yogi who lived in the town. The students of this yogi seemed to have all sorts of health problems from breathing in the smoke. The students noticed that the yogi was full of life and vibrancy and had no health problems, as if the toxic smoke had no effect on him. The students came to the yogi, concerned for their health. They asked the yogi what they could do about stopping the smoke, and they wondered how it was that the yogi was unaffected by the toxic smoke, while they were experiencing illness. The yogi responded that he was able to see the divine, the essence of the creator herself, in everything — even in the noxious smoke. In seeing this oneness and embracing it with love, he was immune to the smoke's negative effects.

I do not recommend that you do unhealthy things and pretend that you will be fine by doing them. I do recommend that you offer no inner resistance to the presence of toxins in our world. This means that you need to feel whatever feelings come up in your body as a result of our toxic lifestyles. When we act or react negatively to pollution in the world, we add psychic pollution to what we see, and thus strengthen and affirm the worldly pollution on the causal level of energy and consciousness.

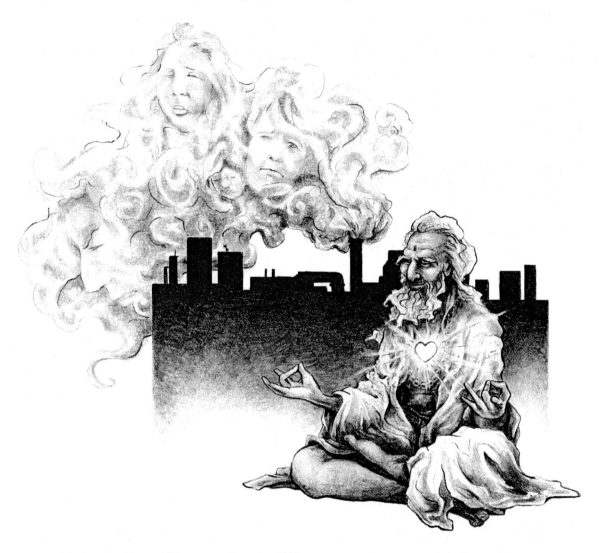

Seeing Light and Goodness in the World. The base metals of suffering and destruction can be turned into the gold of salvation. This in no way implies that we should refrain from saying "NO" or refrain from taking action against the wrongs in the world. It is an inner yes, an inner acceptance to what is.

The yogi embraces life and sees God (goodness) in all things; so he does not suffer. His truthful and positive attitude transmutes the root cause of suffering in all beings, the ones that created the toxins in the first place. His love dissolves the negative energy he sees. He experiences love because he is free from inner resistance to life; he has an unequivocal "yes" to life and thus fulfills his purpose in being here.

The students suffer from the outer pollution. They have an inner "no," an inner non-acceptance of what IS happening in life. They are not aware of this inner "no" and so their health deteriorates from the outer condition. They are at odds with life and add to the collective negative energy field. The result of our collective unconsciousness and negativity is what creates toxins in our outer environment.

Acceptance does not mean pretending you have no reaction, or to censor your reaction to the violence, ignorance, and destruction that is all-pervasive. It means that the destruction we see in the world is also within us as our inner non-loving presence. When we can accept our reactions to life fully, this very acceptance brings the light of love and compassion to ourselves, and therefore to the world. This does not happen through controlling our reactions to life, but by fully accepting them. So if you are angry, let the anger out and yell and scream. If you feel pain and discomfort, feel it; or at least acknowledge it. Moving through the surface feelings, the immediately accessible ones, allows you to uncover the gold underneath the pain. This gold is your (and our) hope and salvation.

You can take action to make yourselves healthier while at the same time accepting what you see in the world.

Summary of environmental toxins to avoid

1. Drink purified water. It can be bottled in glass or filtered, for example.

2. Purchase a shower or bath filter and bathe only in chemical-free water.

3. Use only *organic* soaps and shampoos, as well as organic cosmetics and all-natural sun blocks. A good test to determine safety is if the ingredients are edible (though they may not taste good).

4. Use only all natural cleaning products, including dishwashing liquids and other household cleaners, such as those found at health food stores.

5. If you must have dental work, get non-mercury fillings.

6. Avoid traditional root canals and use nutrition or holistic dentistry alternatives.

7. Do not use birth control pills or the IUD.

8. Do not use **prescription drug**s. Do not use illegal drugs. (Marijuana seems to be unhealthy. However, hallucinogenic mushrooms and other indigenous "drugs" can have significant health promoting and

cleansing effects – use with extreme care.) Avoid even over-the-counter drugs (including aspirin), and avoid vaccinations (see Chapter 11 about vaccines).

9. Live in a non-toxic environment: do not work in a "sick" building; avoid spending time in buildings with new carpets, new paint, newly varnished floors, or new furniture, and avoid driving in new cars. All these items give out toxic gas fumes.

10. Avoid breathing too much exhaust from cars. Fumes from natural gas, such as a gas stove, that are not burned are also dangerous. (Don't hold your breath; just try to limit your exposure. Of course, this is a significant challenge if you live in the middle of a city.)

11. Avoid using, inhaling or touching any pesticides, bug sprays, or any other potentially harmful chemicals including regular household cleaners.

12. Do not touch chemicals, or items that might have chemicals on them, such as gasoline, or car oil. (Consider using gloves or paper towels when getting gas in gas stations.)

13. Avoid toothpaste and all products containing fluoride; use tooth powder, baking soda or liquid tooth cleaners as an alternative.

14. Avoid aluminum (tea kettles, pie and cake tins, baking sheets) and Teflon cookware. Use cast iron, stainless steel, or stoneware instead.

15. Limit your exposure to electromagnetic waves; use a wired or airtube headset with your cell phone and keep the phone away from your body. Limit time in front of CRTs (those big bulky computer and TV monitors), and also limit time in front of plasma monitors. LCDs (liquid crystal) monitors are better than CRTs and plasma monitors because they do not emit radiation. However, the backlights of LCDs are fluorescent and they cause imbalances in our nervous system. I use a low setting so

my backlight is not too bright, and I also shine a standard incandescent bulb behind the monitor to help with eye strain. If you use a computer, the computer case, full of whirring electrical equipment, would ideally be kept some distance away, instead of right next to you through the day. Laptops seem to be okay; they run on less power and put out less electromagnetic waves; their monitors are also LCDs, which produce the least amount of radiation. Do not spend your entire day under fluorescent lights. Use standard light bulbs instead, or as a compromise use filtered fluorescent lights, which are closer to regular sunlight. Finally, do not use a microwave, or stand near one while it is on. And keep electrical items away from your sleeping area.

16. Limit the use of ultrasounds and x-rays.

17. Avoid alcohol (though occasional use of unpasteurized alcohol seems okay), cigarettes and coffee.

18. Avoid commercial tampons; instead, buy organic or natural ones, or preferably use natural pads, or a menstrual cup that is made with only natural substances.

19. Avoid and limit the use of synthetic clothing such as polyester and synthetic "fleece" material. Use natural fiber clothing such as cotton, wool, silk and hemp.

An Explanation for Avoiding These Toxins

I am providing a more detailed explanation of reasons to avoid these toxins. This helps you to be informed and also will motivate you to make changes.

1. Tap water usually contains fluoride and always contains chlorine. Fluoride is a deadly poison; just a small amount, approximately ½ a teaspoon, can kill someone who weighs a hundred pounds. Regularly absorbing this poison through toothpaste, mouth rinse, dental visits, or tap water puts a tremendous strain on your liver. The slow poisoning by fluoride can contribute to the break down of the body's defensive mechanisms and cause a lowering of intelligence. Dr. Dean Burk was a highly respected chemist who worked for the National Cancer Institute. He testified before Congress that he believed fluoridation to have caused about ten percent of all cancer deaths. That's 61,000 people per year.[332] You may wonder why fluoride, if it is so dangerous, has been consistently touted as a beneficial supplement. The partial answer is that putting fluoride in our water promotes a "business with disease," because it makes people more susceptible to disease. It is a profitable way to get rid of industrial waste, as well. But water fluoridation will be mentioned again in Chapter 12, when we discuss social order. It might seem hard to grasp, but this completely insane and violent practice of municipal water fluoridation is even mandated in many states. The Environmental Protection Agency's (EPA) Employee Union (consisting of approximately 1500 scientists, lawyers, engineers and other professional employees) is opposed to water fluoridation. They oppose fluoride due to "the lack of benefit to dental health from ingestion of fluoride and the hazards to human health from such ingestion."[333] If most or all of the employees at the EPA are opposed to water fluoridation, then why does its implementation occur on such a mass scale? Why is it even legal? I have posed similar questions throughout this book regarding other health practices that are advertised as beneficial but which are in reality harmful. Please consider these questions carefully.

According to the EPA, over 700 chemicals have been identified in our tap water, including nitrates, asbestos, and pesticides.[334] Water from plastic bottles loses its energy structure and absorbs chemicals as well (depending on the type of plastic). I am unsure of how good the water is from those large blue plastic bottles delivered by water services. But it is a good idea to have a clean water source. Water filtration is one option to consider. I've enjoyed using a gravity water filter that uses stones in the final filtration stage. This filter is the PiMag™ Aqua Pour. If your water is fluoridated, you need to make sure the water filter removes the fluoride, which requires a special cartridge or reverse osmosis system.

When water passes through pipes its vital qualities are damaged. This is why I like water from the Aqua Pour system: it passes over stones and its structure is restored. There are other systems for restoring water structure (such as vortex devices that spin the water). Previously, we used a sink-hook up water filter using a carbon filtration unit because we were short on money; the water was not too good. But currently we have access to unfiltered spring and well water. Having a good water source is important, so make obtaining high quality water a vital priority.

2. Unfiltered shower or bath water. A significant percentage of pollution enters the body through the skin of children and adults. Chlorine, which I have mentioned is in all municipal water, can promote cancer and heart disease.[335] And studies have shown that fumes from chlorinated shower water are toxic. [336] Take the simple step and get any type of bath or shower filter that removes chlorine.

3. Conventional cosmetics, shampoo, soaps and other body care products. The advent of modern, industrialized civilization brought disease and death to native peoples. One aspect of this modern way of living is the regular application of chemicals, rather than natural, whole, plant-based substances, to the body. The products carried by your standard supermarket or drugstore — unless they are labeled as 100% organic — will contain a variety of hazardous chemicals. Some brands are worse than others, of course, and it is important to use only organic or homemade varieties of these products. According to the US Food and Drug Administration (FDA) 89% of over 10,500 ingredients in personal care products **have not been evaluated for safety**. Many chemicals in shampoos, shaving cream, lotions and lipstick are the very same ones used in industrial manufacturing. Many chemicals marketed to women contain known cancer-causing agents (which may partly explain the breast cancer epidemic). [337] The chemicals used in modern beauty and cleansing products absorb almost instantly into your skin, even though you will not notice it. If you want to know how fast the skin absorbs chemicals, try this experiment: hold a piece of strong garlic in your hand; you

will find that in a very short time your breath will smell of garlic. That is how fast contaminants can absorb into our blood stream through the skin. So, I'll say it one more time: use only organic, homemade, and all natural cosmetic products.

4. Standard cleaning products. Many standard household cleaning products are highly toxic. Read the label of any cleaning agent; it says so right on the bottle. Many common household chemicals are known to cause birth defects, as well as damage sperm, which can result in a deformed fetus.[338] You won't know what effects inhaling even a small amount of toxins might have on an unborn baby. It is best not even to flirt with that possibility. I want to remind you of what I said about birth defects in Chapter 4: a lack of vitamins causes harmful changes that result in birth defects. And the same goes for even regular cleaning chemicals; they have the potential to change the hormonal balance of our bodies and cause damage, which is then passed on to the fetus.

Most dishwasher detergents are highly toxic. Eating from a plate that has been cleaned with dishwasher detergent means you may be eating toxic dishwasher chemicals. Use natural dishwasher detergent and make sure your plates get an extra rinse with plain water.

5. Mercury Fillings— Mercury is a poison, and there is no reason why it should be put into people's mouths. I want to be clear that I am not recommending for or against amalgam removal; that's a case by case issue. If you don't have a serious illness, then it definitely is not urgent that you remove them. In fact, I still have mine. The body has natural protection mechanisms for heavy metals, and if you are in good health, you can remain so even with mercury fillings. Two adults I know who had their fillings removed did not experience any noticeable health improvements. The tricky part of the procedure is that the time most likely for high mercury exposure is when the fillings are put in, and when they are removed.

If you do decide to remove your mercury fillings, it is important to know the best time to do it. A survey of websites and practices in other countries indicates that a safe time for removal of mercury fillings is two years before pregnancy (and even one year before pregnancy might be okay).[339] If you are closer than that, then don't have mercury fillings removed except for an urgent reason.

If you need new dental work while pregnant or close to pregnancy, get non-mercury fillings. If for some reason your mercury filling is deteriorated and needs removal, find a dentist who takes special precautions to limit your mercury exposure, such as dentists from www.iaomt.org.

The best treatment for tooth decay…is to avoid getting tooth decay. I wrote a book about it called *Cure Tooth Decay.* You'll also find that many dietary guidelines that I recommend for pregnancy in this book help mineralize teeth, too. If you need more help with healing cavities, see my book or website www.curetoothdecay.com .

6. Root Canals- A root canal is performed when the pulp of the tooth is damaged. The pulp is removed and for appearance or physiological reasons, a hollow dead tooth is left in someone's mouth. Dentist George E. Meinig was one of the founding members of the American Association of Endodontists (root canal specialists). For a time, he was a great proponent of root canal therapy. He completely reversed his opinion when he discovered and read the 25 years of root canal research carried out by Dr. Weston Price. The research showed that it is very common for malignant bacteria to grow under the root canal, in such a manner that the body cannot clean up the infection. The constant decaying matter weakens the body and can even lead to death. Modern root canal techniques administered by some natural dentists may inhibit bacterial growth, making the root canals safe. Seek a biological or holistic dentist if you have a concern about a root canal making you sick. If you do have an infected root canal you might feel a vague sense of malaise coming from your mouth, or you might note a subtle feeling of irritation under the tooth with the root canal. Of course, not all root canals are necessarily infected; again, you need to take a moment and consult with your inner guidance to sense if treatment or further examination is needed. The idea here is to prepare your body for excellent health for pregnancy.

7. Birth control pills and the IUD. Birth control pills are synthetic hormones that fool the body into thinking it is pregnant. The pill can be highly dangerous and have severe side effects. I will mention just a few: infections, irritability, sore breasts, nausea, weight gain, eczema, bone loss, gallbladder problems, blood clots, strokes, epilepsy, high blood pressure, infertility, heart attacks, allergies, and cancer of the breast, uterus, liver, pituitary, ovaries, and lungs.[340]

We know we need a healthy balance of minerals in the body in order to produce a healthy child, and taking the birth control pill upsets our internal chemistry significantly. It alters our internal levels of copper and zinc. This results in many women starting pregnancy with a zinc deficiency, which can lead to problems in pregnancy or after birth.[341] The pill also causes severe magnesium deficiency, and the pill and the IUD cause copper to unnaturally increase in the body.[342][343] Also, because hormones are used to constantly fool the body into thinking it is pregnant, the body is continuously secreting special substances to prepare for pregnancy, and thus depletes its vital nutrient reserves. It likely takes months or even years to recover lost minerals from the use of birth control pills (depending on how long you use them).

Birth control pills are also dangerous for your health because they increase your risk of cancer by several fold. Dr. Samuel Epstein, in his book *The Breast Cancer Prevention Program*, explains that more than 20 careful studies have demonstrated a clear risk of breast cancer associated with use of the birth control pill. A young woman who uses birth control pills has up to ten times the risk of developing breast cancer compared a woman who does not use them, especially if used for two years or longer.[344]

Finally, an important and yet overlooked fact of birth control pill use is that it alters women's sex drive. The idea of having a birth control pill is to have sex without other barrier methods while preventing conception and pregnancy. But what's the point of this "freedom" if a woman's sexual feelings are diminished or altered significantly by the synthetic birth control pill hormones?

The IUD is a small device implanted in the uterus. It is essentially a bundle of plastic, copper, or plastic-coated copper left in the womb. Its failure rate is higher than the pill for preventing pregnancy. Some side effects include cramping and pain, especially during menstruation, ectopic pregnancy, spontaneous abortion, uterine bleeding, blood poisoning, bowel obstruction, cervical infection, pelvic infections, infections of the Fallopian tubes, dysplasia, cancer of the uterus, anemia, perforation of the uterus, and mineral imbalance.[345]

Ultimately, the problem with both the pill and the IUD is that neither considers the guardian or deva spirit of women and reproduction. Only when this spirit is honored will the potential for a healthy birth control pill manifest. It is also possible that while in communication with this spirit, it will be learned that a healthy birth control pill cannot be created. Only natural plant medicines, or other carefully made harmonious substances, can be used for birth control without harming the body. Meanwhile, while effective herbal birth control[346] exists and has been used in indigenous cultures world wide, I have not seen clear references to what herbs work effectively and safely, or how to use or obtain them. It is to be hoped that someone will study this area and help make natural herbal birth control available in the modern world. Until then, the other effective and safe pregnancy prevention methods that we are aware of are FAM and condoms. FAM is discussed in more detail at the end of this chapter.

8. Prescription drugs. Almost every prescription drug has **not** been tested to evaluate its safety for women during pregnancy, so little is known about the side effects of many prescription drugs on the unborn child. The warning labels on almost every medication warns against use during pregnancy. This is because the harmful side effects of drugs are more severe during pregnancy. Prescription drugs work generally by poisoning the body. The poisoning of the body is what we call a "side effect." The

body responds to the poison and that response makes the illness improve temporarily. Over the long term, such a response is usually detrimental (unless the drug was used in an emergency situation), as the body's reserves become depleted. The toxic substances in the drug many times are not eliminated and stay stuck in the body. I had the experience of valium being stuck in my body for over 15 years; it was later released when I began consuming raw eggs in blended drinks. Also, sometimes when I sneeze I experience the distinct smell of a nasal spray that I used for allergies in college (when I was 19). Part of the chemical spray is still trapped in my body, or has altered some of the tissues in my nasal passages. It seems to be lessening over time, however.

Most or all diseases are the body's response to its environment. But most western drugs inhibit this response (there may be a few exceptions, such as Gaston Naessen's cancer curing 714-X, which, by the way, is outlawed). A cough suppressant is a good example. The body coughs in order to expel some deeply held mucus full of toxic substances. If you stop the cough with medication then you have eliminated your body's healing response and ability to cleanse itself.

Antibiotics have a devastating effect on the beneficial bacteria in our bodies. Antibiotics invade tissues and cause disease. They can turn a healthy ecosystem into a diseased ecosystem in which bacteria that we associate with disease are present.[347] Antibiotics damage our immune system and make us more prone to infections.[348] The much- acclaimed penicillin, for example, is so toxic that the body eliminates it in a few seconds. Penicillin works by overstimulating the already tired glands into action. Thus, a short term "cure" is accomplished while in the long run the body is made much weaker and more prone to future disease.

I have not used any western drugs or medications for over ten years. I do use herbs and occasionally have tried homeopathy. After several detoxifications and cleanses like the ones I have described earlier in this chapter, I rarely

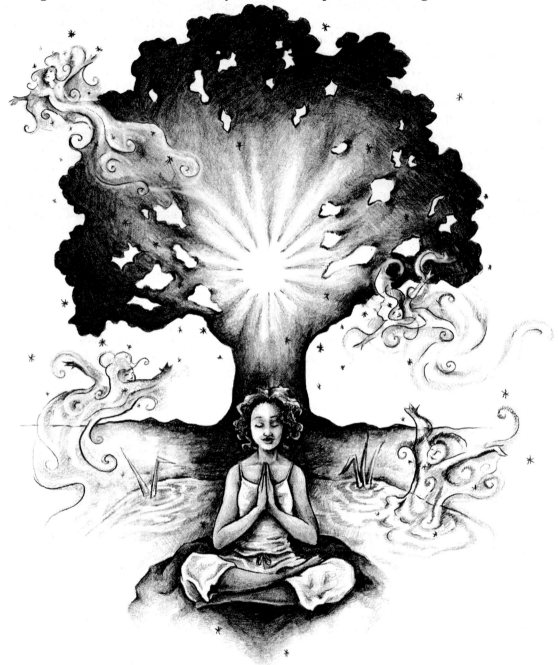

We can create medicines and solve many complex human problems through consulting with the spirit or deva that is in charge of the particular thing we want to create. They exist to love and serve humanity. Few people take advantage of these spiritual energies.

Consulting with Dark Forces (Not Recommended)

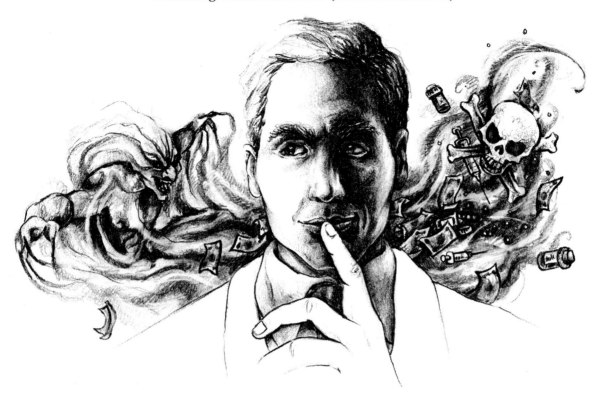

Rather than consulting in a loving manner with the abiding spirit, our culture supports a medical establishment that consults with the spirit of money, greed, and quick profit. The modern drug scientist creates medicines without considering their ill effects, because it is more important that he gets a patent and makes more money, than if he really can help people or not. This is action and work in the name of madness. Non-error drug deaths kill over 106,000 people per year; birth control pills increase women's risk of cancer by up to 10 times; and there are millions of injuries due to known and unknown side effects from drugs. This is the pinnacle of our diseased lifestyle, in which some people knowingly and willingly cause death and injury on a mass scale, while hiding their actions through deception.

fall ill, if at all. When I have gotten even the slightest bit sick, I have been able to correlate the illness with eating a questionable food. Over the years, I have also become more attuned to my body. For instance, I discovered that prior to cleansing and healing efforts on my part, the glands in my neck were constantly swollen; I just didn't notice it until the swelling relaxed. My body was in a hyperactive state trying to fight off disease because it was so loaded with junk.

As a parent, you will be tempted by dark forces surrounding the approach to safeguarding your children's health. Vaccines are one such example. Labeled as a higher good, they appear to promote health. Yet behind this illusion lies the truth — vaccines cause death and suffering. We are lured into making mistakes like these for our health and our children's health because of negative and unresolved feelings in ourselves, which I have already discussed. For example, some will experience pleasure and a feeling of aliveness that come with being destructive. Destructive actions are not themselves good, but energy moving feels good, whether it moves positively or negatively. Of course positive energy flow is much more powerful than the negative flow.

Activity - consult with a deva: Just to warn you, as there are good energies and good spirits, so there are also bad ones. When we do bad things, we usually have a brief interaction with a bad spirit; then we rush off and buy the candy bar (or whatever your favorite bad habit might be). Yes, you do contact and consult with these spirits, it just happens very rapidly and most of us don't notice it. It is very much like in the cartoon with the angel on one shoulder, and the devil with the pitchfork on the other. The cartoon character listens to both voices and then makes a choice. It's okay if you don't believe in spirits; just think instead of thought forms, intentions, higher energies, or creative aspects. Start paying attention to and getting in touch with these different energies. Here are some guidelines. First take a few deep breaths and allow your mind to relax. Feel your feet on the floor and open up to all the energy pulsations flowing everywhere. Become aware of the enlivening cosmic energy flowing through all things, including you. Think of something good you want for your life—better health or healthier children, for example. To contact the guardian spirit of what you are going to create, state your intention through visualization or through saying it quietly (or out loud). In this example, we'll choose the spirit for healthy and happy children. Welcome the spirit here, even if you don't feel anything. Then ask for help. You may perceive guidance through a thought, smell, feeling, sound or taste. Open up to whatever guidance you receive, and begin your consultation. A good question could be "What do I need to learn about myself to be healthy?" You could also ask the spirit what it wants from you. It can be difficult to clearly hear what the energy communicates to you because many of us have noisy minds. Usually, once you contact the spirit, you immediately receive an energetic download of feelings. Even if the feelings don't make sense, the feelings are the communication. This book, by the way, also has a deva spirit. If you want to understand the book several times faster than you would normally, think of and communicate with its spirit, or with my writer deva spirit while you are reading.

9. Indoor air pollution in buildings and cars is a health hazard. The World Health Organization (WHO) estimates that over one-third of new and remodeled commercial buildings are "sick." Over twenty percent of office workers in the United States suffer from symptoms of poor air quality. In some cases the pollution level inside buildings is 100 times higher than outdoors. [349]

A former friend worked in a sick building (of course, it was government building). It was one of those buildings with thick walls, no ventilation and just those horrible fluorescent lights. My friend developed strange growths in her lungs, and then unfortunately took all kinds of medications for it. Knowing that the growths in the lungs were a response to a stimulus, I suggested that her building was making her sick from the toxic air she was breathing. She of course seemed to get better when she was away from work, and became worse when she returned. I lost contact with her so I don't know if she ever recovered. Another friend worked in a building that had mold. The mold triggered a response in this friend that led to severe arthritis and intestinal upset. Not everyone in the moldy building developed illnesses. Only those with already compromised immune systems became sick.

Formaldehyde is another dangerous chemical that we should avoid. Formaldehyde concentrates in the brain more than in other tissues and can cause cross-linkages in the RNA and DNA. Formaldehyde is found in many products: building materials, particle board, glue, paints, carpets, foam pillows, foam mattresses, foam insulation, cosmetics and leather.[350]

Solvent fumes from paint, varnish, newsprint, especially glossy color print, inks and dyes are to be avoided. Inhaled solvents can reach the brain and heavy doses can cause nervous system damage. Moth balls and pesticides are also highly dangerous due to their fumes. I must say that most printed materials, including the cover on this book, unfortunately contain some minor amounts of toxic chemicals. I have found less toxic printing methods, but have yet to find a printing method which is completely toxin-free. I will continue seeking more environmentally friendly printing options for future book revisions. The worst exposure from printed media comes from full color magazines that have a slight ink or chemical odor. Touching these makes my fingers hurt, and after a few minutes my throat starts burning. To limit ink exposure, touch the pages carefully and find methods to minimize skin contact.

There is no reason for us to continue making such poisonous products. Even when we are done using them, they eventually go back into the ground and pollute the earth. And even though these chemical-laden products may have a lower price tag in the beginning, the high cost of ill health effects and environmental poisoning is exacted in the long run. Building methods can be changed to be in much more harmony with nature while still providing comfortable and safe homes for people to thrive in.

10. Exhaust. Carbon monoxide and other substances from automobile exhaust are poisonous. It is also important to be aware that inhaling the unlit gas from gas stoves and furnaces is also hazardous. Gasoline is highly toxic, and its gaseous residue can kill you. Some of our greatest exposure to car exhaust occurs when we are driving with the windows open. It is a really poor idea to continue using gasoline for our energy needs in the long run because it is so dangerous and highly toxic. By the way, ethanol and other biofuels are widely available in Brazil, and the air there is noticeably cleaner than in, say, Venezuela, where gasoline is cheaper than bottled water.

11. Pesticides work by disabling the nervous systems of insects and many pesticides have not been tested for their safety in case of human exposure. It should be enough, however, just to know that insecticides like DDT came from chemical weapon research. They are designed to kill anything. Avoid all pesticides and chemicals, including insect repellent.[351] It is known that pesticide exposure, especially chronic exposure even at low levels, can cause genetic damage, birth defects, defective sexual development, allergies, asthma, cancer and many other health problems. Even one-time ex-

posures can cause hormone disruption.[352] Furthermore, spraying pesticides not only kills the bugs, but also their natural predators. Thus, pesticide spraying is a complete waste of time as crop-eating bugs reproduce faster than their predators, and the original problem is compounded. Safe and alternative methods to dangerous chemical pesticides exist; people merely must be willing to investigate them.

The government has been on a pesticide-happy rampage for some while. We had to move out of our home when the Federal and State governments collaborated on spraying a highly toxic chemical over our city via airplanes, supposedly to try to stop a harmless moth. Other alarming pesticide blanket-spraying programs are for West Nile virus mosquito and any other type of large scale moth, fly, mosquito or bug spraying. I can tell you from first hand experience, and from speaking with others, that exposures to these chemicals can severely damage your health. If you live near conventional farms, spray drift can enter your home and cause severe reactions. Many immigrant farm workers are unethically exposed to chemicals while they work in the fields, tending the food we eat. As a result, there is a higher incidence of sterility, birth defects, miscarriage, cancer, leukemia, and other serious diseases in these workers and their children. Saturating our food with chemicals is a sick idea. Applying it when it can harm humans is even sicker. Don't remain ignorant of the real dangers of chemical exposures, and take any step necessary to avoid being sprayed. Remember, the people who work for the government doing the spraying are still people, and must abide by the laws. Last time I checked, it was still illegal to dump chemicals on someone else. Just because the government has gone mad and mandated mass poisoning doesn't mean it is legal, moral, or that it should be tolerated.

12. Touching Chemicals – Chemicals absorb very well through your skin. Do not touch them.

Male reproductive health. Radiation from nuclear power plants and medical facilities, high voltage areas like power switchyards and communication facilities, paint strippers, and ethylene bromide can all damage sperm cells.[353]

13. Toothpaste– Ever read the warning label on toothpaste? It warns "Do not swallow." Regular toothpaste contains chemicals like sorbitol, PVM/MA copolymer, fluoride, hydrated silica, and saccharin. Many of these can be toxic and are broken down by saliva and absorbed into the body through accidental swallowing and diffusion into gums and the rest of the mouth. As I mentioned earlier, fluoride is a toxin. So, if toothpaste is so dangerous, why even put it in your mouth in the first place? Furthermore, toothpaste contains glycerin, the stuff used in soaps, which coats your teeth and prevents re-mineralization. It can take 27 washes to remove a coating of glycerin from your teeth. Replace toothpaste with any of the following: toothpowder, herbs, tooth liquid and tooth soaps. (www.mytoothsoap.com)

14. Aluminum weakens the gut lining and causes nausea, loss of appetite, skin problems and fatigue. Avoid all cooking utensils made with aluminum.[354] Baking powder often contains aluminum. If the container doesn't explicitly state "aluminum free," there is aluminum in the baking powder.

15. Electrical, magnetic and microwave fields can wreak havoc on our internal body chemistry. The damage is usually in direct proportion to the number of hours exposed to this kind of radiation. If you watch TV for one hour a day then that is minimal exposure and not too much of a risk. If you stare at a huge computer monitor, while sitting next to a big highly electrical computer case all day, then that may negatively influence your health. Our nervous system runs on electrical energy. Unnatural sources of radiation can negatively affect our level of vitality and health. I can feel the harmful effects of many radiating devices, especially cell phone microwaves. Lower power consumption devices that don't have wireless features turned on are the least harmful. Keeping your cell phone on all day and carrying it close to your body (especially in a pocket near your reproductive organs) is a bad idea. Be aware of your daily proximity to high tension power lines (the big towering ones that you can hear buzzing

when you are close to them). Fluorescent lights have a negative effect on our health, too. Avoid them if possible. As I have mentioned before, LCD flat screen monitors emit less radiation than the boxy CRT monitors. Over time this exposure can affect your neurology.

Also make sure to avoid electric blankets, microwave ovens, and sunbeds.[355] Limit your exposure to x-rays.

16. Ultrasound– There is evidence that suggests that ultrasounds can cause mild brain damage and learning disabilities.[356] The technology for ultrasounds has not undergone rigorous scientific investigation for long-term effects on the unborn baby. Clearly, the earlier in pregnancy the ultrasound exposure occurs, the greater the possibility of damage since the fetal brain is less developed. Findings published in the British Medical Journal suggest that the ultrasound is a waste of energy, citing no improvements in pregnancy outcome, false diagnosis of malformations, and the possibility for brain damage.[357] The Foresight preconception program in England advises parents to avoid ultrasound scans whenever possible.[358] Based on these prudent concerns, we did not allow ultrasound scanning when we were pregnant with either of our children, and we didn't know they would be girls until they were born—the old fashioned way!

Doppler radar is another type of ultrasound technology which is used to monitor the fetal heart rate. A growing trend over the past 15-20 years is to monitor the heart rate of the infant during birth with Doppler radar technology, and supposedly this technology is implemented to help limit lawsuits. Doppler was originally promoted because it was supposed to decrease rates of intrapartum fetal death and cerebral palsy. But Robert Resnik, MD, in his editorial for Obstetrics & Gynecology, found that there has been no reduction in the incidence of cerebral palsy of the last three decays.[359] What's more, Doppler radar is likely more dangerous than the standard ultrasound scan. Of course, the effects of the Doppler radar will be proportional to how long it is used. If it is used for one minute it will have less harmful impact than if it is used constantly for eight hours. By now, though, I hope you know that any risk or cause of physical deformity or disease is greatly increased by toxic exposures or nutrient deficiencies in the parents occurring from the time of preconception — and not by a lack of Doppler radar in the birth room.

The use of fetal heart rate monitoring devices during birth has been linked to other complications as well, including increased rates of cesarean section.[360] Traditional midwives use a harmless fetal scope to hear the baby's heart rate, but when interviewing midwives for our second daughter's birth Michelle and I found that a majority of midwives here are utterly attached to using their Doppler heart monitor during birth. Perhaps they feel that they wouldn't have a purpose without monitoring the baby's heart rate. When questioned regarding its use, a few admitted that they were aware of Dr. Resnik's editorial comments, but that they still needed to use the Doppler for the time of transition, when the baby passes through the birth canal. The fear prompting this policy is the belief that one must monitor the level of stress or trauma experienced by the baby while in the birth canal. But if you are assisting a homebirth, what would you do if there was some serious problem that far along in the birth? Really you couldn't do anything. Transporting a woman who is in the pushing phase of labor is dangerous and unwise. At that point, the goal is to get the baby out in a safe and efficient method regardless of the heart rate. Because science has told us that Doppler radar does not decrease the risk of key health problems, I think midwives use it in California due to their fear of lawsuits for personal injury. Midwives fear loss of their practice along with hundreds of thousands of dollars in fines. The standard practice, at least in California, is to use a Doppler under all circumstances. This is fear-based medical practice, and unless there is a pre-existing risk factor, it is simply not needed.

In the next chapter I'll describe to you what happened during the birth of Yeshe. We managed to get by without a Doppler even though the birth attendant brought one. One midwife with whom we stopped service tried to manipulate Michelle into having an ultrasound, claiming that it would indicate whether or not there was a birth defect. Of course, she prefaced her comments with, "You can refuse any treatment." She then concluded with something like, "I won't be your midwife unless you have one."

You can read some evidence of the harm of ultrasounds at www.alternamoms.com/ultrasound.html.

A special note: In a majority of cases, the evidence *is* completely clear that ultrasounds can contribute to a decline in health for the mother and child. However, there might be rare special exceptions when the technology can be used for good. If you are very ill during pregnancy and feel that something is very wrong, you will know you are an exception and will have an urgent feeling to have an ultrasound. Using technology wisely is a good idea. Using technology when the harms outweigh the benefits is not intelligent.

17. Alcohol and Cigarettes

The Foresight preconception program recommends avoiding smoking, alcohol and drugs for four months prior to conception. Alcohol decreases sperm motility and sperm count. Alcohol does not have a safe limit during these times.[361]

18. Commercially made tampons

are made from cotton and rayon that have been grown with pesticides. Commercial tampons may contain dioxins (byproducts of bleaching) which are highly carcinogenic. Organic cotton pads, reusable cloth pads, or a menstrual cup are safer options.

19. Conventional clothing

can reduce your level of health. Synthetic fibers block the flow of life energy that comes into your body, and as a result promotes imbalances. The forest doesn't feel as fresh when I wear a synthetic fleece coat. Occasional wear of synthetic fibers is acceptable. Cotton produced for the textile industry is not a food, so very harsh pesticides not even allowed on conventional foods are used when it is grown. Usually, after cotton is grown, peanuts are planted as the next crop cycle in the same field—in the highly toxic soils. This may explain why peanut allergies are wide-spread. I suggest buying organic cotton, natural wool, or hemp if you can afford it. If you cannot, used clothing that has been washed several times, made from natural fibers like cotton or wool, may have fewer chemical residues than new cotton clothes. Be sure to wash your clothes in unscented, ecologically safe detergents and dry them outdoors!

There are many facets to the disease called modernization. We abuse the environment, and we do not honor its spirit even as we take its fruits. We convert Nature's precious resources unwisely into disposable goods in the name of more profit, for a few elite individuals. We create huge piles of toxic garbage in the process and pollute our precious land, air and water. Cost-cutting methods and other evil influences have added tens of thousands of chemicals into the mainstream. These chemicals and products can absorb easily into our body, which was never designed to handle such large amounts of toxic substances — and ill health is the result. The government doesn't protect us from these chemicals, even when their dangers are well understood and acknowledged. Many more chemicals have never even been studied for their possible harmful effects. It is now up to us to make informed choices about how we live.

On the personal level, there are many alternatives we can use to avoid many of the toxic substances in our day to day life. This decreases the burden that our bodies must bear, and increases the likelihood of creating a healthy, vibrant child. Let us cease poisoning ourselves, and let this be the end of the poisoning of our children-to-be.

A fabulous book that more thoroughly outlines the problems of toxins in our environment (our air, food and water) in relation to our children's health is *The Truth about Children's Health* by Robert Bernardini.

Emotions, Pregnancy and Fertility

Your emotional health does have an effect on your physical wellbeing. Negative emotions can be a source of toxins in your body. These emotions — fear, some forms of anger, greed, hatred, selfishness and so on — are not "bad," however, many times they come from a part of ourselves that is distorted and not harmonious.

They come to life when we try to freeze, control, and block the life energy in our bodies. One's honest level of happiness is a good measure of one's emotional health. If you truly feel happy during at least a portion of each day, then this is a sign that you are emotionally healthy. When examined honestly, most people, at least in the United States, are unhappy and completely disconnected from themselves. In this disconnected state, they pretend to be happy and put on a mask to show the world that they are happy. Underneath, these people are unhappy and feel that they are in a lost and alienated world. Emotional dysfunction usually promotes poor lifestyle choices which then lead to illness and complications in pregnancy, rather than the emotions being a direct cause of the problem. However, in some cases emotional dysfunctions can be so severe that they can contribute to or even result in infertility.

Defense

Our bodies are pre-programmed with defensive measures that help us quickly respond to threats. In an emergency we can run, freeze, or fight back. These animalistic defensive actions are needed, as they are designed for circumstances when we are in real danger. Through a force of habit, however, and because we grew up in an unconscious and uncaring world, many of us have come to live primarily through our defensive postures — we use them too often. When we are overly defensive even trivial matters can turn into a rageful fight. For example, I once had a furious fight with Michelle over turning the light switch on and off.

More often than not, our defense mechanisms are incorporated into our daily lives. Please pay attention here as these topics are important for the parenting chapters and they can help you respond with greater poise to the events in your daily life. We have three main defense mechanisms:

Pride is using the mind to protect ourselves from our true feelings and prevent true contact with others. It is characterized by the feeling of being above others, or above our own genuine feelings. Typically, a result of expressing pride is a temporary withdrawal, in which we distance ourselves from inner painful feelings.

Self will is using our will power to defend ourselves with aggressive or intimidating types of behavior. The expression of this behavior can be active, or passive and subtle. When people employ this defense mechanism, they use their will to control the situation by being intimidating, loud, and controlling, or by physically leaving and passively attacking others.

In fear, we are always habitually running and internally hiding from contact with others, and from any situation that is difficult. The feeling of fear is tangible. People who are in fear mode are shut down emotionally and are hiding their true feelings. Unfortunately, because of this posture they miss out in life, since engagement in life involves fully feeling your feelings.

These defenses intermingle with each other, and we all use various combinations of fear, pride, and self will in our daily lives. Your defensive posture is based on how you responded to an unloving and un-present environment as a child. If your mother yelled at you, you might have used fear, running and hiding from her. If your brothers beat you up, you may have used pride, pretending it did not hurt. On the other hand, maybe you were the one walking around trying to intimidate people, fighting with people all the time to prevent yourself from getting hurt (by hurting others first). This would be an example of an aggressive self will defense. There are many more examples; I'm sure you can think of several yourself.

Traumas stored in our bodies create a type of hyper-vigilance, where we tend to move into defense even in situations when we do not really need to be defensive. This is seen clearly in my silly argument with Michelle over the light. Because of the defensive mechanisms in action, this petty event triggered deeper and more intense feelings from the past, far more feelings than just the light switch could evoke.

The reason I have brought up this topic is to note that when we are in a posture of *defense,* our bodies engage our innate fight or flight response. Poisonous substances are released in our bodies, for example, the moment we are fright-

ened. If this happens naturally, say, once every few months, it won't be a big deal to recover from. But if you are fighting with life, constantly irritated, stressed out at every inconvenience, and about to fall apart, then you are putting a severe physical strain on your body.[362] I do hope that you are not stressed to that extreme, but most of us exist somewhere in the middle of the spectrum.

The child's body is literally formed by the internal environment of the mother. During pregnancy, her defense postures can create a toxic bath that can negatively affect the fetus in the womb. Toxic patterns and habits can become ingrained into the physical container (the body) of your child's soul. Of course, if the mother's body is filled with happy hormones from positive feelings, then some of that good energy might go into the physical formation of her child.

For now, noticing yourself when you are in a defensive pattern is all you need to do. With loving compassion, simply notice and be aware of your behavior. Full awareness eventually will lead to transformation.

Reducing Stress and Practicing Self Care

Stress contributes to infertility. We experience stress when our needs are unmet, when we are disconnected from ourselves, or when our bodies are weak and we have difficulty accomplishing the day's tasks.

Stress is also caused by shutting down to one's feelings. Usually because of imbalanced emotions, we end up creating situations where we have two opposing inner currents, a psychic split. For example, you may feel tired and want to rest, while another inner impulse reminds you that you have many responsibilities and must get to work. You cannot work and rest at the same time, so the result is a feeling of stress. Many of us have several opposing currents going in many different directions simultaneously. We do not stop and consider what is best for ourselves, and go on living with these stresses, tolerating what is not really tolerable, until we fall apart and are forced to make a change.

Activity from Michelle - practice self care: Take a prenatal yoga class (or a regular yoga class if you are not pregnant) and practice deep breathing or some kind of breathing meditation. Spend a lot of time in nature. Our true nature is to be peaceful. Is that peace located in the mall, on television or in the newspaper? No. Those things take you away from peace, and from inner awareness. Peace can be reflected back to us through observing and being with the simplicity of nature. A tree or a mountain, for example, even air or open space, can reflect peace back to us. (These suggestions apply for both the time of pregnancy, or for pre-conception preparation.)

Give yourself regular foot massages. When your belly is getting too big and you cannot bend over, have your husband or friend give you a foot massage—at least once a day every day, for about ten minutes.

Daily, rub oil on your breasts and belly. Organic, cold pressed olive oil can work, or you can find belly oil for pregnancy in a natural health store. This is relaxing and soothing. And we are getting healthy this way as well, as our bodies absorb nutrients through the skin.

Create a favorite spot in your house where you feel comfortable and where you can breathe and relax and not think about anything. Be around positive people with a good attitude and nurturing spirit. Spend time around people who understand you and who can support your soul and spirit.

Healing from Loss and the Emotional Body

Many of us are tied to the past in ways that may complicate our feelings toward our child-to-be. If you have had a miscarriage or abortion in the past, then you may have complex and tangled emotions on the matter. Perhaps no words can be said, and no solace given, to a mother or father who has lost a child, and this of course includes losing a child from miscarriage. The parents' hopes, excitement and anticipation of their child-to-be have been dashed. This may leave feelings of despair, frustration, anger, sadness and grief. As with any emotion, it is important to be honest and truthful with yourself about how you feel. Many times we are disassociated from our true feelings, so it requires honesty, focus, intention, and space to see what is within. Allow yourself the time and space to be with and experience your feelings. When emotions are fully experienced, they usually pass or transform into different feelings. When dealing with deep grief, I find that this Course in Miracles® summary quote is helpful: "Nothing real can be threatened. Nothing unreal exists. Herein lies the peace of God." It is a solace to understand that ultimately some of this experience of loss, no matter how raw and sharp it feels in the moment, will pass. And that nothing that is true and genuine can ever be lost or taken away. Much of what we grieve over is the loss of an illusion, such as the *idea* of having love, happiness or fulfillment. When we feel this loss, we realize that what we have lost in the world can yet be found within us. When we trust that what happens in our life is somehow meant to happen, we may be led to a doorway of peace with what is, even in the face of loss. That does not mean you won't experience pain or deep sadness, but it does means that there can be a space for peace around the pain and sadness.

Many of us have experienced loss in one form or another in life, particularly in intimate relationships. Take a moment to reflect upon any residual feelings of loss that are coming to the surface right now. Sometimes the feelings are vague, as if something indistinct is missing. You cannot pinpoint what it is, but it is as though you are looking for something that has been misplaced. This too is loss, a loss of self. Through feeling and accepting loss, a portal opens to the dimension of depth and spaciousness within.

To prepare your emotional body for conception, take a moment every day (I hope you will do this more often than that) and ask yourself "How do I feel?" Another useful practice is to sit quietly and align your thinking with the intention "I want to feel all of my feelings." The way you feel prior to conception as the seeds of life are being created will be a part of the framework of how your pregnancy, birth, and parenting experience will unfold.

To prepare the mental body read a good book on pregnancy health. You are reading a good book right now, so you are enhancing your mental body! The mental body refers to the clarity and energy of the thoughts and understanding of the feelings that you have. Reading high quality material is a good way to enhance your mental clarity. Talking about your ideas and expressing your thoughts and feelings with others is another way to enhance mental clarity.

Journaling

We are now going to travel down a side stream, on what looks like a tangential journey, by switching gears and temporarily leaving behind the rational mind space. Our purpose is to fill you with energy, to help uplift you, to pull you out of any dark space that you may be in. And for this I ask for help from the highest plane and ineffable kingdom. (As I call for assistance, please do so as well in whatever way is comfortable. You may merely accept the help that is offered, or ask for it yourself.). And if you haven't realized it yet, this book is meant to help you to open yourself to a deeper and more fulfilling experience of being alive.

Many times when we take the wrong actions, the impetus for these actions stems from not taking the time to be clear about what we feel. One good way to clarify thoughts and feelings is through journaling, as described by the Pathwork Foundation, an organization devoted to aiding personal transformation:

The Daily Review. With its help you can find out your true reactions to certain events; you begin to pull off masks and stop pretenses. You can find out where your actions go against a spiritual law. The daily review should be conducted in the following manner: Let the whole day pass in front of your eyes and in your memory; think of everything that has happened and has given you, in some way, a disharmonious feeling or reaction. And no matter how wrong the other person may have been, the moment you have been negatively touched by it, there must be something wrong within you.

Write down in a few words the occasions, your reactions and associations. If you follow this practice through for some time to come, and not just once or twice, but faithfully, you will see after a while a clear pattern emerging. At first, these disharmonious incidents will appear entirely unconnected and isolated; they will be meaningless for you. Later on you will begin to sense and, in time, clearly understand the pattern. This will help greatly.

You should pray for enlightenment and guidance every time you conduct the daily review. Then ideas will flow into you and will eventually furnish you with further clues, though at first they may not make sense to you. Do not discard any of the ideas; do not resist them. Later on, all of them will form a clear picture. As with a puzzle, when you look at the pieces, you cannot see the picture, but if you patiently put them together, you will succeed. Thus you will uncover your hidden anxieties and complexes which are responsible for your disease. Most of it is anxiety or fear. This is true of almost all of them, in one form or another. There might be a fear that you do not permit yourself to acknowledge consciously, that you have pushed down into your unconscious. So now you have to let it out. It takes time and effort before you can deal with it properly in your conscious mind and become aware of the spiritual laws from which you have deviated within your soul. [363]

Sample Daily Review

Occasion	Reaction & Association
Global Warming	Anger, hostility, doubt A feeling of fear in my heart Existential fear: is where I live safe? (I lived very close to the ocean at the time of writing this.) Reminds me of a vague sense of not trusting life
Skipped Yoga Class	Tired, Bored, Unsure, Fatigue Is this right for me? I do not know what to do
Friend did not laugh at joke	I felt ashamed of myself I did something wrong I do not want to be here Why am I spending time with this person Reminds me of being uncared for as a child

This sample daily review is real, taken from my own journal. The aim here is not to pretend to have certain feelings, but to be open and accepting to all feelings that arise, even those that might be considered unacceptable. One's feelings do not have to be logical, and they should not be judged. Any event that is disharmonious, no matter how insignificant, is valid enough to be recorded; it could be as simple as noting that someone gave you a funny look. This practice enhances both the emotional and mental bodies. I strive to faithfully record my daily reviews. Knowing your true purpose in life and understanding your place in the world also help refine mental clarity, and help you to align your intentions with positive energy. While the full purpose of your existence is a complex subject, I will simplify two key purposes most of us share in life.

The first purpose of life is to grow and evolve. Life seems always to bring us lessons. These lessons trigger emotions within us. Through accepting our feelings, we hope to grow into a greater sense of our self. This growth is more of an inward journey, about opening to the inner experience of the life moving through you.

The second purpose of life is to be a parent. Your longing and purpose in this moment, therefore, is to fulfill whatever you desire in relation to becoming a parent. Your purpose is to prepare to be a parent. Don't underestimate the role of parenthood. I cannot think of anything more important. Can you?

Inner Wisdom

Much of what I write about in this book, in addition to what I have learned through research, comes from my own inner wisdom. That being said, a more accurate assessment is to say that I am an open vessel to life and energy, and that an aspect of the force that moves through me enters into this world as wisdom. It is not my wisdom, though; I am merely the gateway for wisdom that is already here and will always be here. So, as you read this book, a pathway can open within you to receive this wisdom, which can then become embodied in you for your use to help you live better. To take the analogy of the vessel for wisdom a bit further, consider that the child being born through you is not your child. You are a vessel that allows one of life's creations to enter into the world. Neither you nor your partner made the child. Nature and life made the child. You simply allowed the seeds to come together, then nourished your body and kept it well. Very little about creating a child is under our control; it is very much an involuntary and automatic process of the body. The ability to procreate, the creation of the seeds and the birth process itself, all happen mostly involuntarily. The child coming through you was initiated by you, but his creation was not your doing. Thus, your child is not just your child, but a child who is a part of life and connected to everything. This perspective makes all children *our* children. Now, of course you feel a special affinity to the child that comes from you, who usually looks very much like you, and you will care for this child in every way whether you want to or not. But the point is that we are vessels for something else, something bigger and greater than the limited sense we have of ourselves. Accepting this helps encourage inner guidance and wisdom.

Every guideline in this book is just that: merely a guide. The guides are not an attempt to tell you what to do, but rather to help you find and awaken the truth — the dormant energy potential — that is budding within you. The purpose of what I write is continually to point you towards your true self that wants to be healthy and knows how to be healthy. The seat of responsibility for your life always resides within you. Not the outer you, the one whom you see in your mirror, but the inner you, the "self" who is all-knowing. I acknowledge that not everything I write will magically create health for everyone. And some of the guidelines I provide may not work for you due to your unique situation. This we must accept, as my real purpose is to remind you of that home which is in your heart, the place where all your inner knowing comes from. So let this small attempt to do good for you be a message of caring from my heart to yours and your family's.

Many people do not live through their real self. The real self or higher self is our divine spark which resides in our earthly bodies. "This is the finest and most radiant of the subtle bodies, with the quickest frequency of vibration."[364] But the higher self is covered by layers of denser matter and slower moving energy, that we call the lower self. These lower energies are distorted, separated and altered, and represent a lower vibrational frequency. The energies of the higher and lower selves mirror each other. While the higher self quality might be love, it can become twisted into fear by the lower self.

Or the higher self energy of enthusiasm and joy might, in its lower self form, become anger. When our individual denser matter merges with the *collective* lower self, we become almost entirely disconnected from our higher self. We then together create the disease of modernization, the modern plague. Remember, however, that the covering of our true nature is never complete, but only partial. When we are connected to our higher self we feel peace, we radiate joy, and we accept the highs and lows of life within a container of a deep and abiding peace.

We usually hide the emotions that come from a darker place, because we believe these emotions are "bad." For example, standing on your roof and screaming how much you hate the world is not a typically accepted behavior, so this behavior and others like it are labeled "bad" and stuffed into the closet. These real and powerful emotions — greed, envy, hatred, resentment, pride, aggression, cruelty, and so on — are destructive forces that are not well tolerated by our culture. We enjoy these emotions vicariously and "safely" from watching the latest violent action film. But in our own lives, many people try to hide these facets of themselves. The judgment of something as "bad" is also part of the lower self. Ultimately nothing within you is "bad" and judging it that way keeps it hidden and stunted in darkness. The lower vibrations stay low and drag you down in life, so you feel as though you are drowning. Of course, there are practical social reasons for containing, hiding and denying the lower self: you control yourself so that you don't wind up in jail after smashing the neighbor's windows because you had a bad day at work. The problem, however, is that these negative feelings are real and need to be released and healed.

We start to suppress our negative emotions when, as children, we learn to label these feelings as "bad" and "wrong." For example, if a young child feels aggression and hits his mother, mom may say, "Stop!" The child feels he is "bad" and shouldn't have had the impulse to hit. The child internalizes this belief, and starts living life by hiding his aggression because he thinks he is bad. He does not separate himself from his feeling of aggression.

As children, we find that many of our true qualities are not tolerated well by the adults around us. We learn to hide, protect, abandon and distort many of our pure and positive feelings. When they are hidden, these feelings become distorted and come out as negative energy. The child who at first just wanted some love and attention may, if his needs are not met, becomes a tyrant or sinks into a shell and never emerge. Over time, we forget that we operate within these negative patterns. As adults, we then experience shortcomings, difficulties, and dissatisfaction in life because this part of ourselves is missing and we have developed automatic behaviors to inhibit our natural responses to life. It is precisely these unresolved hidden feelings that cause many negative effects in our lives.

As we grew up, we began to believe that these dark and hidden aspects were in fact who we really were. In response, we created a personal outer identity that embodied socially acceptable features in order to function in the world while hiding the intolerable and "bad" feelings that lurked inside. This fabricated outer image we call "the mask." The mask functions to make us look good, while hiding our real motives and behaviors. "The idealized self masks the real self. It pretends to be something you are not. The idealized self-image is supposed to be a means of avoiding unhappiness."[365]

Here's a simple example: let's say that while driving on the highway a reckless driver runs you off the road, nearly causing an accident. You are left frightened, shaking and furious. When you return home, an acquaintance greets you and asks, "How are you?" Your automatic reply is, "Fine!" The mask presents a disconnected story centered in a lost realm within us. And part of trying to convince ourselves of the truth of this story is by telling it to other people. The mask is a façade that separates us from others, ourselves, and life itself.

Our hidden lower self is life destroying. It feels good when it gets to break things apart and shatter them — even paradoxically believing this is a constructive movement. Collectively, our modern civilization has destroyed many healthy and happy native cultures around the world and then called it progress.

Rather than avoiding your "bad" feelings, it is important to accept them and feel them. This does not mean to act them out and destroy things. But at the same time, we have energy in us that needs to be acknowledged so that it can evolve. We need to act out our energies in a safe way, without hurting people. For example, you may feel angry and want to hit someone who is making you angry; but you can hit a pillow instead, and in that way the energy in your body is acknowledged and expressed. I have about 50 hours of pillow punching under my belt. If you try it you'll realize you get tired and frustrated after 5-15 minutes.

Maintaining the mask of our idealized self and avoiding our true feelings causes our mind to become constricted and burdened with excessive thoughts. We then act hurried and impatient, moving the focus of our mind from one thought to another because our idealized self constantly strives to avoid the present moment by searching for activities that bring pleasure or let us avoid pain.

Activity - dissolve your inner obstacles: When you seriously ask the universe to help you overcome your inner obstacles, your prayer or request will be answered. Usually the answer comes in some form of a life lesson or difficulty to overcome. A good prayer is "Show me, Father, the real reason for my difficulties, so that I can solve them." I invite in the spirit (referring to the deva or guardian spirit) of overcoming obstacles. After invoking these energies, we simply need to receive their energy and pay it due homage. Just notice the sensations in your body right now. Take a deep and mindful breath.

Increasing Life Force for Becoming More Fertile

Part of the focus of preconception health is to be aware that your level of health at the time you conceive will have a direct influence on the health of your child. The following are some suggestions to encourage greater health.

Movement and change are a part of nature and the universe. The human body stagnates when you do not move, and fluids pool in the body. Many kinds of movement exercise can quiet our minds and increase mental focus. Our lymphatic system is based on a system of pumps which function properly when we regularly move our bodies. Exercise increases our appetite and many times improves digestion. I encourage 1-2 hours a day of movement that you enjoy. It does not have to be strenuous; walking, jogging, or swimming are all excellent forms of exercise.

If you feel you do not have time, then ditch the television news hour, reading the newspaper and other useless "information" collection activities and take just 10 minutes out of your day to start some movement. The important thing is to do something that you enjoy that inspires you.

Hatha Yoga is the practice of physical postures and breathing exercises. *Ha* means sun and *tha* means moon. Together they represent the yin and the yang of nature. The purpose of yoga is to become one with life. Physical exercise, movement and breath move us toward clarity and oneness, but they rarely bring us to the ultimate goal. A daily yoga practice calms the mind, strengthens the glandular system, improves digestion, connects us with our physical body, and clarifies, strengthens and balances our aura (which includes our emotions).

Tai chi is a slow moving art form. It gets our energy moving, and a part of its purpose is to unite the yin feminine receptive force of the universe with the yang active force of the universe. Tai chi builds patience, and strengthens the lower and upper *dan tien*. The upper *dan tien* is located near the thymus gland, just below the bony half-circle that's 2-3 inches above your heart. Within the upper *dan tien* lies your soul's purpose for incarnation. The lower *dan tien* is located 1.5-2 inches below your belly button, in the center of gravity for your body. The lower *dan tien* is your intention to incarnate and to exist. Over time, the various forms of tai chi strengthen these centers and help you become more aligned with life.

Qigong. Qi, or Chi, means energy. Qigong is the practice of moving energy in our body. It makes us healthy and opens up different energy centers in our body.

There are also western traditions and practices that vibrate and energize our bodies. Here are a few.

Continuum Movement is a type of free form movement that is facilitated by music. It is a real practice of being in the formless state and for awakening one's inner instincts and innate intelligence — whose purpose is to create more harmony in life. It has many health benefits. (www.continuummovement.com Click on the teachers link to find a local teacher.)

Core Energetics and Bioenergetics is a psychotherapeutic dynamic healing modality. Part of this modality is a set of physical exercises designed to enliven the body and help liberate emotions trapped in the muscular armor of the body. There are many of these therapists across the country, but not too many classes that focus just on exercise and movement. The book *The Way to Vibrant Health: a Manual of Bioenergetic Exercises,* by Alexander Lowen, contains a list of exercises, some of which, like punching a pillow, are extremely useful. Learn more at: **coreenergetics.org** or **www.bioenergetic-therapy.com**

Dancing– Most styles of dance are an enjoyable way to exercise and feel more alive. Almost every city or town has at least one dance class or studio.

The above mentioned exercises nurture your physical, mental, emotional, and spiritual bodies. They help you feel your physical body and thus feel more alive and connected to life. Regular and frequent movement that involves enjoyment and/or awareness will go a long way to preparing you for a healthy pregnancy and birth.

Activity: Enhance fertility with Kegel exercises & PC pull ups. Kegel exercises (for women) or PC pull-ups (for men) access the muscle between the genitals and anus. This pelvic floor muscle is directly connected with your root energy center, which affects the quality and quantity of your sexual energy. These exercises for men and women can increase sexual pleasure, and help women restore muscle tone after childbirth. The regular practice of these exercises will no doubt help in the childbirth process.

To learn how to do the Kegel exercises, start by restricting and releasing the flow of urine. The muscles engaged for starting and stopping the flow are the pubococcygeus muscles, sometimes called "Kegel muscles" after Dr. Arnold Kegel, developer of these exercises. The principle is the same for men and women. Once you can feel the muscles, you can practice squeezing them several times per day throughout the day to increase their strength and tone.

Spiritual Factors in Conception

The sexual force is an expression of consciousness pulling towards oneness and unity. Its purpose is to regenerate life, to unify the opposites of male and female on the physical, emotional, mental and spiritual levels.

Love is the essence of spirituality; it is the essence of conception. Through an act of love, we create our children.

Many parents at some time intentionally decide that they want to have children. Other parents do not intend to have children and pregnancy happens by accident. But from a spiritual perspective, there are no accidents. Everything in life has a purpose. On the same hand, we are not predestined to live out a certain fate. We have control over the choices we make in our lives and we have a hand in choosing our actions moment by moment, which can affect not only ourselves but the world greatly.

Many parents, even if they actively choose to become a parent, are not fully aligned with being parents. Other parents become parents from a more passive choice, and the child on its way is awaited without 100% enthusiasm and clarity. Some examples include children outside of marriage or even outside of relationships, or when the couple was not planning on a long term commitment or on having children. I've seen many young mothers who seemed as though they weren't quite ready for motherhood. They still clung to their "old" life and identity— their younger self without children. Other parents choose to have children and then don't take much effort to take care of them. They pack them off to day care and give them to other people for large periods of time every day.

Take a moment to look within to hear your inner voice, or to feel your inspiration, to see where you honestly stand with regard to having children (or with your current children). Recall the practice of asking "How do I feel right now?" This looking inward process is not necessarily easy, but it is an important practice. Regardless of the circumstances, if you have decided to be a parent then the child is coming. So you might as well say "yes" to life and to children and align yourself with a positive vibration and energy. Align yourself fully with your intention to parent, **now**! As you do this, notice both your positive "yes" current, and any negative "no" voices or currents. To maintain health we must acknowledge both the good and the bad. Continue to align yourself with your positive "Yes, I want to be a parent," or "Yes, I want to fulfill my role as a parent fully," while being aware of the voices of "No, I can't," or "No, I don't want to," with compassion.

Knowing your goals in life and being clear with at least part of your overall purpose helps you to be a successful parent. When we do not actively state or clarify our goals in life then life will give us goals we might not desire.

Spiritual practices can help you align yourself with being a parent. These include readings of scriptures appropriate to your beliefs, meditating, praying, asking for help from higher powers, mindfulness, selfless service, taking care of your physical body, and other special practices.

Activity - How do you feel now?
What do you feel in this moment? Happy or unhappy? Gratitude or ingratitude— or just numbess? Simply notice how you feel. Noticing, by the way, is the opening to greater awareness.

Natural Birth Control and Pregnancy Achievement

One key to being fertile and to healing infertility is for the mother to understand her fertility cycle. Becoming familiar with your fertility cycle has two advantages: it can help you to achieve pregnancy, and it can help you to avoid pregnancy. You will need to learn this method if you are going to have successful preconception health, as it takes months or years to restore the body from the abuses caused by birth control pills or the IUD. I want to remind you that using Fertility Awareness Method (FAM) is a serious responsibility; one "mistake" with the method and a baby might be on the way.

Since fertility awareness is all natural there are no side effects. As you may have experienced, the birth control pill has many side effects that are undesirable (including headache and weight gain). Other birth control methods can lead to infections and irritations.[366]

FAM is not the same as the Rhythm Method but is based on sound fertility signs. It uses scientifically proven fertility signs, waking temperature, cervical fluid and cervical position.[367]

When the guidelines are strictly followed FAM is virtually as effective as the contraceptive pill![368]

During the monthly menstrual cycle, the egg released remains viable for about 24 hours.[369] That means there needs to be seminal fluid present at the right location within those 24 hours for fertilization to occur. During the fertile phase of the menstrual cycle, women produce cervical fluid to keep the sperm alive, and to create the right ecosystem for conception to occur.[370] Without the nourishing cervical fluids, the sperm die within a few hours or even less. During the fertile phase, cervical fluid changes, becoming egg white-colored and very stretchy, so you can use the cervical fluid to determine when ovulation starts, and thus determine whether or not you are fertile. You can monitor your waking temperature to confirm ovulation as well, and use both observations of cervical fluid and the waking temperature to determine when ovulation has ended. Women can only get pregnant during the fertile times. Since the fertile time is of a limited duration, if you know when you are possibly fertile, you can use this information to either avoid pregnancy, or to get pregnant. Hence, FAM is an extremely effective form of natural birth control or pregnancy achievement.

FAM works by eliminating unprotected intercourse during the fertile times, and adding a little extra room for safety before and after the possibly fertile phase. In safely practicing the guidelines, in a typical month you have about 20 days of possible unprotected sex, and generally 9-12 days of abstinence or use of a barrier method.

Many times, women who are supposedly infertile and can't get pregnant actually are fertile, and it's merely that their timing of intercourse is wrong.

I'll say this twice: there is no room for error. If you make a mistake, or cheat with the rules, the odds of a pregnancy resulting are very high.

Below is a chart on the effectiveness of FAM and other birth control methods. Studies by Contraceptive Technology look at two statistics for judging the effectiveness of contraceptive methods. One is the **user failure** rate which is when a pregnancy results from the user's incorrect use of the birth control method. The other rate is a **method failure**, when pregnancy results from a problem with the method that was properly followed.

	User Failure % for Typical Use for 1 year	Method Failure % For typical use over 1 year time
Chance	85%	85%
Male Condom (no spermicide)	14%	3%
The Pill	5%	Less than or equal to .5%
IUD	Less than 2%	Less than or equal to 1.5%
FAM	10-12% (includes intentional rule violations)	2% or less

*Spermicide, along with any lubricant that is not edible, is toxic. Spermicide is intended to disable or kill sperm. And one study shows that nonoxynol-9, a common spermicide, is toxic to human cervical cells.[372] The gel in nonoxynol-9 products does reduce its toxicity, however.

Let's review the chart. If you have unprotected sex without using any birth control methods, then over a one year period there is an 85% chance that pregnancy will occur. Using male condoms with no spermicide, the condom itself will fail to prevent pregnancy in 3% of cases when used properly over a one year period. Since some users employ condoms incorrectly, they have a user failure rate of 14%. The birth control pill is very effective at preventing pregnancy, with 0.5% or less method failure, although I have met one mother who became pregnant while on the pill. The IUD as a method fails less than 1.5% of the time in a one-year period. Finally, FAM, when practiced correctly, is safer (more effective) than using a condom, at 2% failure rate or less.

This failure statistic of 2% can be improved to well below 1% if women use a third ovulatory indicator — checking the position of the tip of the cervix.[373] A study of over 100 women, published in the American Journal of Obstetrics and Gynecology (October 15, 1981), which involved follow up and interviews with all of the participants, found that even though all of the pregnancies were statistically attributed to a failure of the FAM method, only those couples who knowingly broke the rules became pregnant. In this study, the method failure rate of FAM was 0%.[374]

Some people who rightfully support FAM suggest the use of a barrier method during the approximate 10 days in which women are possibly fertile, because people might be turned away from using FAM if they know they will have to abstain from intercourse for about 10 days. The typical failure rate of condoms (3% over one year) will likely remain unchanged or even increase if they are used during fertile times.

During the schooling years all young adults should be taught the FAM program and its application. This would substantially decrease the incidence of unwanted and unplanned pregnancies among young people, and also limit the detrimental health effects of the pill and the IUD. As a society as a whole, I think we fear our sexual drives and instincts, so we do not teach our teens about how to have sex without having babies (which usually happens beyond parental

control anyway). I also believe that synthetic barrier methods of contraception represent a mechanistic way for us to remain separated from each other. With barrier methods like condoms, even in our most intimate moments we need a device of modernization, a barrier produced in a factory, to keep us "safe."

We do not teach natural birth control to young adults because we try to limit and control their sexual activity. It is completely unrealistic to expect young adults to abstain from sex. Young adults are teeming with sexual energy, and rather than making it taboo we could make it safe and healthy. (In many other countries there are fewer sexual taboos for teens.) By preaching abstinence, we create a culture of fear, and of control. And we only do this to our young adults because we do it to ourselves. Frustrated sexual feelings are driven underground, which leads to more risky and imbalanced behaviors (such as sex while intoxicated). And if you don't know this, once American teens get to college, many do engage in sex while intoxicated. This is usually a result of fears of intimacy and lost sexual pleasure due to our sexually repressed society. Without proper education about sex, young adults cannot enjoy safe and intimate sex with each other. In the U.S. for one year (1990) approximately 1 million pregnancies and 521,826 live births occurred among women ages 15-19.[375] And what is of more concern is that 95% of these pregnancies were unintended.[376] That is over 950,000 unintended pregnancies per year. About half of those teens chose to become mothers. A study of over 1,000 teens found that 30% of women aged 15-17 have had intercourse and 46% of teen men of the same age have had intercourse.[377] I don't necessarily wish to promote teenage sex, but we need to be honest with ourselves. Many teenagers are not responsible about their sexual behavior because we have failed to show them how to be responsible. It is time to bring this issue out of the closet and create a safe space for teenagers who wish to be sexually active, without them producing babies when they don't want them or aren't ready. We also don't want to start them on birth control pills, because introducing synthetic hormones while their hormonal systems are still maturing will not only increase the risk of cancer and other diseases, but it will ruin Nature's wonderful maturation process. We need to start looking at, paying attention to, and treating teens as equals, as humans. That means loving our teens. We can then begin to take steps towards healing them.

Menstruation and the Divine Feminine

The menstrual cycle connects women to the divine female energy. Allowing the natural fertility cycle to unfold, without synthetic hormones to control it, is a way for women to be naturally in contact with their femininity. Women are the manifestation of the divine feminine (both men and women possess divine feminine energy; however its physical manifestation resides in women). Perhaps birth control pills have arisen from a denial or betrayal of the divine feminine. Cycles of creativity and heightened sensitivity move in accordance with the cycles of ovulation, which is itself connected with the moon and the cycle of life.

I pray for more natural methods of birth control in the future, in addition to FAM. We can increase the use of natural pregnancy prevention while encouraging intimacy.

A full guide to the practice of FAM is beyond the scope of this book. In other words, don't attempt the FAM protocol by merely reading my brief summary of it. If you intend to practice FAM, I recommend that you purchase one of the following excellent books, and plan to attend a class in your area if there is one available.

Taking Charge of Your Fertility by Toni Weschler – **www.ovusoft.com**

Garden of Fertility by Katie Singer – **www.gardenoffertility.com**

Beyond FAM: SFAM

Spiritual Fertility Awareness Method (SFAM) is in some ways a humorous way to point out that sometimes children come when they want to,

and many times it is beyond our control. One example of the SFAM is a couple who both had surgeries to make sure that neither of them could produce offspring. Then sometime later in their life they got pregnant and had a baby boy.

The reverse scenario is also possible. If conception is impossible, it must be the will of the divine. All pregnancies, including unplanned pregnancies, serve some higher purpose, or plan, no matter what type of painful feelings or what difficulties in life they may bring up.

Conception by the future parents cannot happen unless it is the will of God. If a conception today is not to serve a definite purpose for the entity to come into your world, it will be prevented by spiritual means, though it may take place next month.[378]

Preconception Health Conclusion

Why is it that we in the west have come to conceive and raise children so haphazardly? Why does our culture neglect one of the most valuable health practices conceivable?

We have lost contact with ourselves. We have lost contact with what truly matters, and allow ourselves to live in a way that promotes sickness and disease. But this can be changed. Indeed, it is changing.

A high force has given us a type of manual for preconception health. Its ancient wisdom was passed down through countless generations of indigenous peoples, who knew to eat special foods and how to provide adequate spacing between their children's births. We must consider our practice of conception carefully, following the examples we see everywhere in nature. Animals naturally practice preconception health in harmony with their environment, as their mating cycles peak when their food has the highest nutrient content. In our modern world we act less intelligently than animals, because we take no special care for preconception.

In the U.S. there is no clear health program or protocol for preconception health. In some crevices of our culture there still exist natural health care practitioners who are successful in restoring health to the body prior to conception. Good natural health practitioners will aim at diagnosing and healing glandular imbalances using natural supplements and health therapies. They will also use methods to remove and de-toxify chemicals and heavy metals trapped in the body. The International Foundation for Nu-trition and Health maintains a list of practitio-ners, many of whom will fall under this descrip-tion (find the list at www.ifnh.org, if it is not online, then call or e-mail them). While I cannot vouch for them, I am certain that some practi-tioners available through this organization are excellent. The Price-Pottenger Nutrition Foun-dation maintains a list of health practitioners nationwide, some of whom may be helpful for preconception health: www.ppnf.org. In the menu click "Health Professional – List of PPNF professional members." There are many holisti-cally oriented medical doctors, naturopaths, acupuncturists, osteopaths, chiropractors and more who specialize in effective healing modali-ties. See Appendix A for some additional online resources to help you find such a licensed pro-fessional.

The moment of truth. Now a greater plan has been carefully studied, and special preparations have been made in the world be-yond the physical earth world. The being who is about to come waits for that special moment of conception to take place. Astrological signs and other factors are taken into consideration, as well as a vast number of minute details. Then at the moment of conception, the entity coming to earth becomes unconscious and a part of its vast knowledge hidden. At the time of birth, spirits come and assist the being to enter the baby's body.[379] And your new baby is born!

Part III
Healing Our Children

8

Childbirth
Enabling the Divine Purpose of the Universe

Through birth you experience your divine purpose.

> *You are here to enable the divine purpose of the universe to unfold. That is how important you are.*[380]

I want you to take a moment to acknowledge that you are important. Even if you think you are not important in other people's eyes, think about how you are perceived through your new baby's eyes. You are vitally important to that child. **You are the entire world to that child**. You are here to enable the divine purpose of the universe to unfold. That is how important you are. Apart of that divine purpose…is parenthood.

Intention: To learn how to have a healthy birth, and learn why and how our modernized ways are the source of birth difficulties. To awaken the spontaneous feminine energy in you; to make wise and empowered birth choices.

The Divine Human Form

The human form is a state of existence based on separateness. This separated existence is earmarked by the division of the sexes into male and female. In a unified existence male and female would be one and there would be no longing or need for the opposite. The two sexes are both longing for oneness with each other. Each side wants wholeness and completion. When these two separate beings, male and female, merge in the divine act of love, then their two separate beings become one.

In that state a new life is created.

Two beings create one new being.

Their child is therefore a symbolic and actual realization of the oneness and unity in the universe.

As a result, when a child is born he experiences life in a unitive state, at one with life and at one with the Universe. **Gaze into a new baby's eyes** and you will see in their depths the divine aspects of the universe: infinity, and eternity.

Women are the divine vessels through which this new life enters our planet. And men make it possible for the creative act to happen. How could such divine aspects exist in a human form? Eckhart Tolle writes in *The Power of Now*,

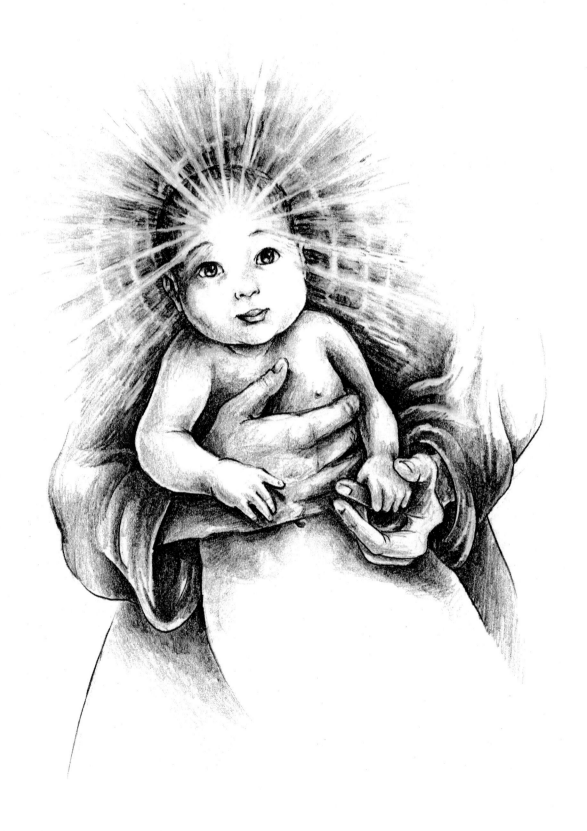

Go out on a clear night and look up at the sky. The thousands of stars you can see with the naked eye are no more than an infinitesimal fraction of what is there... And the greatest miracle is this: That stillness and vastness that enables the universe to be, is not just out there in space - it is also within you.[381]

We are able to touch and taste this creative force in the process of conception and birth.

Indigenous Wisdom for Healthy and Safe Births

In several tribes visited by Weston Price, he noted the "ease with which childbirth is accomplished"[382] and how birth is looked at as an "insignificant experience."[383]

Something has radically changed. Dr. Price observed with the Canadian Indians that:

The grandmothers of the present generation would take a shawl and either alone or accompanied by one member of their family retire to the bush and give birth to the baby and return with it to the cabin. A problem of little difficulty or concern, it seemed...Today the young mothers of this last generation are brought to [Dr. Davis's] hospital sometimes after they have been in labor for days. They are entirely different from their grandmothers or even mothers in their capacity and efficiency in the matter of reproduction. He stated that that morning he had had two cases in which surgical interference was necessary in order to make birth possible.[384]

Dr. Price observed the same situation among the Eskimo people.

*A similar impressive comment was made to me by Dr. Romig, the superintendent of the government hospital for Eskimos and Indians at Anchorage, Alaska. He stated that in his thirty-six years among the Eskimos, **he had never been able to arrive in time to see a normal birth by a primitive Eskimo woman.** But conditions have changed materially with the new generation of Eskimo girls, born after their parents began to use foods of modern civilization. Many of them are carried to his hospital after they had been in labor for several days.[385] (Emphasis added.)*

I have been advised that [a comfortable and rapid birth] is a relatively normal occurrence so long as they are in that excellent physical condition which is found to be present when they are on an adequate native dietary.[386]

In rats fed a diet deficient in fat-soluble vitamin A, the same vitamin whose absence led to birth defects as discussed in Chapter 4, prolonged and difficult labors were common.[387]

What It Takes For a Natural Birth

As seen in Chapters 2, 3, and 4, people eating a modernized diet do not develop proper bone structure. Many photographs illustrated improper development and poor bone growth, which resulted in narrow faces and narrow spaces for the teeth (dental arches), which in turn led to crowded teeth. I also illustrated that these conditions **are not genetic** aberrations but caused by a blocked (intercepted) genetic potential.

Let's digress and talk about a subject that is sensitive in nature, the pelvis.

*Activity - What's going on down there?*Our culture has a habit of ignoring that lower part of our body which goes to the bathroom, that we sit on all day, which gives us pleasure, which makes babies and is their portal to the world. Why is that the case and how did it come to be? Many of us have been acculturated with feelings of shame or humiliation surrounding our sexuality. The lower body is associated with enjoyment in life, the ability to get our needs met, and our connection to the Earth and to all things. During childhood many of us did not have our sexuality honored. It is a common experience for both women and men to have had been subjected to some type of abuse related to their sexuality, whether it was physical or emotional. When our physical boundaries have been violated in some way in the past, it is hard for us to feel safe or comfortable in the world, or to let life energy flow through the pelvis. Uncomfortable feelings can also be associated with medical procedures like abortions. All you need to do right now is just notice how your pelvic region feels. How do you feel in relation to it? Try not to censor any feelings whether they may be deemed positive or negative; just notice them. Then if you are feeling up to it, invite in the deva, guardian spirit (or a related spirit) for sexual healing. This energy helps us feel grounded, safe and accepting of our sexuality.

In the climate of fear and mistreatment of our sexuality, discussion of the physical form of women becomes a delicate topic. This discussion is not meant to add to any collective pain that many women already experience in some way about their bodies or sexuality, but to help clarify something very important: what it takes to have a safe birth.

In a healthy new baby, the largest part of its body is the head. The head is soft during birth and the cranial bones are made to mold to the interior shape of the birth canal. During birth the head usually appears first and for birth to occur the baby's body must pass through the pelvic bones. One can then reason that if the opening for the baby's head and body (the pelvic brim) is large relative to the baby's size, then the birth will be rapid. If the opening is very small relative to the baby then birth will be difficult or even impossible.

Imagine for a moment that you are Nature. You want humans to survive and to thrive. If birth is too difficult, humans will stop making babies and soon disappear, so you design the process of making babies to be a pleasurable act, and you make the process of birth a pleasurable experience as well in order to encourage the practice. You, as clever Nature, therefore create a blueprint for an easy and rapid birth, by designing a pelvic shape that easily accommodates the baby's body and makes childbirth "an insignificant experience."

The pelvic brim is the circular shaped space that the baby's head must pass through during normal vaginal birth. The ideal shape is round, and of course of the widest diameter possible. The enlarged pelvic bone structure which makes space for a baby to pass through is why women's hips have curves. But the outer curve of a woman's hips is not as important for birth as is the inner spaciousness. As in the disturbed facial and bone structures we've seen, the shape of the interior of the pelvis, the pelvic brim, is influenced by diet.

If you can use your creative visualization for a moment, it should be clear that the rounder the pelvic brim, the easier childbirth will be for the mother. The heart shape of the pelvic brim and other varieties of pelvic shapes are now the norm in our modern culture. Some clever people experienced with birth will say that the pelvic shape does not in fact seem to relate to the ease with which women give birth. This observation may appear to be true since not only is the shape of the pelvic rim important, but so too is the relative diameter of the pelvic brim compared to the diameter of the baby's head. In this case, a birth may be easy even with a heart-shaped pelvic rim, provided that the baby's head is relatively smaller than the opening.

Dr. Price described how many native groups prepared their growing girls for the process of birth by feeding them special foods high in activator X. These foods support complete bone growth in the pelvis as well as proper hormonal development. These native people knew that special foods were essential to produce safe births.

I presented data indicating that the Peruvians, who were descendants of the old Chimu culture on the coast of Peru, used fish eggs liberally during the developmental period of girls in order that they might perfect their physical preparation for the later responsibility of motherhood... They were available both at the coast market of Peru and as dried fish eggs in the highland markets, whence they were obtained by the women in the high Sierras to reinforce their fertility and efficiency for childbearing.[388]

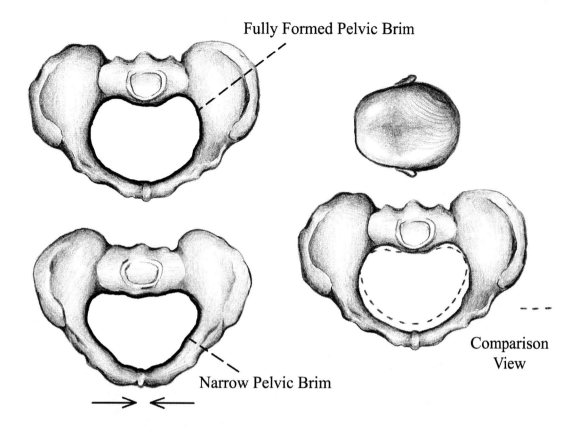

Fully Formed Pelvic Brim

Narrow Pelvic Brim

Comparison View

Notice the difference between the round pelvis above and the heart shaped pelvis below. The darkened inner lining of the pelvis is the pelvic brim. The heart shaped pelvis represents a narrowing caused by malnourished physical development.

By feeding girls according to special guidelines, Nature's blueprint would fulfill itself to the maximum potential with the most complete bone growth, producing a well filled out face with enough space for all the teeth to come in straight, and a pelvic brim that was wide and round in shape relative to the size of the baby. Fulfillment of Nature's plan made birth for native people, in general, of little difficulty.

Dr. Kathleen Vaughn, who studied the births of women in rural India, identified three keys for a successful and safe childbirth:

1. round pelvic brim;
2. flexible joints;
3. assuming a natural position for birth (for example, squatting).[389]

The creation of a round pelvic brim is begun in the womb, when the pregnant mother consumes special foods that support healthy bone growth and a balanced body structure in her developing daughter. Later, as this girl grows, and especially during periods of rapid growth, she eats special foods such as fish eggs or high vitamin summer butter, to allow her body to develop to its full, natural potential with ideal childbearing hips.

Dr. Vaughn found that "In practically all countries a restricted sedentary indoor life greatly increases the complications associated with childbirth."[390] For example, reclining daily on a couch could lead to the baby being in a less than ideal position for labor.[391] Dr. Vaughn further showed that in all primitive tribes living an outdoor and active life, childbirth is easy and the labor is short. She also demonstrated that even small distortions in the pelvic brim, such as a narrow or kidney shape greatly reduces the ease with which the baby's head passed through the birth canal.[392]

The Shape of the Body Distorted by our Modern Foods

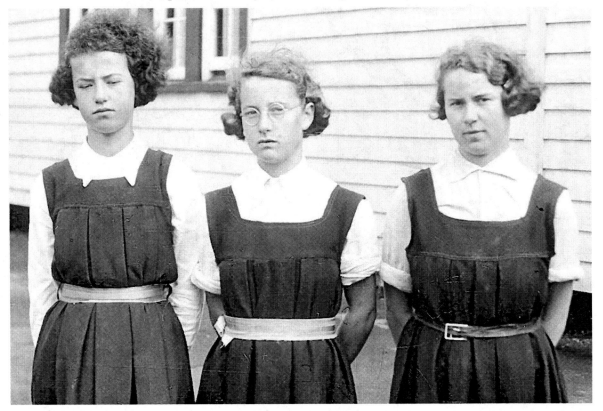

© *Price-Pottenger Nutrition Foundation, www.ppnf.org*
White Girl Scouts, New Zealand. Note the progressive lengthening and narrowing of the face and narrowing of the hips in the younger girl at the left.[393]

In these pictures of the girls, you see two girls on the right nourished by a more natural diet, whose bodies have squarish proportions; they have broad shoulders and broad hips. The girl on the left has an elongated structure that is a result of imbalances which began during the phase of preconception and carried through childhood. As a result, she is taller, but her body is thinner and her hips are narrower, resulting in a figure that is more boyish. Narrow hips likely mean a narrow pelvic brim, such that later in life, birth for this girl will be more difficult.[394]

In the past the estimated shape of the pelvic brim was wrongly used to indicate that a cesarean was needed or might be needed. Midwife extraordinaire Gail Tully explains on her website www.spinningbabies.com (which I highly encourage you to visit and read) that the only way to tell if a baby fits or not is to try to have the baby naturally. That includes a labor which encourages vertical positions (standing, squatting, etc.) and free access to food and fluids.[395]

With the coming of the *white man* and modern civilization came a plague. Once

healthy and relatively disease free, native groups began to suffer from diseases never before known to them. Now we add to the list of modern diseases birth difficulties and birth complications.

Birth complications and birth difficulties are not normal aspects of the human condition. They are only normal to the imbalanced conditions that humans have made with their "modern" lifestyle.

Now that we understand the cause of the problem, we can address it at its roots, so as to eliminate it forever if we want to. Women are not helpless victims of the curse of painful and complicated childbirth. Far from it. Our modern culture has created birth difficulties from an improper childhood diet, and from a lack of proper birth education for older children and teens. Most problems in birth, even those that seem out of our control such as improper birth position, abnormal placenta and so on, are nearly always a direct result of an imbalanced internal chemistry of a mother who did not prepare her body for birth. Whether from drug exposure during childhood and the teenage years, extended use of birth control pills, or a diet filled with toxic foods, additives and too much sugar and white flour, it is modern humans who have set the stage for every major birth complication that is so common today. Birth complications could be vastly reduced if we realized how we cause them, albeit in ignorance (until you read this book). Why resort to heroic surgeries and dangerous birth interventions when we can do something much better? That something is to prevent the need for them in the first place.

What It Takes To Have a Safe Birth

What was once a commonplace event of little difficulty or concern is now an ordeal that for many women is very difficult and daunting. Pleasurable births in modern countries are now rare and there is a great deal of fear of childbirth in our culture.

Activity: write down your fears about birth. Record all your fears associated with the birth process. If you feel brave, read the list to a friend. Make sure nobody tries to talk you out of your fears. Yes, fear is irrational; at the same time, you only realize that the fear is just an idea and not real by **first** feeling the fear.

Several factors weigh together to affect a women's ability to have a safe and rapid birth.

- The storage of nutrients in her glands, to support a strong and steady flow of hormones.
- The overall tone of the uterus which is in part determined by the supportive ligaments such as the round and broad ligaments.
- The strength of the pushing muscles, which include the psoas and the pelvic floor muscles.
- The shape and relative diameter of the pelvis.
- The position of the baby during birth.
- The size and proportions of the baby relative to the mother.
- The overall health of the mother.

Take note of these factors because you can significantly influence a majority of them. Over the course of a woman's life the various possible birth experiences she could have are significantly, if not completely, determined by her nutritional status — particularly during her growing years. What people often fail to understand is how important the nutritional and glandular health is for the mother during pregnancy. Having adequate nutrition before and during pregnancy, as described in Chapters 6 and 7, will support good muscle tone and nourish the glands, which provide hormones for the growth of the baby and for birth. Furthermore, a good diet will provide energy for birth, help the baby's body grow into proportions ideal for birth, and support healthy ligament stretching. Conversely, weak contractions in labor, an excessively slow labor, a baby whose size is out of proportion, and tears and other complications are more than likely caused by a poor diet that began at the time of preconception and carried on through pregnancy.

A Program to Encourage a Safe Birth

The primary factor in creating a safe birth is the nutrition of the mother-to-be.

Preparing the Physical Body
- Follow the Preconception health guidelines from Chapter 7 prior to pregnancy.
- During pregnancy follow the diet for pregnancy and lactation in Chapter 6.
- Exercise in order to stretch the ligaments around the uterus and pelvis, as well as strengthen the pelvic floor, and stay physically active. Some chiropractors and doctors can also help gently release stress on these ligaments.
  - Kegel exercises described on [page 149]
  - Pelvic Tilt
  - Inversion
  - Rebozo Sifting
  - Yoga

Preparing the Emotional Body by Creating Safety
- Find a birth care provider with whom you feel comfortable.
- Journal, talk, and draw pictures in order to learn about your personal fears associated with birth and pregnancy.
- Ask yourself, "What do I need to feel supported?"
- Watch videos, take classes, or do anything else to help you feel prepared for birth, and to help you explore your fears about childbirth.

Preparing the Mental Body
- Visualize a safe birth, read other women's birth stories, and read and learn about healthy birth practices.
- Prepare for possible complications, and know and understand what they mean.

Preparing the Spiritual Body
- Pray, and ask for spiritual help and guidance

Labor Tips
- Avoid drugs.
- Avoid or minimize time spent in the supine position (for most cases).
- Use special foods and herbs if necessary just prior to or during labor.
- The mother needs to feel comfortable, safe and have privacy respected.

Preparing the Physical Body

We can substantially influence the likelihood of a healthy and uncomplicated birth through preparation with nutrition and physical exercises. Weston Price writes:

> Many workers among the primitive races have emphasized the vigorous health and excellence of the infant at birth. We have here, therefore, emphasis on the need in the interest of the infant that the mother shall have an easy and short labor. Both of these factors are directly influenced by the vitamin content of the mother's body as supplied by her nutrition.[396]

It is therefore vitally important for women to be physically active prior to and during pregnancy, so long as the exercise is harmonious with pregnancy. The baby needs to be in the correct position in order to be delivered with the least amount of resistance. If the baby is not in the ideal position, labor becomes far more difficult or even impossible. The ideal delivery position for the baby is encouraged by the mother's engagement in appropriate physical activities.

Activities that encourage joint flexibility

- Walking
- Hula-hoop-style big hip circles while sitting on an exercise ball
- Prenatal yoga (regularly, ideally 20 minutes a day)

- Belly dancing
- Inversions (when appropriate; see below) or use of a slant board
- Pelvic tilt

The Pelvic Tilt

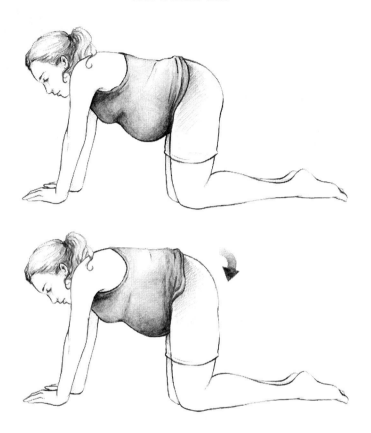

The Pelvic Tilt

The pelvic tilt encourages the baby to be in the correct delivery position; it also helps relax the lower back and pelvic joints. Practice daily in the middle and later stages of pregnancy.

1. Lift your lower back up towards the ceiling. (Don't arch the shoulders.)
2. Then straighten your back. (Don't ever dip your lower back as it can strain muscles, keep it level and parallel to the floor, and don't go lower than that.)
3. Repeat steps 1 and 2 about 40 times. Curl the lower back, and straighten the lower back.[397]

Inversions

Performing an inversion helps relax the involuntary muscles. Do not perform an inversion if you have excess amniotic fluid, high blood pressure, a sinus infection or loose ligaments from a previous birth or **if your intuition suggests that you should not perform this stretch**. To do an inversion, carefully lift your knees and hips higher than the rest of your body. This can be done, for example, by placing knees on a couch and hands on the floor. This is somewhat similar to the downward dog yoga position. Practice at least one time per day for 30 seconds to 2 minutes. During late pregnancy do not practice this pose for too long. For instructions, video, and precautions, visit: spinningbabies.blogspot.com /2007/02/how-to-do-inversion.html

Body Work

A first-time mother or a mother who has not had a natural birth may benefit from body work such as massage. Other forms of gentle chiropractic adjustments such as offered by Network Chiropractors, craniosacral therapy, pregnancy massage and Maya uterine massage can all help create an easier birth.

The rebozo method, not described in this book, is a method for promoting a safe birth through helping release tension in the mother's involuntary muscles. To learn about the rebozo method, go to www.youtube.com/spinningbabies, and/or spinningbabies.blogspot.com and search for rebozo scarf in the search window.

Poor Posture

Our posture affects the positioning of our infant. Do not sit slouched for extended periods, as we often do in bucket car seats or on couches, and don't lie down improperly such that your body is twisted in an awkward way.[398]

Birth Position

The pelvic size changes with various birth positions. A hands-and-knees position, or a squatting position, can add two centimeters of space by allowing freedom in the sacrum. Lying on one's back disables this extra space.[399]

Prenatal Yoga

Yoga can help improve strength and joint flexibility. Take a prenatal yoga class if you feel even the slightest bit inspired.[400]

Nutrient Depletion

The picture above demonstrates the "borrowing" process that can occur during pregnancy. After a difficult birth in which this woman nearly lost her life, her body began to show signs of severe deficiency. Various deficiencies become pro-nounced when the mother doesn't have an ideal diet during the late stages of pregnancy, as well as during lactation.

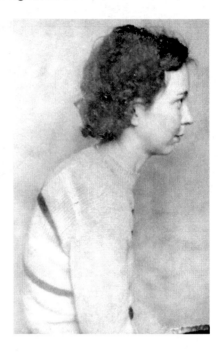

© Price-Pottenger Nutrition Foundation, www.ppnf.org
She nursed her baby for some time but the overdraft of reproduction on her frail body was so great that she aged rapidly, her back weakened and she stooped forward as shown.[401]

Diet Before and Immediately After Birth

These guidelines are primarily for the time leading up to the birth, three weeks prior, and four days after.

Three weeks prior to birth, Dr. Bieler recommends:

1. Omitting starchy foods (potatoes, bread, pastries, crackers, etc.).
2. Eating raw and cooked vegetables, raw milk, and fruit.
3. Avoiding strawberries, seedless grapes, cranberries and cantaloupe.[402]

Dr. Bieler suggests not eating during labor [403] and then not eating immediately after birth.[404]

This guideline applies primarily for women who are in excellent health and have been eating a building diet for quite some time. Women with less than ideal health can benefit from eating during labor. Trust your instincts on this. If you are not hungry during labor or after birth, that's fine; don't force yourself to eat.

Moisturizing Formula (Begin three weeks before birth, once or twice daily.) Drinking the moisturizing drink daily 3 weeks before the baby is due helps ease birth and prevent tearing of tissues during birth.[405] The following recipe helps moisturize and lubricate the whole body, especially the skin, and is reproduced here from *The Recipe for Living without Disease* with permission of Dr. Aajonus Vonderplanitz, Ph.D. Nutrition.

1-2 raw organic eggs
2-4 ounces raw butter
1-2 tablespoons lemon juice
1-2 teaspoons unheated honey

All ingredients should be at room temperature. Warm all ingredients in a jar with the lid on, immersed in a bowl of mildly hot water for 5 minutes. Blend on medium speed for 10 seconds. The formula is most effective when consumed with, or shortly after consuming a meat meal.[406]

Five days prior to the due date begin adding 2 tablespoons of bee pollen with about 2 tablespoons of unsalted raw cheese to the lubrication drink.[407] (Some people could be allergic to bee pollen.) For many women this formula is pure gold, and should greatly enhance the body's lubrication and aid in an easier birth, as well as make the skin more elastic to prevent tearing. (**Raw egg note**: Make sure your eggs are organic and preferably farm-direct, from chickens with access to grass. If you feel awkward taking this every day, take two days off every five days. Some people avoid eating raw egg whites; if you are one of them, consume only the yolks.)

Beef heart contains important amino acids including l-carnitine for muscle tone and will help you keep your strength up during labor.[408] I suggest consuming beef heart two to four times per week in the final three weeks before birth. Even just a few ounces per meal will be beneficial (lamb or bison heart can be substituted). Of course you don't need to wait to consume beef heart; start eating it much earlier, as it is a great boost to health If you are eating a good diet, such as described in this book, and include beef heart in the weeks before labor, your chances of failing to progress in labor will be minimized.

During labor a hot tea with ghee (clarified butter) added to it is believed to make the birth canal more slippery so the baby will come out more easily.[409] In traditional cultures midwives knew of special herbs to help aid and prepare the mother for birth. Many times these methods are far safer and more effective than western drugs, with their harsh side effects. If our modern culture was intelligent we would more often utilize herbs, and not drugs, when help was needed in the labor process.

Labor fatigue is dealt with in the hospital by administering I.V. fluids or other nutrients in the form of juices or electrolyte mixtures. These mixtures likely offer little true nutritional support for the body, and simply over stimulate the laboring woman's already over-stimulated glands. Women in labor who need more energy need to get it from real foods, not from concoctions created in a lab, or from pasteurized juices (though freshly pressed juices may help). Dr. Bieler suggests diluted unheated honey for labor support: one cup of warm water mixed with two full teaspoons of honey.[410] Foods that help in labor will be fresh whole foods that are easy to digest. Stick with foods that are as wholesome and pure as possible. Unless it is an emergency, make sure not to choose foods from the "avoid" list such protein shakes, pasteurized juices, and "health food" bars.

After birth it is important to be extremely watchful of what you eat. According to Dr. Bieler, avoiding solid food after birth is what animals in Nature do (except for consuming the placenta itself).[411] After birth, the womb must shrink from the size of a watermelon to the size of a pear. You don't want to burden your body at this important time of healing. Fruit juices made with pineapple, apple, grape or papaya and diluted with equal parts water can be helpful at this time.[412]

Fish soup taken after birth is a traditional practice in some cultures. In Japan, carp fish is cooked with all the organs except the gall bladder, for four to eight hours, with barley miso and burdock root. It is taken for four days in a row after birth. Make sure you get wild carp, not farm raised. You can also use other white non-oily fish for soup stock.[413] For a few days after Yeshe, our second daughter, was born Michelle didn't have much appetite, but she drank fish soup several times per day. In about two or three weeks' time her energy was normal and she seemed to be completely recovered.

After the mother returns to full eating habits, raw milk and raw butter are good choices. In the Chongqing province in China, mothers consume up to ten eggs per day and eat large amounts of chicken and pork for the first four weeks after the birth. This diet is rich in saturated fats that help nourish the body.[414] Eating oily fish during the first weeks and months after birth is also a good idea.

There is a modern traditional Chinese remedy called *Yunnan Paiyao*. This remedy was created in 1902 to stop excess bleeding, and is made from several ginsengs, sweet potato, and other ingredients guarded in a secret formula. It might be good to have on hand for a homebirth, but use it at your own risk. Several teaspoons of ground cayenne pepper chugged down in a glass of water has also stopped hemorrhage.

Nutrition plays a significant role in the process of birth. Dr. Price described a woman whose first labor took 53 hours; she became a partial invalid for several months following the birth. No special effort involving her nutrition was made during her first pregnancy. However:

> *During the second pregnancy the selection of foods was made on the basis of nutrition of the successful primitives. This included the use of milk, green vegetables, sea foods, organs of animals and a reinforcement of the fat-soluble vitamins by very high vitamin butter and high vitamin cod liver oil.* [415]

Her second birth, which followed these special nutritional fortifications, took three hours. Dr. Price remarks,

> ***It is a usual experience that the difficulties of labor are greatly decreased*** *and the strength and vitality of the child enhanced where the mother has adequately reinforced nutrition...*[416] *(Emphasis added*

I want to emphasize this point because it is part of the reason why I have written this book. I want you to know effective ways to improve your labor outcomes and your newborn's health. Most people and most medical authorities do not possess this essential knowledge, which for millennia has helped create healthy children and ensured rapid, easy births. Improving your diet won't guarantee that you'll have an orgasmic 30 minute birth. However, it does promise to reduce the chance of labor difficulties, and shorten the duration of labor.

Special Foods Eaten During Pregnancy Support an Easier Labor along with Supporting Proper Development of the Child in the Womb

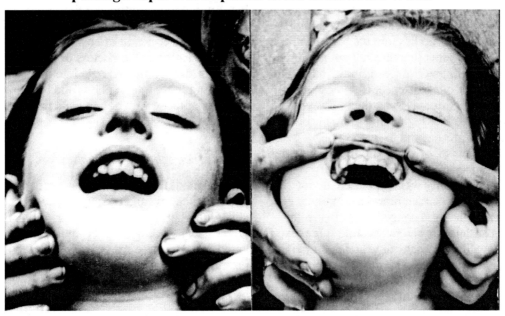

In this family the first child to the left was most injured in the formative period as shown in the form of the face and dental arches above. The first child required fifty-three hours of labor and the second three hours, preceded by special nutrition of the mother.[417]

These are the children of the mother who had a long first labor and a much shorter second one, as was just discussed. Notice how the younger child pictured at the right, who had improved nutrition in the pregnancy phase, has straight teeth. There is a wider space for the teeth to come in. She also has wider nostrils than her older sister (a sign of good nutrition). This is proof that not only is physical disease and degeneration caused by improper nutrition, but that through a proper diet we can reverse these problems.

Emotional, Mental and Spiritual Health for Pregnancy and Birth

Following the guidelines for emotional, mental, and spiritual health found in the Preconception Chapter 7 will also help to create a safe birth.

Activity: a prayer for trust and safety with birth. A feeling of safety seems to be missing as a regular part of women's birthing experiences today. I want to invoke the spirit of trust and safety for all the births on this planet, both now and in the future. Please join me energetically for a moment, if you will. To create this spirit of trust connect the feeling of safety in your physical body—the feeling that it is safe to be here and that it is good to be alive in your body—with the feeling of surrender to a greater will. Combine the feeling of personal bodily safety with the knowledge and the sense of a greater plan for our lives. This plan has our best interests at heart, and we can surrender and relax into this plan. Invite in the deva for safe and comfortable births. I pray for and invite in healing for mothers, babies, and for healing the distorted principles that continue to create violent actions towards women and their children.

Reading **www.spinningbabies.com** during Michelle's pregnancy was enlightening to me because Gail Tully, the site's midwife-author, truly feels this safety and trust surrounding birth. It has also come to me to share with you my experience of a state of being that can be called faith. Faith comes from being rooted through our legs and lower bodies into the earth, while at the same time connecting through our minds and our higher intelligence to the infinite and greater possibilities for our existence. If you can energize yourself in this state, and then open your heart, you can invite higher and more beautiful realities to be present and to live in you.

Part of the lack of safety around birth comes from our propensity for violence against women, and not only women, but the divine female energy that women represent. Women embody a transcendental connection between the earth that sustains us and the cosmic force that creates new life. Women are vehicles for beings to enter into this world. The modern plague is based on the destruction of all that is good and important in the world. In order for the modern plague to fulfill its aim of making this world into a war zone and destroying all life, women's connections to themselves and to their children must be severed. Our western medical system, which is a large part of this disease-causing entity, furthers this life destruction as it contributes to violence against women in birth. When you step back from the narrow focus on birth, it is clear that this violence is a part of the larger attack on women and the divine feminine.

The medicalized management of birth frequently involves cutting and other forms of invasion of the body. Cutting, in the form of episiotomy and cesarean surgery (especially when not necessary), is a thinly disguised form of violence. After the baby is born, it is still common for the baby to be stolen from the mother to be cleaned, suctioned, and handled according to hospital protocol. If the baby is not stolen it is tortured with needles piercing its skin, and its foot being cut for other medical rituals. Please refuse these barbaric treatments.

In our modern world, because we have made Nature (in this case, women's bodies) into the enemy, we have destroyed the spirit of safety that guides the process of birth. The spirit of childbirth safety does include cesarean section, because this surgical procedure does create safety in certain emergencies, when it is medically necessary and a natural birth is not possible. But the indiscriminate use of interventions which attack, mutilate, and drug women's bodies is a clear reflection of how sick our society is. And it isn't just the doctors or hospitals doing this; it is also women who do it to themselves by permitting these interventions and by using the services of those who do not have their best interests at heart.

Labor Health through Midwives

One essential factor in ensuring a safe birth is a positive, healthy, and communicative relationship with your birth care provider. While midwives usually seem to be the choice for the best care for labor, there are some doctors who also provide excellent care; don't unnecessarily limit your choices—remember to be open minded.

Activity: Choosing your birth care provider. I discovered a secret a while ago for making good choices in the world. The secret is listening to my heart. I simply feel my heart and ask it what choice is best for me. When you drop into the feelings of your heart, you can also feel or sense with an open mind where other people are coming from. You also want your birth care provider to be centered in his or her heart. Your heart knows what is best; if you find it difficult to choose your midwife, doctor, birth facility, etc., then just ask your heart and be open to its sometimes unorthodox answers.

Whomever you choose for your birth, you need to be able to trust that person and her intuition and decision making ability. When interviewing midwives, we asked what their rates of transfer and of cesareans were because we wanted to be sure they were committed to the natural process of home births. The average transfer rate to hospitals for certified nurse midwives in the U.S. is 12.1% for homebirths, and their average cesarean rate is 3.7%.[418] You want to trust your care provider, to feel a personal connection, and to sense that they will act in your best interests. An effective birth care provider will help the labor flow smoothly, and be able to help should a complication arise.

Statistics show that midwives will increase your chance of a safe and natural birth. In one study, neonatal death was on average 26% lower with midwives, and the likelihood of a low birth weight was 31% lower with a midwife providing pregnancy care than with a physician.[419] These studies indicate how crucial emotional care is for the mother. The mother's feelings influence her choices and therefore her health. Some midwives are very caring and supportive. They act like mothers to the mother. Many mothers-to-be did not receive the full nutritional or emotional support they needed as children. This can have effects later in life, and make the birthing process more difficult. A good midwife can fill in this role, and the mother will feel cared for and supported. A mother-to-be who is cared for will feel that it is safe to give birth, will make good choices for herself, and will love her new baby dearly.[420] Another study showed that women attended by midwives are 30% less likely to undergo cesarean section, and the diagnosis of fetal distress is made 50% less often in babies delivered by midwives, compared to those delivered by physicians.[421]

One midwife we interviewed made an interesting remark. She said that in a large hospital that had a special intensive care unit for infants, in which heroic procedures and technologies were used to save infants' lives, this unit was in continual use. In a smaller facility which did not have an infant intensive care unit, infants rarely or never needed intensive care. It is not so much a factor of one hospital attracting different patients from the other; however, if the technology is there, the hospital staff feels that they need to use it. Modern procedures and technologies have replaced patience, intuition and good care for our newborns. To some extent, this explains why midwives have a cesarean rate which is on average seven times (786%) lower than physician-attended births. Since midwives cannot perform a cesarean, they make the most effort for a natural birth, usually with the desired result.

One point of interest here is that many insurance providers do not encourage the use of midwives. In California, it is practically impossible for a homebirth nurse or midwife to be "qualified" to be used and still be covered by conventional insurance. I assume this is the case in many states. Why do insurance companies not support many midwives, when the evidence suggests that midwives are ten times safer to use? Safer births mean fewer expensive procedures whose costs must be covered by the insurance company. Wouldn't you think that health insurance companies would want to save money by promoting fewer treatments? That insurance does not cover midwives in some areas indicates that this is not a scientifically based decision. This decision is surely a part of a cleverly designed system that profits from medical interventions. Birth is a profitable industry, especially when something goes wrong or if a cesarean is performed. This is a sign of a great sickness (the plague) in our culture, where financial greed supersedes the compassionate impulse for us as a culture to usher babies into the world safely while supporting their mothers with care and respect.

If you choose to look more deeply at what is happening to birth care in our culture, and at how poor the level of care really is you may find that the motivation to profit from unnecessary procedures is not the only culprit. At a deeper level, these haphazard medical decisions are made by people who are numb to their feelings and to life. When we carry unacknowledged pain, our souls manage this pain by creating numbness to life. The self-anesthetized pain can only attract more pain, as part of a self-fulfilling prophecy in order to amass enough pain to break at last the cycle of numbness. In chapters that follow, we will see how this tragic and unconscious way of living is acculturated into our children through poor child-raising practices and through our educational system. The result is that as adults, children raised in this way will many times not be able to make the best choices for their health or that of their own children. The real cause of birth violence is the loss of love, faith, hope, and the loss of our very humanness.

Where No Midwife Would Go: Yeshe's Birth

During Michelle's pregnancy, we were forced to evacuate our Santa Cruz home due to widespread chemical spraying by the government. We stayed in my parents' home for several months, and we didn't know where we would live or where our coming child would be born. My parents were adamantly opposed to having a home birth in their house, and we were opposed to giving birth in a hospital. There are no birth centers close to the area. Finally, about two months before the due date, we found a home: a small cabin in the forest in a peaceful setting; in other words, the perfect place for a homebirth. The home is 15 minutes from town, and 30-35 minutes from two major hospitals. For most places in the country, 30-35 minutes from a hospital is the usual distance. To reach our cabin, you drive four miles on a windy but completely safe road. We also have a mile-long dirt driveway, and the final approach is a steep but perfectly navigable hill.

We were absolutely determined to have a midwife. After a short while we thought we had made our selection; our midwife had been practicing for over 30 years, was from another country, had attended thousands of births, bragged about how natural she was (what we wanted), and promised "You can refuse any treatment." She visited us to see where we live, and drove up to our front gate in her fancy Mercedes. Then a few days later, she declared that Michelle would have to have an ultrasound to check for birth defects, because of how far we live from a hospital. (Mind you, there weren't any other suspicious health indicators.) We refused the procedure, and were at once dropped by her as clients, so we were left stranded without a midwife about four weeks before the due date. We continued to interview other midwives. One midwife didn't want to drive her BMW sports car on our dirt road. (That's not a joke.) Midwives either refused to work with us, or they couldn't because they were already scheduled. One newer midwife drove up to our house and then had a panic attack on her way back down because she was certain that a fire truck would not be able to drive up the steep driveway to rescue Michelle in the event of some rare emergency requiring paramedic assistance. (That's not a joke either.) All during this frustrating and occasionally farcical time, I held inside me the

space and intention and feeling of a safe birth. I was partly scared, because I was concerned about there being complications without the presence of a professional, but another part of me felt safe, and I felt the safety throughout my body. Then, one week before the due date, we met a woman in a natural clothing shop who had a new baby. She said her good friend was a doula. The doula felt very confident with the birth process and had always wanted to attend a homebirth. She drove up to our place at 2:30am to help with the birth and she did a great job. We had Yeshe at home, 4.5 hours after contractions started. After Yeshe was born she did not cry. She made one brief and loud sound as she took her first breath, and that was it.

Both Michelle and I felt very disappointed in the midwives we'd talked with. They really could not have cared less about us; they seemed only to care whether they would have enough paperwork to protect themselves in case of a lawsuit. No midwife called us for a follow-up, and they generally seemed to lack respect or compassion for parents seeking childbirth support. In retrospect, as much as we needed help with the birth, we also did not need the presence of negative and unconscious fear-based energy. I have heard the midwife and doctor situation is better in some states, so I hope that you find someone you mesh well with.

Pre- and Postpartum Doulas and Labor Doulas

A doula can help a mother feel supported and not abandoned during her challenges with pregnancy and the arrival of her newborn. This support may be needed even during labor. Ideally, excellent labor support would be provided by the mother's family members, but many times family members are either unavailable, or un-equipped to provide that support for a variety of reasons. With the support of a doula, the father can relax more and focus on his relationship with his partner rather than assuming the role of doula himself.

When the mother feels secure and sup-ported, the baby can feel safe and bonded with the mother. Doulas can help the mother and father feel safer with the energy of birth. They can encourage breastfeeding, and support a nurturing family environment. A good midwife can do all of this as well, but sometimes extra help is beneficial.

Some women might think that they should sacrifice fulfilling their needs for the sake of the family, or for anything else. Some women believe that their real needs are not that important. But pregnancy and birth are not a time to be self-sacrificing, nor is it a time to consider yourself unimportant. Take care of yourself, because you are the center of your baby's life, and your new baby needs that caring energy. Give yourself the full support and nourishment you need for pregnancy. When you take care of yourself, the energy of caring radiates via harmonic induction throughout the entire world.

Now, do not mistake my recommendations for self care as selfishness, or as the dualistic conflict which places the mother's needs above the baby's needs, and results in neglect of the baby. The unitive concept is that the mother's and the baby's needs are one and the same; this is beyond the either/or dilemma. I recommend that you take care of yourself by honoring your body and honoring yourself as a human being and as a mother in a way that is inclusive of your newborn.

Unassisted Birth

Unassisted birth refers to a delivery without the presence of professional helpers. Some mothers will feel really inspired to do this, and if you are one of them, then go for it. Proceeding without professional help has many drawbacks and I do not recommend unassisted delivery for the majority of mothers. A good midwife can help reposition a baby if it gets stuck, for example, or revive a baby or administer other emergency procedures, and can also diagnose problems such as excessive bleeding or blocked progress. If you had to get help for some reason, being alone or with your partner does not give you the best odds, and having at least one other person there is a good idea so they can flag down the ambulance, or drive you to the hospital. But the positive possibilities for your birth are endless.

Don't fall into rigid mainstream beliefs of how it ought to be. Make it how you want it to be so that you can have a pleasurable and satisfying birth experience. Let courage rather than fear inspire you. A fearless birth isn't necessarily done by yourself alone, but is one in which you feel safe and comfortable bringing your new baby safely and sanely into this world. Remember, it is your choice.

The Modern Birth Scenario

Since the early nineteen hundreds when negative influences took over Western medicine, the predominant treatment for what is labeled as disease has been drugs and surgery. Modern doctors are taught that drugs and surgery are essentially the only treatments for disease. It is actually illegal to claim that a remedy cures a disease if it is not an FDA-approved drug. The irony of this state of affairs is quite stunning in light of ongoing evidence that FDA-approved drugs often cause disease and even death themselves (we call these *side effects*).

Western medicine typically views birth as a medical emergency. Our modern medicalized approach to childbirth evokes a war zone. The enemy is time, and the baby is but a passenger-at-risk carried by the mother. But birth is usually not an emergency, even if it does involve surgery. It is a natural process of the body. Western medicine nevertheless tries to cure the "medical emergency of birth" with drugs and surgery. If you choose to give birth in a hospital, be prepared to be offered drugs and surgery, except in those more rare instances when you have secured the services of really good and caring doctors and midwives.

Toxins in Labor

Modern doctors and even nurses are taught how to administer drugs and perform surgery. If you want drugs and surgery, then go see a conventional doctor. We are brainwashed by the news media to believe that pharmaceuticals will cure all of our problems.

Let's review what we know about Western drugs: they turn a healthy ecosystem into a diseased ecosystem, and they don't cure disease. Drugs are so toxic that some, like penicillin, are eliminated from the body in a few seconds. In Chapter 1, we learned how disease is our body's attempt to eliminate toxic material. Western drugs are highly toxic. **The last thing you want to do during labor is put a toxic burden on your body.** And when drugs enter your body during labor, they enter your baby's body, too. This is likely to greatly increase the chance of additional complications for your baby, and for that matter drugs are dangerous for babies. Drugs are poison, so don't put poison into your body during labor. When Sparkle was born, the doctors tried to push antibiotics on us for some unclear reason, claiming that if we didn't take them she would get an infection. DON'T ALLOW THIS TO HAPPEN TO YOU! We accepted no antibiotics and Sparkle did not contract any type of infection. If a baby does get an infection the mother can take echinacea tincture which will usually resolve any minor type of infection. If you want to make your child sick, then give him antibiotics and injections. Remember, in a hospital you are at the mercy of a national medical system that is negligent in the deaths of 783,936 people per year, at a cost of $282 billion per year.[422]

Informed consent is given by a patient who is clearly aware of everything involved in a course of treatment, including the risks, benefits, and possible alternatives. Consent is the permission given by a person before surgery or other kinds of treatment. The patient, or a parent or guardian, must understand the potential risks and benefits of the treatment **and legally agree to accept those risks.**

In plain English, you are the final authority of what happens to you at the hospital. If you do not want something done to you then do not agree to it. The proper phrasing is, "I do not consent to _____ treatment." If someone administers a treatment without your consent you can sue them, and probably win in court.

While on the topic of consent, an epidural anesthesia manufacturer's label contains information about the possible effects of an epidural injection. It explains the same things that you should know from reading this book; namely, that modern drugs are highly toxic. It states that local anesthetics "can cause varying degrees of maternal, fetal and neonatal toxicity," and that adverse reactions can affect the central nervous system of the baby.[423]

Cesarean Delivery

Cesarean deliveries have saved the lives of many mothers and babies. The medical procedure itself, which I believe could be vastly improved, has an aspect of good in it. It can prevent an outcome that might otherwise result in death for the mother and/or the baby.

In the U.S. in 1970, the average percentage of births resulting in cesarean sections was 5.5%; in 2004, the average percentage was 29.1%.[424] Do you see a problem with this figure? I sure do.

Here are a few examples of when a cesarean is likely necessary. If the baby is in a sideways position, or if the head gets stuck and labor positioning strategies cannot correct it a cesarean may be the only option. Placenta previa, in which the placenta blocks access to the birth canal, and rupture of the uterus and cephalopelvic disproportion (not very common), when the baby's head absolutely won't fit through the pelvic brim, as well as a few other cases may call for a cesarean to be performed.

According to a scientific study published in *Social Science & Medicine*, at least half of cesareans are performed unnecessarily, because medically verifiable conditions requiring a surgery were not present at the time.[425] The medical industry profits from these needless surgeries to the tune of approximately $1,000,000,000 (one billion dollars) per year.[426] As of 2008, there are approximately 1,300,000 cesareans performed yearly in the U.S., and thus 650,000 cesareans are performed unnecessarily per year. Based on the comparison of 2004 and 1970 cesarean rates, let's assume for now that 5.5% is a reasonable rate for cesareans. The actual figure, then, of unnecessary cesareans is more likely to be over 944,000 per year. Here we can clearly see an anesthetized form of violence against women and their children. Birth physicians just can't seem to keep their surgical knives away from the womb.

About 294,000 cesareans are performed yearly due to lack of progress during labor, and an estimated 24% or 70,560 of those are done for the wrong reasons — for example, because the woman's cervix was not even given a chance to dilate (open).[427] The real diagnosis of lack of progress, according to the American College of Obstetricians and Gynecologists, is that "women be in the active phase of labor and show no change in cervical dilatation or descent of the fetal presenting part for at least 2 hours."[428]

If our birth culture was based on wisdom and intelligent foresight we might expect the following to occur:

1. Herbs and acupuncture would be used instead of drugs for pain relief and pain blocking to prevent the "side effect" of groggy, anesthetized newborns with their higher risks of complications.
2. Special foods would be eaten during preconception and pregnancy to help ease the birth process and strengthen the mother and baby for birth. Deleterious foods would be avoided.
3. The mother would perform the special exercises as discussed earlier in this chapter, and receive massage and chiropractic adjustments to release tight ligaments, along with other activities that help the baby enter the ideal birthing position.
4. The mother would be highly encouraged to keep active and to exercise daily.
5. In nearly every case, labor would patiently and lovingly be allowed to progress before surgery was considered. The mother would feel free to yell, scream, and walk around during labor. There would be no planned cesareans for twins, breech presentation, and so forth.
6. Labor attendants would be trained in every natural positioning technique to help with labor difficulties.
7. Growing girls would be given special foods to ensure their bodies develop properly to make birth easier later.

If many or all of these conditions are met, then I estimate that the rate of cesarean deliveries could be reduced to less than .5%. That is ten times less than it was in 1970. In the coming generation, we can reduce the need for cesarean births to close to 0.0% *if we want to*.

There are many benefits to experiencing an active labor even if it seems that a cesarean will be needed, as hormones which help the baby adapt to normal respiration are released at this time.[429]

An elective cesarean is when the mother chooses to have surgery but doesn't need it for medical reasons. Elective cesareans result in twice as many infant deaths as vaginal births.[430] A cesarean delivery is not necessarily less painful. The surgery severs blood and lymph circulation in vital areas, scarring nerves, veins, muscles and skin.[431] It is, after all, major abdominal surgery. While labor pains are circumvented by this procedure, the pain of recovery from surgery is felt for days and weeks later. Women who have the highest risk for complications are the least likely to receive cesarean operations. And those who are least likely to benefit from cesareans often have them for the wrong reasons, which commonly include breech presentation, slow or difficult labor, and supposed fetal distress.[432]

A doctor deciding whether to perform a cesarean or not is guided by another disturbing factor — the economic condition of the family. But it's not what you are probably thinking. **The more affluent the family appears, the more likely the doctor will want to perform a cesarean to avoid lawsuits**. If you are seeing a regular sort of cesarean-happy doctor, and I hope you are not, you may consider showing up in clothes with holes in them and flip flops. You might get better (i.e., less heavy-handed) service because the doctor will think you cannot afford a lawyer to sue him. Apparently, the courts consider cesarean delivery to be the appropriate childbirth choice, and if the doctor doesn't perform one he may be liable for any complications that occurred during the birth. I have heard and seen from other health care professionals that part of their decision regarding which treatment to use is based on whether or not they may be sued by the patient. If they think they might be sued, they will use the most legally defensible procedure, which usually has nothing to do with what is healthiest for the patient.

Make your baby fit! Our bodies operate with intelligence. Growing a baby that is too large and won't be able to be born naturally would be evolutionary incompetence. Yes, it does occur, and in most cases there is a clear reason for this. Can you guess what it is? Yes, you probably guessed correctly: our modern way of living can create babies with disproportions. How does that happen? Just look around at people the next time you go to the grocery store. Many people are bloated and overweight. The cause of this unhealthy enlargement is due to consumption of modern devitalized foods. How the baby grows is a factor of the glandular health of its mother. If the mother has healthy glands, shuns modern foods while eating the especially nutritious foods for pregnancy, and avoids western drugs and other negative health influences, then the fetus will grow to its ideal proportions in the womb. When the mother subsists on a poor diet, especially one that includes the excess consumption of sugar or processed grains, then the baby's growth mechanisms become *intercepted* and do not function properly. **The result is that the baby can inflate to a larger size, or its body can become slightly imbalanced. A poor diet also can cause wider shoulders or other proportional imbalances which can make birth significantly more difficult.**

Our first daughter, Sparkle, was born long and skinny; we were not practicing special food guidelines. Our second daughter, Yeshe, was born more compact and her body had ideal proportions. We were practicing special dietary habits, and her body looked very balanced and well developed. Many birth complications are caused by the baby being in the wrong position and getting stuck. Many of these imbalances are not normal, but are caused when the glands controlling the baby's growth, and the growth of the

mother's belly, are not properly nourished. The result is a baby that is too long and skinny, shoulders too wide, or a body that is too big. And take special note, a big belly does not mean a big baby. During Michelle's second pregnancy, her belly was so huge people joked that she was carrying twins. Yet when Yeshe was born, her body was dense but not especially large. She was about the same size as Sparkle was during birth except that her body had noticeably more even proportions. As Yeshe has gotten older, she has become very dense and strong. While she looks like a normal baby, she is significantly heavier due to the nutritional density of her body. She also is extremely strong and resilient. She can grab onto things tightly, kick, and even jump out of our arms, so we have to hold her carefully.

Preventing Harm to Your Child in a Cesarean Delivery

Using herbal pain-blocking medications so that the baby and the mother are not so heavily drugged would probably help improve many cesarean outcomes. Allowing the newborn to remain connected to the placenta, and having a family member there to hold the baby after he is born might also improve the cesarean experience. The Nature and deva spirits for healthy births and cesareans could be contacted and one could find innumerable ways to improve and limit the need of this medical procedure.

There is a real danger to cutting the umbilical cord too soon in a cesarean delivery, as well as after a non-surgical birth. According to www.lotusbirth.com, C-section babies can be removed without clamping the cord. Babies who are drugged from the pain-blocking medications given to the mother can have prolonged umbilical cord pulsations lasting up to twenty minutes, whereas the typical umbilical cord pulsations stop much sooner than that. If the cord is cut before twenty minutes, the baby will lose critical blood. Parents have a legal right to stipulate that their baby not be endangered by blood loss in a cesarean delivery.

As the placenta is pulsing it is feeding the infant with nutrient-rich blood, which has been temporarily stored in the placenta in order for the baby to be more compact for the birth process. After the birth, the placenta automatically pumps and returns part of the infant's blood to the infant. It takes a lot of work and physical energy for the infant to create blood, and **it is completely insane that we ever cut the umbilical cord as early** as so often happens today, unless it is required by an extreme emergency.

Only in rare cases is there <u>any scientific evidence</u> to support early cutting of the umbilical cord. If the cord is torn or there is placenta previa, it may be a good idea. Otherwise, such intervention is but an example of egoic excess, in which doctors attempt to exert their superiority over Nature by cutting, stitching and clamping in unnecessary ways. You can obtain a court order prior to birth, if necessary, to ensure that the baby stays connected to the placenta in the case of a C-section. A letter from your attorney may also help.

Here are some links to help you become further supported in your birth rights and awareness.

www.aimsusa.org - Alliance for the Improvement of Maternity Services (AIMS)
www.ican-online.org - International Cesarean Awareness Network

Premature Birth

Kangaroo care is a method of care for all newborns, but especially for premature babies, which supports skin-to-skin contact, exclusive breastfeeding and emphasis on non-separation of mother and baby. This method is a wiser practice than use of infant incubators for a significant majority of premature babies. One probably cannot imagine a more painful experience for a premature newborn than to be put into a lifeless box (incubator) like a little chicken, away from his mother. The incidence of premature births will be decreased when more parents-to-be follow the preconception and pregnancy health guidelines in this book. Premature birth

occurs when the mother's body is out of balance, again due to toxic environmental factors, toxic foods, and western drugs including birth control pills. When following the health guidelines carefully, the baby will be more developed at the time of birth, meaning that even if your baby comes early his chances for good health will be radically increased. With modern technology we can keep babies warm, but they can be held by their parents instead, and we don't have to put them in cages. Learn more about Kangaroo care at **www.kangaroomothercare.com**

Michelle says: "The labor is important. When we don't go through labor we don't get to feel as connected to what we've created. Women who want to avoid labor when it is not a medical emergency really want to avoid feeling their feelings because the labor can be so intense.

Women! Let's get wild, crazy, and return to our spontaneous selves. It is wonderful to be a woman. Women are beautiful and birth is a beautiful thing. A hospital cannot give us the space to be this way. The theory of a hospital as a healing space is a good idea. But the reality of hospitals is that they are uncomfortable and the people who work there are like zombies.

The problem I see is that women are not looking out for each other. We have lost our sisterhood. We are betraying other women when we allow them to make poor choices, and thus encourage them to harm themselves and to harm their babies. We support women living toxic lifestyles. Women are looked down upon for being and acting empowered, for being assertive, and for making positive choices. But being assertive and empowered is part of what being a woman, and a mother, is all about."

Activity: Practice Self-Healing During Pregnancy. I want to share a simple self- healing practice that you can do during pregnancy. You can also do it together with your partner in different and creative manners.

A Mother Practicing Self-Healing with Love

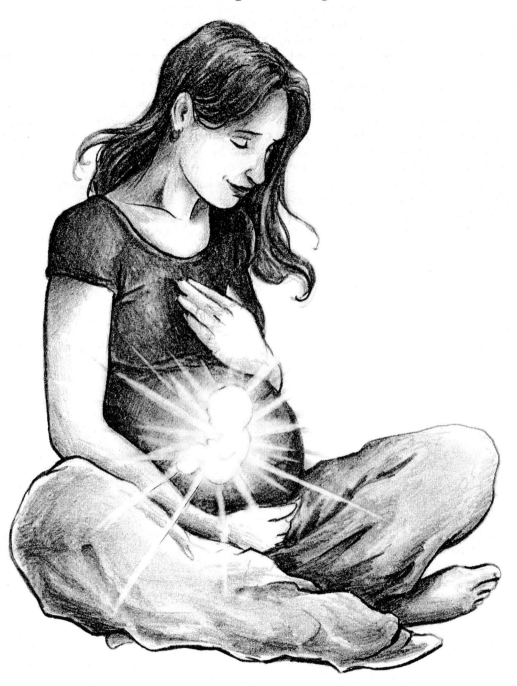

See, feel and hear that you are one with life, that you are one with the creator of life. We errone-ously believe we live in a painful and separate existence. And yet, the unification between a mother and her child is physical evidence that <u>this separation is an illusion</u>. Nurturing and loving yourself is the essence of motherhood, since the degree to which you have those feelings in you is the degree to which you can transmit them to and embody them for your child.

1. Align yourself with your intention for self-healing through love, compassion and acceptance, and invite in the deva for healing.
2. Place your hand on your belly.
3. Connect with your soul, and then connect with the incoming soul of your child.
4. Invite in any other spiritual support from the highest plane of spirituality; also consider inviting in the presence of the Divine Mother and the Divine Father.
5. Share this divine presence between yourself and your child.
6. See, feel, and immerse yourself in the divine presence of the life flowing within you, which is manifested in your child; connect your awareness with this being. The spirit of the being may or may not be in your belly, but may be somewhere nearby.
7. Allow light and earthly and spiritual energies to resonate within and fill the cells of the growing infant in your belly, as well as your whole being. If you have difficulty with this, visualize something that inspires love in you—a favorite pet, a flower, something beautiful and hopeful—and transmit that feeling to your child and yourself so that you both are suffused in its warmth.
8. Continue this practice until you feel fulfilled.
9. Thank the spiritual support and help, and thank yourself.

Repeat this healing method, or your own version of it, as often as possible, even several times per day. Do not forget to frequently ask for spiritual help and guidance from your spiritual teachers, guides, guardian angel, or other higher power you feel an affinity with. This asking helps you be in alignment for pregnancy health on all levels of your physical, emotional, mental and spiritual being.

The Principle of a Painless Birth: Not My Will but _Thy Will_

One can hear stories of women who have had ecstatic births highlighted by joy and pleasure. On the other end of the spectrum, one hears of childbirth experiences that were unrelieved pain- and fear-filled traumas for the mother. Somewhere in the middle, it is reasonable to expect that many women will experience at least some pain during the birth process.

I want to preface what I am going to say next by admitting that to actually practice the theories I will discuss is not easy. But at least you will have some framework to help you handle the pain you might experience, with the hope that you may have a liberating and pleasurable birth, and at the least, a less painful one.

Pain is created when we have two or more opposing forces of energy, such as when the creative force moving towards union and oneness is opposed by an internal force which is moving in an opposing direction. The Pathwork explains it:

> _Pain is the result of conflict. It is when two opposite directions exist in a personality that pain comes into being. One direction -- the direction of the universal, creative forces-- strives towards light, life, growth, unfoldment, affirmation, beauty, love, inclusion, union, pleasure supreme. Whenever this direction is counteracted by another direction, a disturbance is created._ [433]

The disturbance is not the pain. Pain is caused from two directions, when we pull away from this positive life current and when we struggle against our inner life-negating currents. So when you deny your own inner negative aspect, then that aspect actually creates and perpetuates pain. We have the inner direction towards love, and another inner direction towards hate. When we are at once pulled in these two different ways and fight from within the split place, we feel pain. Many times we repress and ignore that part of ourselves **that does not want health**. Meanwhile, we are struggling to feel healthy. We are struggling because a part of ourselves does not want to be healthy, but we are blind to it. Once you can find the negative aspect of the self, the part that doesn't want health for example, the struggle ceases and the pain can dissipate.

But when what goes on is fully understood and the temporary, still unavoidable, consequences of the negative wish accepted, and one lets oneself go into this now existing pain, the pain must cease. This is not necessarily a destructive way of embracing pain or a masochistic, self-punishing element that in itself harbors and perpetuates a negative wish. What I mean is a full acceptance of what is -- and with that, pain ceases. It is the principle, for instance, of painless birth. It is the principle of non-struggle. [434]

In other words, you have to yield to pain, you have to unify with its flow, to become one with it. That intention to unify with what was previously not accepted by the psyche can dissipate pain, or even turn it into pleasure.

If you cannot overcome pain by finding the internal attitude that does not want health, the part that creates the inner opposing force, then you can also surrender to the pain. This is another perspective of what has just been said. When you feel totally helpless and in great suffering, there comes a point when you might realize that this suffering is not yours alone. "**Not my will, but thy will be done,**" can help open a portal to deep surrender. At this point, your very suffering, which is a part of being here on earth, can become an opening to the divine.[435]

If during the birth of your child you experience pain you may think, "This should not be happening to me." You can choose to give that life-negating thought away to a greater power. This happens only when you have an inner "yes," and an inner acceptance to your suffering and your life circumstance. This suffering must have some purpose. Overcoming suffering comes in that moment when you realize your true nature, even if only temporarily.

A Child-Centered Birth

The newborn human being is a very small and extremely sensitive person, still very connected to his mother. Dr. Frederick Leboyer, author of *Birth Without Violence,* pointed out the trauma that regularly occurs to babies as they enter the world. The tiny creature, new to life, is born to loud noises, blinding lights, removed from a warm, soft nest and laid upon cold metal surfaces, and even poked and prodded with cold and sharp instruments.

This insensitivity occurs because people mistakenly believe that babies and mothers are just a part of a faceless and nameless medical procedure. The principles of a mindful and loving birth should include a sensitive and unobtrusive style of care, which is deeply respectful of the natural process and maintains a peaceful atmosphere at the time of birth, with low lights and little noise. After the birth, the baby is brought unto the mother's belly and then allowed to suckle. Placing a hand immediately on the baby's back helps him feel secure and safe. The cord to the placenta is not cut until all the blood, which the infant needs for its life, has been pumped into the child. The baby should be given an opportunity to breathe on his own without being painfully rubbed to induce crying. If a C-section will be necessary, then many of the same steps can be taken to ensure that the child is cared for, according to your desires and wishes after the delivery.

Many mothers have toxins circulating in their bodies which cause mucus in the baby's nose and throat. Excess mucus can be cleared using suction by the mother's mouth.

Your New Baby Comes To Earth

While there are already many theories about whether or not the child is conscious in the womb and perceives what is happening, I have to add my own opinion here. Most of the time while in the womb the baby's spirit is not in its body. The spirit may pay brief visits and its physiology may be imprinted. Memories of sounds or voices, for example, may be naturally recorded by the brain's memory. The soul of your child is accessible through delving into your heart. The new baby may be close to the parents in the parents' aura, or visit the parents prior to birth in dreams or visions, but the baby's soul does not reside in the womb.

I will tell you the way it is. You can believe it or not. It is not correct that the spirit takes over at the time of conception. The movement in the womb is an automatic one. [436]

From my own observations of my daughters' births, the spirit enters either right before or right after the point of transition, when the baby's head is emerging from her mother. Ye-she's head came out and the spirit was not there; it was waiting. For a few moments as I was supporting her head on the way out, her body, alive and well, was spiritless; it had no animation. When her entire body emerged, I immediately handed her to Michelle so I didn't exactly see what happened. The soul sort of slides into the body, and then spiritual forces infuse the soul into the body. Birth is just the beginning of the entry of your child's soul substance to Earth. It will take between twenty one to twenty five years for the human aspect of the soul to be fully incarnated.

Mother Roasting

Mother roasting refers to an ancient health-restoring practice for the postpartum mother. Perhaps this is not the best name, but it is practiced all over the world. This practice actively warms the mother using heated stones, leaves, herbs, sand and/or oil applied to the mother's abdomen and often her whole body. [437]

By keeping the mother especially warm, her internal organs can rest and the healing mechanisms in the organs of the body can devote more of their energy towards healing and repairing, rather than towards producing body heat.

Traditional Chinese Medicine provides a simplified version of mother roasting using moxibustion therapy. The process utilizes moxa,

or dried mugwort herb (*Artemisia vulgaris*), which is ignited and the practitioner applies its radiant heat near acupuncture points to stimulate circulation.

For more details on its use, and information about post-partum massage and special herbs for belly wraps, see *Natural Health after Birth*, by Aviva Jill Romm.

Time of Rest and Bonding

In the West we often under-emphasize or just plain forget about our real needs. We generally try to rise above our needs; this is an act of pride. We try to live up to an idealized image of ourselves. In reality, unless you have an extremely active lifestyle, and have been following a superb nutrient-dense diet prior to giving birth, you will not be able to promptly recover from childbirth and return to your normal life. And why should you want to return to a "normal" life anyway? Childbirth is a transition to parenthood and your "normal" life is no more. You are now beginning a new and enlivening phase. Giving birth is an opportunity to experience the oneness of life, and to experience yourself as one with life. Taking time and space for yourself and your new baby is an opportunity to be at peace; it is an excellent reason to take time out of your "life" and to start experiencing real life. Your son or daughter made a long and difficult journey to be with you. Take time for the two of you to bond and to rest after the birthing experience. Do not be afraid to ask for what you need. Even take one year or more if you want. Who is to say what is right or wrong or how much is enough, except you? In rural India, forty days of seclusion typically follows childbirth. That is forty days when the mother is supported by the other mothers around her. [438]

While you have just experienced a transcendental experience of feeling very connected to the force of life, perhaps the people around you have not, or they do not understand what it is like. This is a good time to practice your assertiveness and ask for whatever you need.

Conclusion about Birth

It is no longer a mystery why there are so many birth complications! The problem is solvable in the coming generation. Take the power away from the false authorities and reclaim your own unique feminine power for birth. You don't have much of a choice in the matter, because the modern medical system for birth promotes disease and suffering. If you remain weak and act out of fear, expecting others to make choices in your best interest, you may not get what you hoped for. Michelle brought up the important point of the lack of sisterhood in our culture. Don't let another woman fall into the void. Do your best to prevent her from making poor choices about her pregnancy care. We can take more responsibility for our births to ensure that our babies arrive safe and sound. When mothers follow these guidelines and their own intuition, they will be clear and present during and after the birth, open and ready for the rich reward of bonding with a new baby. We should not continue to place our faith in the marvels of modern technology, but we can place our faith in ancient wisdom. Ancient wisdom can help show us how to make birth safe and natural, as it was meant to be. Medical interventions should be an ally in emergency situations and not the norm, as it now is.

Difficulties in birth are not inherent in the way Nature designed our bodies, but are inherent in our diseased way of living. We have unknowingly violated Nature's laws and now women and children suffer as a result, from complications resulting in unnecessary pain and literally millions of unnecessary surgical births. It doesn't need to be like this.

We are now being urgently called upon by our mothers-to-be, and by our new babies who want to be born here, to make birth safer and less difficult, as it once was for all mothers and babies.

Mere words cannot convey the importance and the gravity of the situation we face. There is a great urgency for us to ensure safer and healthier births for mothers and newborns. It is time for each of us to take responsibility for our health. It is time to examine closely, and consciously, the possibilities for your child's birth. You have the right to treatments which are safe, supportive and health-giving for you and your new baby.

Your child does not come to you by accident; his coming is part of a larger plan. Who your child is, how they come into the world, and how they affect your life is a part of a greater scheme whose exact plan we seldom clearly glimpse. We can only breathe in the experience of being in life.

May I open myself to being a vessel through which the cosmic, warm and welcoming arms of a loving embrace extend to you and your family. May this loving energy welcome the new babies, new fathers, new mothers, and new families into this world. The world greatly needs a safe and loving protector to safeguard us from evil, and that brings us joy and grace. May that feeling of safety and protection be in you and surround you.

9

Only To Be With You: Your New Baby's Perspective on Life

A message **from your new baby:** If I could speak, I would say, "I love you." If I have any wish in the world it is only one thing, and that is to be with you. If I have any desire or motivation in life, it is you. I am but a newborn baby, so helpless in the world. You are the light of my life. Hold me close to you, never leave me, never forsake me, and never let me out of your sweet nurturing arms.

Intention: To really care for your new baby you must understand her—who she is, why she acts the way she does, and her inherent design. The purpose of this chapter is to motivate you to raise your children the healthy way and to learn about your child's innate expectations and how to fulfill them.

Those first precious weeks and months are when you can influence your child in a positive manner. This is the time when you can show your newborn that the world is a safe and loving place where he is welcome. This is also a time when a hidden tragedy may play itself out, a tragedy that our fast-moving culture is unable to properly witness. With our modernized approach to child rearing, newborns typically suffer a loss of love, a loss of hope, and a loss of faith. That is because in the "normal" modern way of parenting, our babies often miss out on what they want and need most — us.

Resting in God

When a child is born she experiences the unitive and undifferentiated state of consciousness. The baby's energy field is soft and highly sensitive, without a protective layer. She experiences life from the perspective of being merged with the world. Anything that happens in the world instantly enters the newborn's field of awareness. And without any filter the outer world affects her greatly. The mother and father, but primarily the mother, provides for the child a protective physical and energic layer that is like a second skin. Whoever is physically holding the baby, especially when the baby's chest is pressed against the parent, shields the baby from outside energies and forces. As a result, the baby feels safe. When a child is held by her mother, she experiences the fullness of life. It is as if she were being held in the arms of God. She experiences complete peace, surrender, and bliss.

The Pain of Separation

The most pleasurable feeling for a new baby is physical contact with his family, and especially the regular experience of breastfeeding. Conversely, the most painful sensation for the newborn is the denial of this fundamental close contact.

When a child is left alone, ignored, not tended to and not fed from the breast, he experiences a tear in the fabric of his fragile and limited reality. A baby's suffering goes largely unnoticed by most adults, because they themselves may be disconnected from their own bodies and sensations. Typical parents today believe it is normal to ignore their baby's cries.

Resting in God

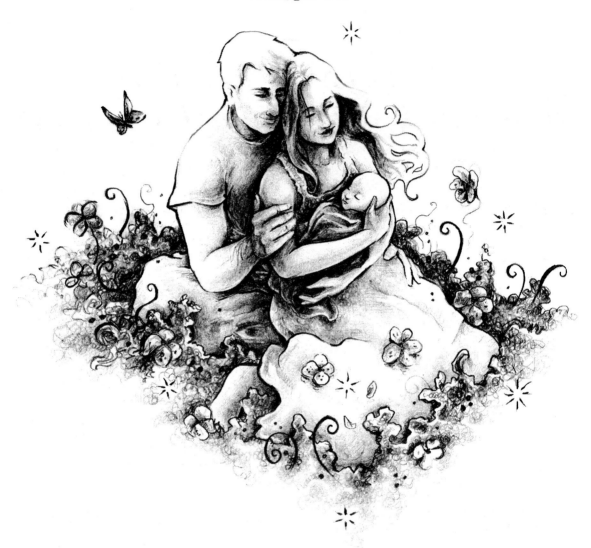

When an infant is held in your arms, she feels as if she is being held in the arms of the Creator. There can be no higher experience of peace and bliss than for a child to be held tenderly in the arms of her mother.

Nature gave us a blueprint of how to nourish ourselves in order to be healthy. The guidance provided in the laws of Nature is transmitted through ancestral knowledge. Other animals also provide role models to show us which foods are healthy and which are not. Now I want to take these laws one step forward by suggesting that

there is a healthy way to raise children, too, as well as an unhealthy way. These guidelines are not my guidelines, but are a result of my observations of Nature's rules. The rules are easy to follow and feedback is prompt. When your newborn is happy she looks content and at peace. After a short time she can smile, and coo and share her happiness. When your newborn is un-happy she will cry, scream, and complain. The parent has a choice in each moment to listen to her baby's communication, or to ignore it. Within your heart, each and every one of you knows Nature's rules and can feel their effects. But many of us have forgotten these rules and have mistakenly chosen to ignore them. **Your choice is simple: abide by them, or you and your children will suffer.**

In our modern world, most parents do not choose the noble path of abiding by Nature's principles. They create suffering for themselves and their children. With the advent of modern civilization came a plague that infects not only the physical bodies of those who live under its regime, but the hearts and minds of them as well. For the majority of us, our separated way of living started from the first day we were born. Soon after birth, parents begin "teaching" the newborn of life's realities, influencing how their child will perceive the world by caring for him in certain ways. They are not teaching their children of how life truly is, but rather are show-ing their children how they *believe* life to be.

I know these lessons. I was raised in an un-conscious way myself. I was breastfed for only a few months, attended day care at an early age, probably before the age of two, and had a nanny take care of me part of the time. I went to pre-school, briefly attended private school, and spent most of my primary education in public schools. I was spanked as a child, punished, sent to my room, made to stand in a corner and hu-miliated in various typical ways — all in an at-tempt to control the behavior my parents labeled as inappropriate. By the time I was in high school I spent most of my time playing video games and using the computer. I haven't met anybody yet who had a happy childhood. I know that happy childhoods do exist. However, most people who think they had a good childhood are in total denial of their feelings. They are trapped in a cage, and yet they don't know it.

The positive side to the suffering I felt as a child is that I still remember what it feels like. I do not have too many memories but I have enough. I remember being left in cribs and car seats, and I have a vague memory of being

dropped as in infant. I can remember how diffi-cult it was being unable to communicate with my parents. Once when I was less than a year old, my parents were feeding me. I remember how much I enjoyed it. Then, whoever was feeding me hit my lip with the spoon and it hurt. I felt how insensitive they were to me. Because it hurt, I became upset, but I couldn't communi-cate what had happened or what I was feeling. I didn't want to eat anymore, so they punished me for refusing to eat and turned my chair away from the table. I began to scream. I remember that faint thought in my mind, "They just don't understand me." Remembering all this has given me an innate sense of compassion for children. And as a parent, when my daughter is hurting or upset, I do not fight her or defend myself against her cries or expressions. I really understand how she feels and I let her know that. Being rejected by one's parents out of anger is very painful. Babies and children are still in contact with their feelings and scream as a result of the pain they experience. The screaming is a desperate at-tempt and plea for the adult to make right what the child has no power over.

I want to share two more personal stories that illuminate the infant's view. I have a mem-ory of being held by my mother when I was very young. Her silky black hair looked like so much fun to touch. Oh, what a delight — I could reach out and play with it. Feeling such joy and pleas-ure I grabbed her hair, and then I pulled it. I got slapped, and started to cry. As you can imagine, I did not understand why I had been struck.

When I was a little older but still quite young, only a few years old, my favorite object was my little blanket. I think I latched onto a piece of fabric because I hadn't been held as much as I needed to be. As an adult I have seen pictures of me being held as a youngster, but I can rarely remember such occasions. At any rate, as a toddler I didn't know that my favorite blanket was just a cloth diaper. I thought there was only one, and it was that precious one that I carried with me every day. Then one day it was time to travel to Hawaii. My parents wanted to wash my blanket before they went since it was fairly dirty. Perhaps they were embarrassed to bring their child who carries a blanket around into public. I thought they wanted to take away my favorite blanket, and I did not understand that they intended to give it back again. I believed they were taking it permanently. They threatened to leave me alone at home, because I wouldn't give up my blanket. Eventually I made a choice (a bad one in retrospect) to dishonor my blanket connection to be with them. Years later, after I had begun my healing and growth journey, I realized that I still felt upset at them for taking my blanket. I was then around the age of 20. It was a traumatic experience for me, even though they claimed they didn't know how hurt my feelings were. With a casual attitude, someone might say that children need to obey adults, or that they need to understand the adult world. But this is really a cruel attitude that allows the adult to inflict pain (abuse) upon their own children.

The same natural force that created the planets, the sun, the stars, the trees, and the flowers also has a plan for your newborn. This creative force equipped your baby with certain needs. The baby needs food, warmth, physical and emotional comfort, and sleep. These needs must be fulfilled promptly, as waiting too long will cause babies physical pain. The problem is that modern parents often have very strange ideas about how to respond to these needs, and often act as if they are incapable of meeting all of them. Or even worse, they act as if it is a good idea to *deny* their child's needs. Most modern parents are simply very lazy, and these are the "lessons" they want their newborn to learn.

The biological blueprint in you is designed to enable you to feel capable, equipped, happy, and have time to fulfill ALL of your baby's needs. This blueprint has nothing to do with the modern and ignorant way in which we live, with parents in a continual rush, unable to ever take a deep breath, spending most of the day separated from their children while barely managing to pay the bills. When parents choose to fulfill the baby's every need, the baby is happy and content. I can hear the groaning already with the words *every need*, but it really is important. The problem is most parents have convinced themselves that their babies are not sensitive and delicate creatures who need all the warmth, nurturance and care possible.

Activity: The health matrix. There is a plan for you and your child — to be together in happiness. There are also other possible plans for you and your child, as you can also suffer and languish in misery. Which plan do you want? You have the power to choose. If you want the healthy plan, then feel relaxed in your body and try the following. Feel, hear, smell, taste and in every way imagine a crystalline, vibrant, dark blue grid. It is a matrix upon which your worldly actions, thoughts, relationships and feelings fit. Connect yourself with the grid for the most vibrant care and communion with your child right now. Do this at least one time per day. It has a slight feeling of structure. It feels as if everything is right in the world. This is the matrix for health.

When parents choose not to meet their babies' innate needs they create pain for their babies and themselves. This is always a choice. When your baby experiences emotional pain for too long, or if it is too intense, then their fragile sense of self can weaken, or even crack and break. This does not happen as often with physical pain. If the event is repeated often enough then their life force, the current moving through them, becomes split, because their existence becomes intolerably painful. They attempt to control the pain, because the emotional pain and longing is so intense they feel as though they might die. Rather than die, they choose to live, but as a result, learn to hide, control, and avoid the pain that they feel. This is the fall from grace, and this is the pain of separation.

In other words, your baby can whine and complain a bit when she's uncomfortable; that's normal. But often times, when there is prolonged or very intense crying, it is from something that is beyond a simple physical discomfort such as fatigue or indigestion. The baby is expressing a deep pain and sadness. If what they need does not get fulfilled, or if they are hurt in some way, then as a survival mechanism they split off from their own needs. Let's look at an example.

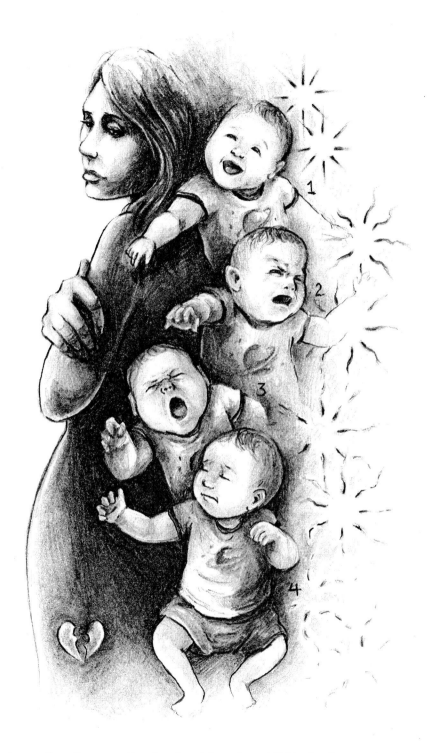

A sad part about a mother disconnecting her bond from her child is that her motivation many times is just a pile of green pieces of paper (money), or that increasing number on her bank account statement.

The story behind this picture is a mother working from home temporarily while she recovers from birth. She is very happy her new baby is sleeping soundly, as she just spent an hour tending to her. The mother's goal in life is to serve a company so that she and her husband can have more money to buy nice cars, live in an upper-middle class house and vacation twice a year. She believes that her job, how she makes money for the corporation, gives her a purpose in life. Her home office is downstairs with a microphone monitor to hear if her baby upstairs wakes up.

1. Need. At first, the baby wakes up from a nap. She is happy, but needy. She feels good. She expects her mother to come running to see her.

2. Pain. The mother is engrossed in her work and has an important deadline. She promises herself that the baby will not interrupt her work. She hears some funny noises coming through the baby monitor but she wants to finish her report by noon so she keeps working. She wants her new baby girl to learn not to interrupt her. After a short time the baby's need is not being met. The baby begins to feel upset, sad, and hurt that her mother didn't know she woke up. Her lip starts to quiver and involuntarily she starts to wail.

3. Screaming. The mother knows her baby is tired and that she'll soon cry herself back to sleep. The mother is hungry herself and is trying to finish this "important" report. She continues to work while her daughter starts to scream. At first the infant was sad, but now she is in deep pain and distress; her mommy is gone. She wonders if her mother is dead, and if she'll ever come back. How can she live with this pain, she wonders. It would be so miserable to live without mommy. She feels her intense longing to be held by her mother, and feels sick and angry that she is not being held. To her, one minute is a thousand years of waiting. It is an unending misery. She has no concept of time and space and doesn't know why her needs are being ignored.

4. Withdrawal. The pain becomes too intense; she has been ignored too many times before. The infant gives up on getting her needs

met. She starts to try to control herself by clenching her entire body to control the feelings of pain and hunger. She starts drifting off almost automatically into a fantasy world that is more pleasurable than her painful earthly life.

Perhaps less than 10 minutes go by in this scenario. The mother finishes up her report, and rushes upstairs to her baby. The baby appears calm; she is just lying there limply, not fussing. The mother has a flash of intuition that something is wrong, but ignores it. She is happy her report is done and is now happy to see her new baby. The mother believes her daughter is so intelligent and helpful, because she is being a "good baby" and learning how to keep quiet. At this stage of withdrawal the baby has split off from her own life force. Part of her has gone numb and dormant. It will stay numb and dormant for years and will never revive unless, as an adult, this child takes efforts to heal and to reconnect with herself.

False Belief Systems

Many parents subconsciously believe that they need to teach their new baby lessons in life. They may believe that the baby needs to learn how to control and soothe himself, not be too needy, to be quiet at certain times, and not to touch certain objects. The deeper lessons the parent is trying to "teach" is that the baby should learn that life is difficult and that people have to work hard and struggle to get what they need and that they should not feel the simple pleasure of being alive. (Perhaps you can feel yourself how convincing this truth sounds; you might even think, "Of course, that is how life is.") Parents typically teach the baby to learn to take care of himself because no one else is going to take care of him. "It is a cruel world out there," the parents think, and they believe they must instruct their child in these cold facts so that he will be prepared and won't be hurt by the world. The means of teaching their children this world view includes constant commands of "Do this but don't do that," or "This is good and that is bad," and so forth.

Another key distortion to this style of instruction is the belief that in order to be prepared for life's hardships our baby must be tempered by various deprivations early in life. A parent may believe that his child's needs should be controlled and restricted. (I am not talking about false or petty needs such as TV or candy.) Parents think this approach teaches children about discipline, boundaries, and earthly limitations. Perhaps these examples are ringing familiar tones in you, reminding you of how you were raised. Maybe this is how you see your own children. **How we treat our children is largely a reflection of how we were treated as children.** Even if you believe that you are not such a parent I still urge you to look for that quiet hidden voice that says something like, "I do not want to give my child what he needs because I am not getting what I need." Or it could be a voice which reflects a negative belief about the world. "Life is full of suffering, so I will teach my child about suffering, and I will show him how terrible life is. I will show him that he only gets attention when **I** feel like giving it." The voice might also say, "I do not want my child to be disillusioned about life when he is older, so I will show him now what life is about; I will teach him about suffering, failure and aloneness, and how to manage those feelings." These voices or other similar voices arise out of a secret part of the parent that wants his child to suffer. In our conscious minds we might think that we are truly loving parents and doing what is best for our babies. But under that image lies a different energy, and our children will suffer as a result.

To suggest that ordinary parents actually want to inflict emotional pain on their own children, even if unconsciously, may seem blasphemous. But ask yourself if you experienced pain in your own childhood. Did you sometimes experience your childhood as not being loved fully? Were you abused by someone you loved, or not protected from abuse? Where you yelled at, punished, threatened, hit, or spanked? If these examples do not ring true then look out into the world. Do you see a dog-eat-dog world run by a survival-of-the-fittest mentality? The best and strongest survive, right? It was normal just a short time ago to hit children with rulers, to spank them and even to beat them. It seems a little less common today, but corporal punishment of children is still a widespread practice. Even a slap, a pinch or a prod are just less overt forms of the same abuse. Many well-intentioned parents will resort to locking their child in his room, or purposely ignoring him in order to "teach him a lesson." These are examples of many types of pain that parents unconsciously but voluntarily inflict upon their own children. While the parents might be convinced that they are doing the right thing, in reality their behavior is a form of violence directed towards their own child. People do not behave this way for no reason. Parents will only act negatively if they believe that their child will benefit from their behavior. It is as if the parent himself is acting not like an adult, but like a small child. Many adults don't even speak with their parents, their relationships are so frayed. Or parents have a policy that once their child is 18 the child is divorced from the parents, and so they see one another once a year and pretend that everything is okay.

The life force streaming through you is clear about your role as a parent. This life force says to your child unconditionally, without hesitation, "Yes, I will take care of you." This life force says, "We will rejoice in life together. I will do anything for you, I will sacrifice my selfish needs and wants for you, I will transcend my limitations, only to enjoy one more moment with you." The life force says, "We are one." Take a moment to find your own feelings or words that reflect your pure intention towards experiencing life with your child. Many parents don't experience this part of themselves until a crisis arises, such as when their child is very sick or gets hurt. We forget how important our little people are, and how much we care about them in our day-to-day routines. This forgetfulness is really our unconsciousness. You can open up to this life force energy and allow it into your body, heart, and mind.

Many parents are in a hurry for their young children to grow up. They may also be in a hurry to get back to work, or in a hurry to resume the "normal" patterns of life they had before their child was born. In this hurry we stand to miss entirely the most important moments of our lives, when we can make the greatest difference in our children's lives through the influence of our loving presence and attention. These moments that we choose to spend with our children are precious, and valuable beyond calculation.

Many parents pattern their behaviors on what other parents do, or on what their own parents or other respected relatives tell them to do. If they cannot get good advice from their immediate friends or family then they may consult a doctor or other authority and ask for advice. In case you are wondering, I don't consult with any relatives about any child raising advice and hardly ever have solicited anybody else's opinions on almost any topic. When you stop listening to what other people want you to do and start looking deeply within, you'll know what to do. The process does not involve rational thinking exactly, such as "I'll do this because this is the correct action." Rather, it is a spontaneous action that reflects how you feel about life; it reflects your intentions in being a parent. Sometimes, to help you know how to act, you will sense how to move in the right direction to find the information that can help you. When you are aligned with your inner truth, however, you won't need any book, authority, or anything else to know what is right. You will know what is right. I hope that these words will communicate to you that deep loving presence that resides in you so that this presence will come to the surface for the benefit of your child. I hope to point you towards what is healthy and right in you, and toward opening up to a more joyful and fulfilling life for you and for your children.

Many of us have our gaze directed only to the world outside. We do not act as our own authorities and thus we must be subject to inner voices that say, "I do not trust myself. I need help." In Chapter 8 you'll recall that I connect many difficulties in childbirth with the fact that modern women do not embrace their divine feminine selves. Part of the divine self is authoritative (yet not controlling) and embodies leadership. When you look outside of yourself for advice on how to parent you are going to have to look long and hard to find something that you can feel compatible with and benefit from. That's part of why I have written this book. I want to share with you how Michelle and I have parented our two daughters in a very caring and nurturing way. Both of us want the best for you and your family.

Close to the time of Sparkle's birth, before I became a parent, I knew that the way most people were raising their children was wrong. It took some grace for me to find an outside role model with whom I felt an inner "yes." It was the wisdom within me that pointed me towards principles more aligned with my own— principles that would guide me in my daily experience as a parent. Beware of the trap of looking outside yourself too frequently, however, as you can become lost in this search. I am often frustrated, for example, when people tell me that my dietary advice isn't working for them. My response is, "That's right, it won't work for everyone exactly as it is described here. You must alter the program to accommodate your particular situation." These people expect me to make the changes for them. They wish to deliver the authority for their actions onto me but I want nothing to do with it. When acting as your own authority, resist the hasty act, but instead take one conscious inhalation, and then one conscious releasing exhalation, and acknowledge what is bubbling up from within you. And if you find that it's not the advice you want to hear right now, good. I didn't want to hear it either when I heard it the first time. I wanted someone to tell me what to do, and I wanted someone to tell me what is right and wrong. Now I understand that we make our own rules. We create our own lives, and we make our own choices. Letting someone else make choices for you, or approve of your choices, is a passive way of relinquishing your power. It is a sign of inner weakness, and a sign that you are not willing to live fearlessly as a parent. You alone will have your own best interests at heart. Start to practice making choices and taking authoritative action. Power comes to people when they make an important choice in their life, such as "I choose to make a difference in the world," or "I choose to make my life purposeful." If you choose to be completely present for your child, I cannot think of anything that is more meaningful.

While we limit our life experience because we disowned parts of ourselves when we were hurt as children, our own children typically do not limit their life experience. This creates a fissure between your limited belief system and your child's expansive beliefs. Their expectations for life are designed by Nature, which has few or no boundaries. It is usually not the child who has to "learn." But as adults, we need to learn how to release our love, compassion, and humility, to be able to meet our children in the state of consciousness that they are experiencing.

Michelle says: "My father always said, 'Children are resilient.' The implication was that you can hurt them and they will recover from it. But no, when a child is hurt an imprint is left on them.

I never thought I wanted to be a mother. It looked so uncomfortable. I would see all those kids in strollers, crying, wearing plastic diapers. The parents always seemed stressed out. That's not what I wanted. I could see and feel how uncomfortable those babies were and I didn't want anything to do with it. At the time, I didn't realize there was another way to raise children."

Two fundamental beliefs underlie parental negative behaviors: the fear that "I won't get my needs met," and the belief that "Life is suffering." When we tell this story quietly to ourselves, it blocks us from the enlivening feelings of sadness, grief, remorse, and anger that are lurking underneath our façade. We repeat the "I won't get my needs met" mantra because we have experienced this often enough that we believe it is true. "Oh here it is again, another disappointment." Then, in the midst of our internal conflicts and struggles, along comes this little being, so tender and full of life. While you may subconsciously seek your missing fulfillment in this child, you also come with your baggage from the past, your pessimism and your distorted beliefs about life. These parts of you act towards your undefended infant with the intent of teaching them that "Life is going to hurt sometimes, and that is just how life is. Life is painful, so you better get used to it." These ideas

and beliefs are subconsciously expressed and prevent you from feeling fulfilled as a parent. Fulfillment must come through allowing the enlivening power of the universe to move through you as a parent, and as you relate to your child. The life energy will fulfill you, but it is up to you to let it in. This life current is constricted and even cut off in many of us because we do not allow our energy, our enthusiasm, our feelings or thoughts to move freely into the world. **Parenting is a gateway in which the experience of fulfillment through opening to the life force is possible.**

It takes tremendous energy and force to avoid fulfilling our children. It takes a lot of misplaced strength to show our children a continual state of deprivation, to convey the belief that "In life you don't get what you need." If you pay attention to many modern parents, you see them ignoring their screaming child, or becoming impatient or irritated with every little thing their child does. As you watch these scenarios you might feel how much energy is wasted in the parents' struggle. I believe it is our natural state as parents to fulfill and honor fully our children, and I also believe that it takes a great effort to avoid fulfilling this promise, <u>even if done unconsciously</u>. And we do have a promise to fulfill. It is a promise whose fulfillment your child innately expects. He has faith that his parents will love him without conditions, protect him, and provide him whatever he needs.

Very few parents are bold enough to tear through the veils of this unconsciousness. It takes courage and strength to step out of the old and worn societal molds and to firmly grasp your child and say, "Yes, I am here for you. I want to give you what you need, and I will do it now and always." You must be bold enough to say "I will never leave you!" and really stand behind this statement. It requires a parent who is willing to look inward and who can feel and acknowledge herself and her own desires.

If you do not believe your child is born with the ability to experience God, to experience life in physical, emotional, mental and spiritual contact with you, then you have only to observe what happens to infants when they are denied this experience; the results speak for themselves.

The cries of the child tell you that something is deeply wrong. It is a genetic knowledge speaking to you, asking you to change your behavior. The crying child feels pain and suffers greatly. The world is not how it should be and he knows this in his body, but he does not understand why. He does not understand why he is in a basket or a cage (i.e., crib, playpen, stroller) when his body naturally expects to feel the contact of his mother's body. He was born in a body which expects nurturance, which expects satisfaction of hunger from the breast. He does not understand why he is hungry.

What is this force in us that causes this suffering for our children? The Pathwork explains:

The child who feels hurt, rejected, helplessly exposed to pain and deprivation, often finds numbing of his feelings the only protection against suffering. This is often, quite realistically, a useful protective device. The same applies to circumstances in the life of a child that it cannot understand. When it is confused and perceives contradiction and conflict, equally contradictory emotions result in its own psyche. The child cannot cope with either. Numbness is also a protection against its own contradictory responses, impulses, and reactions. Under such circumstances, this might even be a salvation. But when such numbness has become second nature and is maintained long after the circumstances have changed, and when the personality is no longer a helpless child, in the smallest measure it is the beginning of evil, and this is how evil is born.

Numbness and insensitivity towards one's own pain in turn means equal numbness and insensitivity towards others...The numbness, instituted for oneself, must be continued towards others just as every attitude towards the self is bound to expand towards others.[439]

Once this numbness exists within us we feel apparently safe, but also separate. The separation then spreads to others like a contagion. Consider how your child is affected by your numbness. To begin to work through your own anesthetized emotions it is important to honestly acknowledge your behaviors, attitudes, and what really motivates you to act the way you do.

Negative Pleasure

Parents sometimes do not listen to their children because their numbness makes it difficult to really hear anything at all. It's rather like living underwater—you can't clearly communicate because the sounds are all muffled. I have already spoken about the constriction of your life force, which leads to this numbness. An important mechanism which causes this constriction is a distorted current of pleasure called *negative pleasure*. Allow me to speak about negative pleasure by giving another example.

I have seen many mothers, even mothers who promote conscious child-raising habits, who leave their babies at home. I believe that a mother who leaves her eight-month-old child at home in order to do something else is acting unconsciously (especially if she is going out to promote motherhood). Why do we do this to ourselves and to our children? Why do mothers and fathers choose to leave their babies?

The above example is real. The mother who leaves her baby at home to go out and promote healthy mothering practices seems to be unaware of how leaving her baby is detrimental to the cause of motherhood. In her mind motherhood is an idea rather than a direct experience or action. This mother's thoughts are separated from her actions. She is fueled and motivated by a negative force that is stimulated by the freedom she'll feel in leaving her baby — *negative pleasure*. Negative pleasure is the sort of good and satisfying feeling one has from doing something wrong. An excellent illustration of negative pleasure can be found in the movie *Pirates of the Caribbean*. Every act of the pirates is twisted and backwards; they enjoy causing pain, betraying loyalties and foiling justice. And the audience enjoys their actions, too. Like the pirates, we all feel a pleasure from acting in an unhealthy manner. If there were no pleasure attached to our negative actions <u>then we would have no impetus to perform them</u>. Therefore anytime you do anything negative to yourself or others, deep down there is always a seed current of moving energy — negative pleasure — fueling the behavior.

Positive pleasure is when you feel juiced and excited on the inside and your <u>energy flows in an unimpeded cascade</u>. **Flowing energy brings pleasure, which feels good.** That's why people like to engage in exciting activities like sky diving: they become very stimulated, which moves lots of energy, and pleasure is a result. Sky diving is a good example of an outer world stimulating activity. When we don't feel sufficiently alive, we often participate in risky or dangerous activities in order to amplify our sensations. When you normally feel vibrantly alive, then your need for outer excitement becomes less. A more positive example of pleasure is when you are doing something you really enjoy and energy is moving and flowing within your body — dancing, for example, or sports or artwork. Pleasure is the pulsation that is a spontaneous result of our life force moving unimpeded in healthy directions.

Negative pleasure is what we experience when our life current has a knot or kink in it, sort of like a bent garden hose impeding the water flow. The positive pleasure cannot flow freely out, and only a bit of pleasure energy leaks out, like water trickling from the bent hose. In this state the person feels dull, bored, and numb. Numbness is an unhappy state. It is not a healthy way to go through life, so the pleasure current tries to create enjoyment. Because of its repression it comes out the wrong way; it comes out negatively.

In infancy, everything you experienced was a pure emotion. Whether it was joy and love or sadness and pain, your internal energy flowed so well and unrestrained that every experience involved a type of pleasure. You may observe this pleasure flow in children exploring the world; they will do whatever feels good to them. Young children almost always seek pleasure, through letting their life force move them. Watch young children at a playground as they laugh and cavort with apparently endless energy. The only time they stop is if they accidently get hurt, or when it is time to go home. The worst thing for them is the seeming end of carefree pleasure. As a parent you are capable of rapidly understanding and responding to the needs of your child but when some inner impulse in you blocks that response your mission (if you choose to accept it) is to find what that is.

To see a typical example, think of a toddler moving his hands through that plate of food just set in front of him. He experiences pleasure from the feeling of the warm food oozing through his fingers. In his excitement he discovers that he can direct his arm and make the food fly. He must think how amazing and pleasurable this world is! With great humor and enjoyment, the warm mushy stuff goes everywhere. He is so excited. Then angry mommy comes. Mommy has just cleaned the kitchen and doesn't want food everywhere. Mommy grabs the food out of the baby's hand and yells, "You are bad, NO!" The child doesn't understand what made mommy angry and unhappy. From his point of view there is nothing inherently wrong with throwing food compared to other behaviors he might have engaged in. At the moment of punishment the child is still full of the pleasure of being alive, exploring his environment and playing. But he wants to listen to his mommy, who is so important in his world, and his pleasure is shut down and he thinks he is bad. The pleasure of being alive is now tied into his mother's angry reaction, and the belief that he is bad. If this confusing message continues from the parents, then when the child is older he will try to engage in pleasure but end up doing bad things. He will seek to recreate his childhood feelings — both the good and those bad associations about the good feelings. Suppression of children's energy, punishment, and anger directed at them all lead towards instilling patterns that cause them to express reckless and destructive behavior as teens and adults.

Amoeba Principle

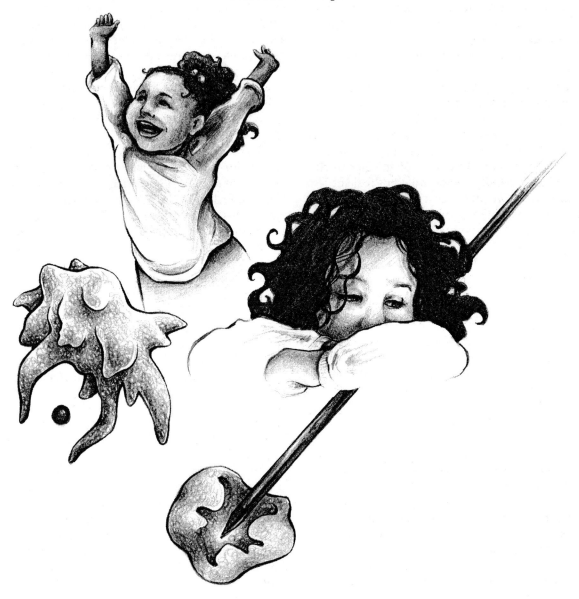

Left: *When the amoeba senses food it reaches out and expands. This is the pleasure of reaching out and expanding into the world.*

Right: *When the amoeba is poked it experiences pain. It contracts and shrinks inwards to avoid being poked. Children are the same way, responding to the food of love (left image) and contracting from pain (right image) and rejection of separation.*

Our children's responses to life are no more complicated than the way an amoeba behaves in its environment. The amoeba expands towards food, and the child reaches out towards love, food and breastmilk, and warm and caring attention. Children literally open their arms to you and to life. They open their hearts to the world. The child, like an amoeba, constantly seeks food, constantly reaches out for pleasure, joy, and relationships. Conversely, when the child gets jabbed or is told that he is bad while in that state of reaching out he will contract. If children are told that what they are doing is wrong, they slowly stop exploring the world. If an amoeba is poked once it contracts a little bit and changes direction. If it is poked repeatedly, it will stop moving entirely, contract inwardly, and wait until it is safe before moving in any direction. In the same way, if a child is emotionally attacked or otherwise denied love, his natural impulses to reach out will lessen and lessen. Eventually he will stop trying. The child in this case would become partially resigned to life.

The amoeba illustrates a universal concept. Love and pleasure are foods that encourage us to expand; whereas pain, negativity, and hatred are the foods that cause us to draw in and protect ourselves. The child naturally responds to how he is treated, just like the amoeba. This is a law of life.

Negative childhood events are wrapped around a negative pleasure current. Parents who were emotionally abandoned as children will actually feel a negative form of pleasure from similarly abandoning their own children. And in fact, any negative form of parenting is fueled by a distorted pleasure current. These parents will not even feel that abandoning their children is wrong and maintain that their behavior benefits their children. They will defend their actions if confronted. These parents will deny that their negative pleasure exists and then create justifications for their positions. Since almost everyone is inharmonious in one or several aspects of parenthood, it is easy to make excuses for doing bad things in relation to children. In every moment that you are not present for your baby; in every moment that you do not recognize his divine nature; in every moment that you ignore the transcendent nature of your child's existence you have abandoned him.

Transcending Negativity

I hope at this point that your negative pleasure has not engaged you to withdraw from reading this book. Some uncomfortable feelings may have come up in the last sections, but you have stuck with me. I hope that you want to understand how to heal the distortions of negative pleasure. If you want to just get rid of the response and forget about it…well, that's negative pleasure fueling your unconsciousness. We cannot just rid ourselves of negative pleasure, but we can transform the negative pleasure back into its positive origin, and thus do good in the world.

To transcend negativity requires being utterly and totally truthful with our hidden agendas and emotions. And not just to yourself: you must be able to admit your negativity to someone else, or at least write it in your journal. You must look beyond the immediate and short-lived pleasure of the negative behavior. Looking at the bigger picture, seeing what type of destruction or hurt it causes, can help you begin to tune into your true feelings which will begin to break up the negative cycle. For example, eating unhealthy junk food seems to provide an immediate pleasure. But when you consider the indigestion and poor health that will result, the longer term effects of your action will help you see that eating junk food doesn't really seem that pleasurable after all.

Activity: dissolving negativity. Consciously look for and try to catch your feelings of negative pleasure. Looking for these feelings or recognizing them in the moment they appear helps you to dissolve the negative pattern. Anytime you are upset, seek inwardly to find the origin of your unhappiness. Once you've found it and felt more clearly, with awareness, your negative feeling, the next step is to decide to change it. Set your intention and align yourself for a positive change. Ask for deva spirits, or whomever you connect with spiritually, to help you change the negative behavior. Ask to feel the true positive pleasure rather than the distorted negative one. As a reminder, don't suppress or attack your negativity. You have to court it and dance with it until it is willing to finally transform itself. And change does take time; be kind to yourself and be patient.

If you are interested in further exercises to help transform your negativity, I suggest *The Undefended Self* by Susan Thesenga.

The Second Womb

Why does the infant experience pain when left alone? In Nature, animals raise their young in many different ways. Some animals can simply leave their eggs somewhere and when they hatch they are on their own. Other animals are born immediately equipped to survive and they can run almost instantly after birth. Kangaroos, on the other hand, carry their tiny young in a pouch until they have matured enough for life away from the mother.

Full-term human mothers look like they are about to burst. Nature keeps the infant in the mother for the maximum length of time the mother's physical body can tolerate. Yet at birth, the physical and emotional development of the newborn is minimal. The infant is helpless after birth and is still growing and developing. **So Nature created a second womb.**

Although you may not be able to see the second womb with your eyes, and although it is possible to separate the infant from this second womb, the second womb is real and does exist. A transition occurs at birth as the infant moves from the physical womb to the etheric, second womb. In this transition, the infant shifts from getting nutrients from the placenta to feeding from his mother's breast. The infant shifts from being inside of the mother to being outside of the mother. Now, in addition to physical nurturance, the infant needs her mother's energy and protection for survival.

In the first womb the infant experienced Nature's perfection, as food was constantly channeled into her body through the placenta. The child resides in the second womb until she individuates from her mother. Although the child will pass through many levels of individuation, I believe that the child resides in the second womb for about 6 years.[440]

The presence of the second womb explains why babies can experience pain when separated from their mothers. They lose their feeling of the safety of this close bond, which to them is as if they are lost in the world.

Michelle says: "In the second womb, babies and children need lots and lots of love. Children learn the virtue of patience through experiencing the mother's patience with them."

The Second Womb: Mother and Child

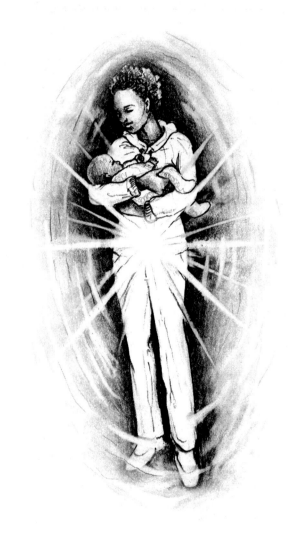

In the second womb, the infant feels safe and trusts life. The mother radiates warmth of presence and comfort. The mother's womb is the actual source of this radiant energy.

Imprinting the World

When a baby is born his brain is essentially blank, except for a few minor imprints of some sounds and movements from his time in the womb. The brain does contain pre-programmed functions to interpret its experience, but your **baby does not have life experience** when he is born. The child's brain is a biological organ that evolved inside the womb. It evolved from the basic seeds — nutrients, energy, consciousness, the intention — of both the parents, as well as from the creative force of Nature. The newborn's mind is like film in a traditional camera. When you open the shutter of the camera light burns an imprint onto the film. In the same way, the eyes, ears, nose, mouth, skin, and emotional senses of the baby begin to open and they are constantly recording and taking imprints of everything around them. The imprints are stored not just in the brain, but in the entire body through the autonomic (involuntary) nervous system. We experience imprints as adults when we remember things. In particular, a certain smell can remind us of an event that happened to us 10 or 20 years ago.

Nature designed infants with the ability to have life experiences imprinted in them. Imprints build on top of themselves and create an interior map and system through which we interpret the world. The earliest imprints form the base of the pyramid of memories and our voluntary and involuntary responses to life. Everything about those early days, months, and years forms the template for how your child will perceive and make sense of the world. In other words, as the child ages, the child will subconsciously believe that the world **is** how it **was** when she was an infant. Her internal map of the world in her mind will be how life was for her in childhood. As an adult, she will censor and perceive the world through the template created in infancy and childhood. The world your child sees—much as the world you now see—is not in fact the real world out there, if such a world even exists. The world we see outside of us is our interpretation of the energy streaming into our sensory receptors. But there is more. You may be familiar with the scientific tenet that the observer always influences the experiment through his observing. The world we see outside of ourselves is not really static. It is a world that is within us, projected outward. What we see as separate from ourselves is actually an outer reflection of what is separate within. Our view of the world bends to the beliefs we have about it. We cannot ever separate our perceptions from the world out there. The conclusion, then, is that **our perception of reality creates reality.** Whatever your child experiences in childhood will become his reality in adulthood.

Many child raising concepts are based on faulty and distorted models of parenting. "Modernized" parenting is based upon parents controlling their child's feelings. Parents withhold love from their children, for example, or control their will through punishment; parents also control their child's behaviors by emotionally leaving the child. "Modern" parents believe that **by <u>not giving</u> to the baby**, they will effectively "teach" the infant "lessons" that she needs to learn about life, and that successfully learning these lessons is necessary for their child to succeed in life.

Typical parental withholding patterns include giving infant formula made in a factory instead of breastmilk, and feeding the infant from a plastic nipple instead of the breast; others include hauling them around in plastic car seats instead of holding them, putting them to sleep alone in a crib instead of with the parents, leaving them with unfamiliar caregivers instead of staying with them themselves, putting them in day care with other children their age instead of caring for them with the help of older children.

Whatever world the parent creates for the child, the child will believe that this is how the world is. Your child becomes an imprint of life as he experiences it. When you leave your child alone in his room to cry himself to sleep you may believe that this "lesson" will teach him how to go to sleep by himself. In this example, the subconscious mind of the parent abandons his child and feels negative pleasure from it. The child, however, does not cheerfully learn to go to sleep by himself, but rather learns that life is full of aloneness and cruel isolation. The experience of being forlornly alone is imprinted, rather than an experience of being held with care and helped to sleep by a loving parent.

Activity: Are you withholding love from your new baby? I expect that the typical reader of this book understands that babies need extra care, and that they are more than objects to gratify the selfish needs of parents. Even so, I have rarely seen a parent who provides the level of care for his children as Michelle and I do for ours. And we are far from perfect in our level of care. Day after day, Michelle and I both realize different ways that our unconsciousness influences our parenting — preventing our love to pour forth into our children fully. This happens through our thoughts, behaviors and interactions. People tend to create internal justifications to convince themselves that their parenting practices are correct or at least adequate. However, parents too easily withhold their love from their children by not being present. Try to search for ways in which you are being dishonest with yourself regarding the care you are giving your child. There is <u>always</u> room to improve, so take a moment and ask the Universe to show you the ways in which you avoid being present with your children. Part of you longs to become a better parent, and desires to improve your parenting habits; otherwise you would not be reading this book.

A mother's love is expressed through her positive and active attention, and the second womb is embodied through the mother's physical holding and breastfeeding. When the infant is <u>not given</u> his mother's full love, that raw experience of being unloved is imprinted. It only takes a few minutes for a young baby to feel abandoned. It is the imprint of the abandoned child which says, "When I am needy I do not get what I want." Based on this repeated trauma the infant concludes that he should cut off his feelings of need. His imprint becomes the belief that "When I scream and cry, and when I want to be held and nurtured, instead I feel pain and aloneness." The imprinted feelings of pain and aloneness, which is what he experienced in infancy, will create the later beliefs that **life is filled with pain and aloneness.**

When this child grows up it will be difficult for him to feel fulfilled, and he won't understand why he can never satisfy his needs in life. His relationships will be filled with rejection, or he will treat other people exactly the way he was treated. He will seduce people, making them need him and then reject them in an endless cycle. All of these patterns just seem inherent to

him, or seem to happen *to* him, and he cannot understand his unluckiness in life. These patterns occur because of the imprints of his early childhood experiences; as he grew, he became unconscious of their original source. He believes he is acting the right way and in goodness, just as his parents believed when they ignored his early needs. As an adult, this abandoned child will believe that "Life is about denying people what they need." When he has a child and his child cries, he will respond in exactly the same way to his child, and the cycle of deprivation will continue. Many of us come from long family lineages and patterns of deprivation. One method for healing these conflicts as adults is called Hellinger Family Constellation work. www.hellinger.com (Make sure to find a trusted and recommended facilitator if you try this.) During the Hellinger Family Constellation process, the individual chooses members from a group of participants who volunteer to assume the role of their family members. The imprint of our childhood is so strong that when these volunteer family members stand in the physical position of one's parents, it can trigger the release of childhood pains even if they don't say a word. The volunteers can even feel as if they were the individual's parent. They become conduits for the source of the person's imprint. People around us and in the world subconsciously react to our imprints of childhood, and we react to theirs.

And after many years of helping people heal their childhood wounds, Bert Hellinger has come to a conclusion about the role of parents. Quite simply, he states that the role of the parents is to give; it is the role of the child to receive.[441] Modern parents have it backwards, thinking their children should take care of them and give to them. And what you give to your child not only will come back to you when they are grown up, it will spread out to the rest of the world through them. The child who is well cared for will, as an adult, care the same way for himself and others, because his imprint was of being cared for. The child who was scorned and not wanted spends his adult life hating himself, others, life, and his parents because that is how he believes the world is. The positive side to Nature's principle of imprinting is that you have the power to imprint a positive experience of life for and with your infant. When you fulfill your child you will be deeply fulfilled as well. You will feel full of joy and a peace that transcends your limited human self. When you hold your child and give to your child unconditionally from your heart, then she will grow to believe that the world is about being held, cared for, and accepted. When your infant cries and you tend to her, and you give her what she needs, she will believe that "When I am needy, my needs are fulfilled. When I need love, I will be loved and nurtured. When I want to be held, I am held. When I am hungry, I will be satisfied." For an infant, needs are the physical and emotional comfort of breastfeeding, and of being held. How will this child be when she becomes an adult? As an adult, she will feel capable and self-assured; she will find it easy to satisfy her needs because she knows in the deepest way possible that when she is needy she will be loved. As an adult, this child will get what she needs from life because she loves herself enough to bring all her creative forces into fruition. Even when she is alone as an adult she will feel her aliveness, joy and excitement about life. When she is in relationships or friendships with other people, she will not be stingy or greedy; she will be warm, open and generous just as her caregivers were to her. She will treat the world in the way the world treated her during infancy. She goes about her days spreading love and goodwill to others, regardless of whether she is conscious of it or not and regardless of her active effort to do anything. She emanates human kindness and warmth as her natural birthright.

You can actually make an enormous difference in the world by simply taking that one small moment with your newborn baby. When you love your new baby tenderly, you infuse love not only in her. You are infusing love into all of the relations she will have in her entire life, even in people who merely look at her as they pass in the street or happen to stand nearby. Her experience of the world, of being loved, spreads and radiates. That tiny little shared experience, those many personal moments when it is just you and your baby — they are not insig-

nificant. They matter more than you can even imagine. They make every difference to life on this planet.

As a parent, you are deeply responsible for the health of our world. By offering unconditional love and service to your children, by taking every effort each moment to give to them and to be present for them, you are creating people who have a capacity to shape our world for the better. On an energetic level, you set the template for other parents—even those whom you'll never meet—to give their children more joy and fulfillment. Your actions will ring harmonically throughout the Universe and bring a much needed stream of positive energy, and a consciousness of peace, to our Earth.

That is how you can transform our world. And through you, you can transform the world of your own son or daughter. In this way, you are like a god to them. You can be vengeful and inflict untold amounts of suffering, or you can be benevolent, and be a carrier for a high frequency of love. The choice and attitudes begin with your own mental and emotional makeup. It begins when you take care of yourself, when you are aware of your actions and feelings and when you truly desire and choose to make a new Earth for your family. This is not an easy task. Your friends or relatives might think you are crazy because you are breaking out of the familiar mold of suffering and deprivation. But then one day they will say, "You know what? Your child looks so happy, and she behaves so well. I see other children all the time who are not so happy." They will wonder how you did it. Even if you feel totally unsupported by the world around you, even as if it were a crime to love, I want you to know this: I support you. One day you will receive the quiet but profound rewards of your hard work. Your care for your baby is not done in service to them, but it is an opening and an expanding into life, in which your consciousness and theirs become one. Remember the opening of Chapter 8, "You are here to enable the divine purpose of the universe to unfold. That is how important you are."[442] To your new baby, it is beyond mere words and facile explanations how important you are to them.

An Infant's View of the World When his Mother is Present, the World Arises

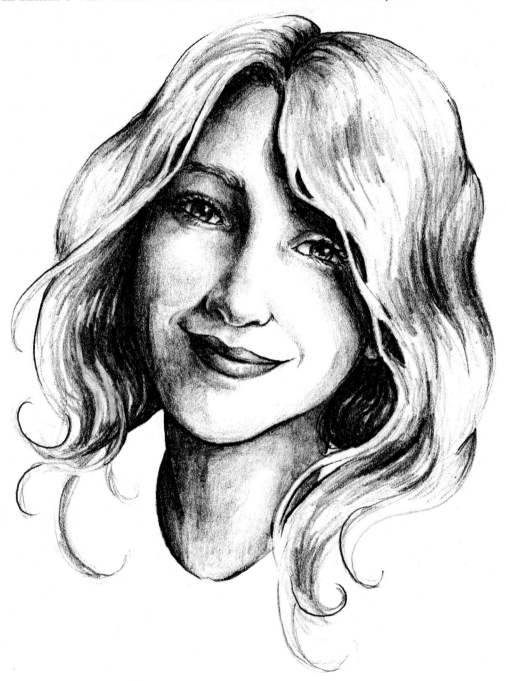

To your infant, you are the world. You are their creator. This is how your child sees the world when you hold her, when you are right there with her. Your child memorizes your features, and your face becomes the face of the divine. The child's first impressions of the world are the shapes of your face. Seeing and recognizing this landscape becomes her center, her home, her beloved. When you are there holding your child, she feels a sense of aliveness, purpose, and rightness about the world.

An Infant's View of the World:
When the Infant is Left alone even for a Short While, the World Disappears

*When the mother is away, **the infant sees nothing** and his world has disappeared. The lines of love from her face will not be imprinted into his memory. This is not a printing error, this is the emptiness an infant feels without his beloved. The infant feels unsure of himself and he does not understand what happened to the world. He is floating, lost in a vast Universe of pain. He is alone, empty. Life has failed him. He even loses his will to live. Where did his life go, he wonders? He experiences himself as his mother in the early stages of his life. Without his mother present for him, he falls into an abyss.*

Your Child's True and Innate Needs

Love is what creates and sustains the Universe. Many modern mothers have forgotten how to love. They have forgotten how to be mothers. They have lost touch with their own divine feminine nature (which includes the animalistic self), because as children they were not loved and their true self was not nurtured and encouraged. Their early childhood experiences did not provide the imprints of care, honoring and acceptance. As a result, most mothers are thrown into motherhood without ever having satisfied all of their own childhood needs. Most adults are like children, except bigger, more complicated, and more confused. Many of us haven't even got a clue about what our purpose here on Earth is. In that emptiness, it is really challenging to be a nurturing mother in the way you need to be for your children. The Pathwork explains some of your child's true needs: love and closeness.

> **Love.** *More often, however, both parents are emotionally immature and cannot give the love the child craves — or only in insufficient measure. During childhood, this need is rarely conscious. The child has no way of putting his need into thoughts. He cannot compare. He does not know that something else might exist. He believes this is the way it should be. Or in extreme cases, he feels especially isolated, believing his is the only lot. Both attitudes are not according to truth... Thus the child grows up never quite realizing or understanding why he is unhappy nor even that he is unhappy. Many of you look back on childhood convinced that you had all the love you wanted just because you actually did have some love, but rarely all that you wanted.*[443]

> **Closeness and the Divine Feminine.** *In the infant closeness is an entirely passive experience: the child takes in, receives, soaks up as a merely receptive organism (the feminine principle) while the mother is the giver and dispenser (and in that capac-*

ity the truly feminine woman expresses her masculine principle).[444]

Indigenous Child Raising

I am very thankful that a friend suggested I read *The Continuum Concept* by Jean Liedloff before the birth of Sparkle. Liedloff came into contact with a tribe called the Yequana, who live isolated deep in the Amazon in their native way. The indigenous method of child raising among the Yequana is based on a continuum of care in which **the children are never abandoned**. I admit that this came as quite a shock to me when I first read of it. Since the mother leaving (abandoning) her child is such a part of Western parenting behavior, I didn't even consider that it was possible to *not* abandon one's child. In countless tribes worldwide it is the norm that during his infancy and early years, the new baby is never, ever kept away from his mother when he has even the slightest interest or desire to be with her. This treatment continues until the age in which the culture deems the child ready to spend time with others (6-13 years old, generally).

Sound impossible? Do you want to try it? When a newborn is imprinting the world in the very tender early stages, part of that imprint is the delicious and highly pleasurable act of breastfeeding. This contact enforces the already primal bond between mother and child. Part of this early imprint is the development of the self. The infant's gaze and attention become focused singly on his mother. In so doing, the child seeks to find his own self. Yet as an infant he has very little self, so he starts looking for it. In the early weeks and months, his mommy is his surrogate self. He believes that he is his mother. Over time, being merged into the second womb, in the ideal situation, the mother reflects the child's self back to him, like a mirror. The child learns about himself through his mother. When the mother is happy and nurtures her baby, and the baby feels loved and cared for, then all is right in the world, because all is right in her tiny world. If you watch toddlers, you will see that if they are allowed a secure bond with their mothers, they will always want to know where their mother is. As the child grows, they embody how their mother took care of them and eventually that caring mother lives inside of them and becomes incorporated into their being. This reliable pattern of transfer is observable to anyone who looks for it, and has been studied in various disciplines, including in certain branches of psychology.

As a side note: Because most men didn't get their mother's full love as babies, they are still looking for it, trapped in infantile consciousness. Women do this, too, making men into their surrogate mothers, expecting their husbands or boyfriends to take care of them in the ways they desired in childhood. Most men are quite incapable of fulfilling this role, however, first because testosterone tends to make men not terribly maternal, and second, they weren't well cared for as children either. This might explain the stereotype of the "sugar daddy" who provides the male version of breastmilk or nurturance: money. Both men and women often find themselves stuck as they seek relationships to satisfy their unfulfilled childhood needs. This is why very quickly the happy marriage becomes a painful divorce. If one or both members of the couple in childhood had an imprint that was filled with pain, then that is how the person believes the world is, so they continue to create or attract pain. At the same time they try to satisfy their unmet needs through different methods. I know of several couples with young children who have separated in very negative and painful ways. In the end, the only way to grow out of these patterns is to feel the loss of love. For me, I started noticing this loss of love when I kept falling in love with beautiful women but then, for whatever reason, I could not continue the relationship. This happened many times: once in elementary school, twice in high school, once in college, and once after college. My imprint was of a mother who was unavailable but at the same time desirable. So I would fall in love with a surrogate mother. Of course one's drives are not quite so uncomplicated, but you can see that early impressions have powerful influences in adulthood. Somehow my early imprint directed me in my search, for as soon as I met a certain type of woman I

would begin the chase, because it was so pleasurable and exciting. Sometimes these women would unexpectedly chase *me*. The relationships would then end rather rapidly and seemingly out of my control. A great deal of crying on my end would follow. The last time I experienced this "crash and burn" disappointment, about six years ago, I cried several hours a day for two to three months. I didn't have any intelligent support at that time. People didn't really understand what was happening to me. They just saw a miserable and lifeless blob. But this recount gives you an idea of how painful it is for a child to become disconnected from his mother. It might take several months or years of crying to recover from this loss. Crying, by the way, is almost always a good, healthy exercise for adults. That is what frees us up, makes us whole, and brings us back to our center. The tears are not just tears of pain; they are also tears of freedom and redemption. Tears have streamed from my eyes when writing many portions of this book. Those tears represent the hope, care and salvation that I did not receive as a child. This redemptive energy is illuminating the dark places in my soul. As a result I experience more freedom, bliss, and the possibility for mature relationships.

The Continuum of Care

The basic provision of the "continuum of care" simply involves a mother holding her child continually from birth until he begins to crawl away of his own accord, sometime around six months of age. After this point a mother can always stay nearby until her child is sufficiently older, and really able to be out on his own. It is best to also hold babies while they sleep, but this is not always possible or convenient. If they wake up while you are not holding them, you must attend to them immediately. After the age of six months the very lengthy process of natural maturation begins. The baby is still held and attended to by his mother, but this now includes longer and longer periods of not being held. Sparkle, at four and a half years, is still held often by her mother or me, and is gradually becoming her own person. Again, I feel very happy that she is allowed to be a child, that she is frequently held, and that she also likes to hide and be shy. That is a part of her learning and growth, and we always provide her a safe space to go to when she has overwhelming feelings about the environment around her.

For four and a half years Michelle and I have maintained the continuum of care for Sparkle. She has never ever been without access to her mommy when she needed her. For a time, I would take her on walks and we would be away from Michelle for up to 30-45 minutes a day. But that was it. Whenever Sparkle said, "Go home," which sometimes took only a few minutes, then home we would go. And there was mommy, waiting for us. The continuum of care is not merely physical, but emotional. A mother can be continually in the same room as her child, but if she ignores her child she is completely emotionally absent. The continuum of care on the emotional level involves always being present and attentive to your child's emotional needs. This bond unfortunately has been broken many times on the parents' end. But we do our best to make each mistake, in which the emotional bond was damaged in any way, into a learning experience. And our intention is to maintain the continuum of care on the emotional level. Our society takes negative pleasure from trying to disrupt the continuum of care between the mother and child. This is generally done through what we call having work responsibilities or pursuing a profession, and attending school.

We first maintained the continuum for Sparkle by never physically abandoning her, never going on a date, out to dinner, or to the movies without her, and we did not know what the results would be. I can tell you that Sparkle is capable of feeling great happiness. And people comment that she is so "well behaved," which really means that she doesn't have to create chaos — yelling, screaming, and pouting — to get attention because she already receives the attention she needs. She still does those things sometimes, but not in public and not all the time. She feels very free and at ease in being herself. And she has a very strong bond with her mommy. Rather than say what Sparkle can do, I will say as a father that I feel very happy that she can simply be a child. I find I remind Michelle many times that Sparkle is just a few years old, that she is still new to the world. So if Sparkle is needy, or acts like a baby, then it is my pleasure to give to her, because she matters to me, as do her needs, wants, and desires. I cannot always fulfill them, and sometimes it is impossible to do so, such as the time she wanted to take home a giant plastic statue. But I can give her the imprint, the sense and the feeling that my intention is to fulfill her needs anytime it is even remotely possible, which, happily, turns out to be most of the time. The more Michelle and I give to Sparkle, paradoxically, the less she needs and asks for, and the happier and more pleasant she is.

I strongly support, encourage, believe in, and live the continuum of care for children. You will find that the positive results of practicing the continuum of care on the overall health and wellbeing of your child will be phenomenal. Some people may be able to perceive the subtle but profound differences between children who have and haven't been raised with the continuum of care. I know a family of holistic chiropractors who raised their children this way. They say that "conventionally" raised children's bodies (children who are not held all the time) are hard and spastic. However, the bodies of children who have been raised in the continuum method feel soft, supple and receptive. This couple's children had a particular and subtle glow to them which I have only very rarely seen in children. It was as though their skin was translucent. One could feel that their children were intimately cared for.

Humans have evolved under exactly the conditions that inspire a continuum of care. This is also seen in higher animals like gorillas and chimpanzees. The Bonobo chimpanzees, for example, carry their young for five years. Holding and carrying babies is naturally part of the primate evolutionary pattern since both monkey and human infants cannot fend for themselves. Therefore, holding is a biological need and requirement for survival.

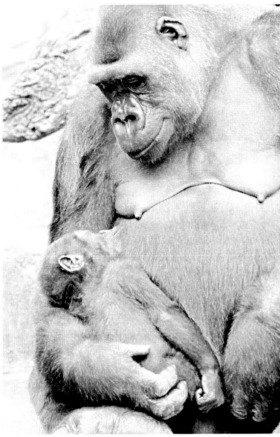

Gorilla mother feeling love for her baby.

There is a big difference in the experience of a child when he is held close to his mother and when he is stuck in a stroller. The continuum of care includes:

- **Constant physical contact with his mother** (or another familiar caregiver as needed) starting from birth.
- **Sleeping in his parents' bed**, in constant physical contact, until he leaves of his own volition (this takes several years).
- **Breastfeeding "on cue"** which is nursing in response to his own body's signals.
- **Constantly being carried in arms, or otherwise** in contact with someone, usually his mother, and allowed to observe (or nurse, or sleep) while the person carrying him goes about his or her business — until the infant begins creeping, then crawling, on his own impulse, which usually begins at approximately six months.

- Having **caregivers immediately respond** to his signals (squirming, crying, etc.) without judgment, displeasure, or invalidation of his needs, yet at the same time showing no undue concern, nor making him the constant center of attention.
- Sensing and fulfilling his parents' expectations **that he is innately social and cooperative** and has strong self-preservation instincts, and that he is welcome and worthy.[445]

Weston Price also noticed the superb treatment of children in indigenous groups. He wrote, "I have been continually impressed with the great infrequency with which we ever hear a primitive child cry or express any discomfort from the treatment it receives."[446] This is not because native parents teach their babies not to cry, or punish them for crying. It is because the babies are content, so they do not need to cry.

When a mother truly bonds with her child she won't want to leave him. Breaking the bond is painful, and preserving the bond feels good. The bond becomes solid, real and concrete when you do not leave your baby. This is how Nature intended for us to raise our children. Out of this bond between mother and child, the child forms his sense of security and peace about the world. Such children believe in a world filled with love, communion, connection and unity, because this was the emotional imprint of their childhood. The practice of holding children throughout the first 5-8 months is an embodiment of the second womb that I have mentioned earlier.

An important note about the continuum: in tribal groups young children learn how to be parents by holding and caring for the infants. When the baby needs his mother, the child immediately brings him to his mother. Sparkle loves to hold and play with Yeshe. Sparkle feels and knows that she is an important part of the family when she holds Yeshe, and Yeshe loves to play with Sparkle and be held by her. Sparkle is learning how to care for a baby and always likes holding, hugging and carrying dolls around with her. Sparkle wants to have a baby of her own to take care of one day, because of how much love she feels from being held and cared for. Her yearning is to repeat this experience with her own child when she comes of age.

Tribal In-Arms Phase

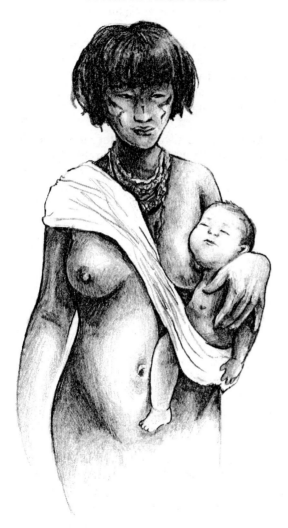

Tribal mother holding baby.

Your Child's Real Needs

Care,

Nursing,

Love, Good Feelings,

Attention,

Appreciation,

Holding/Bonding/Closeness

A child needs to be taken care of; it needs to be solely a recipient in care, nursing, good feelings, attention, appreciation of its own uniqueness. If these needs are not fulfilled, the child must suffer. [447]

Many parents are confused about what their child's <u>real</u> needs are. They treat their child as if he were all grown up, and so the parents miss out on giving the child what the child truly needs. Many parents are so eager for their children to grow up that they tend to rush through the developmental processes of their children, and do not honor the slow crawl of development which Nature intended for their children.

Michelle says: "It is a common experience for mothers or parents to say, 'Oh, they grow up so fast.' Mothers who have older children usually beg to hold other women's babies. That is because their babies 'grew up too fast.' Let's hold our babies as much as they want to be held and let's cherish each moment of their growth so that time does not slip away. You can really be here and take the time to enjoy each stage of your child's development. Then mothers won't feel an obsessive need to hold other people's babies, nor will we feel that they 'grew up too fast.'"

Traditional Child Raising Method

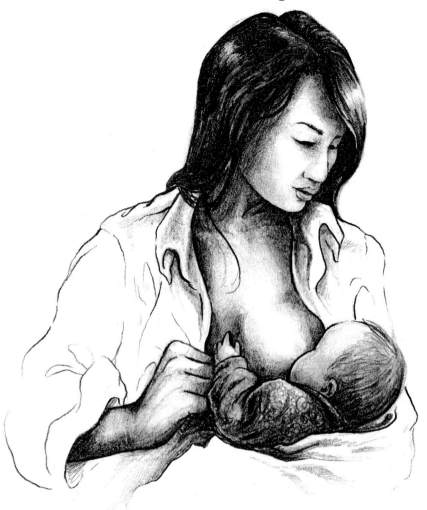

This is an example of a mother following the traditional child raising method. She holds her baby in close physical proximity until the baby begins to crawl. She feeds her baby whenever the baby is hungry. She experiences the energy of divine love flowing through her, and she honors the essence of her child and thus her own essence. She feels good, and enjoys life. This mother is in contact with what truly matters.

With the traditional method, you can sense the ease and peace that comes from giving one's full attention to the child. Since her baby is always with her, her baby feels content and at peace. Together, the mother and child experience the flowering of love, and they fulfill each other. This method of child rearing requires much less stress, strain and struggle. The mother does not need to control or manage her feelings to be with her baby; she can allow life to flow. She never has to worry about her child, because her baby is there with her all the time. Great joy and peace are possible.

The Tragic Child Raising Practices of the West

An important piece to keeping the *modern plague* alive is our diseased child raising practices. Our "modern" uncaring child raising habits are a reflection of our inner misguided ways of living and being. They stand in stark contrast to the method common among indigenous folk, just as the native nutrient-rich diet stands in bold contrast to the white-bread foods of our modern times. For the infant, the so-called "modern" way involves:

- **Traumatic separation** from his mother at birth via medical interventions, and placement in neonatal wards isolated from his mother. The majority of male babies are further traumatized by unnecessary circumcision surgery.
- **Sleeping alone and isolated**, often having to "cry himself to sleep."
- **Scheduled feeding**, with the infant's natural nursing impulses ignored, punished, or "pacified."
- **Being separated** from normal adult activities. Spending the important impressionable moments needed for bonding alone for hours on end in nursery, crib or playpen, where he is inappropriately stimulated by toys and other inanimate objects.
- Parents and caregivers **ignoring**, discouraging, belittling or even punishing him when he cries or otherwise signals his needs. When his needs are responded to, the response is colored by anxiety or irritation.
- The belief that babies are innately antisocial and that they cannot maintain their personal safety. As a result, modern parents implement strict behavioral controls through threats and a variety of manipulative "parenting techniques" that undermine his exquisitely evolved learning process.[448]

Evolution has not prepared the human infant for this kind of experience. He cannot comprehend why his desperate cries for the fulfillment of his innate expectations go unanswered, and he develops a sense of wrongness and shame about himself and his desires. If, however, his continuum expectations are fulfilled — precisely at first, with more variation possible as he matures — he will exhibit a natural state of self-assuredness, well-being and joy. Infants whose continuum needs are fulfilled during the early, in-arms phase grow up to have greater self-esteem and become more independent than those whose cries go unanswered for fear of "spoiling" them or making them too dependent.[449]

Ms. Liedloff expertly describes the pain and the shame which the infant experiences at his own parents' hands. Evolution has NOT prepared the human infant to experience this kind of abuse.

Opposite page: *The "modern" mother is constantly feeling drained (because she doesn't eat nourishing foods) and wastes more energy living a fast-paced, stressful lifestyle. She easily tires of trying to take care of her baby, who constantly seems unsatisfied. She wants to withdraw to what she believes is more important. She only feeds her baby when she feels like it, and she uses bottled milk because she thinks her breasts are not meant for babies. She is deeply unhappy. In the above right of the image, the baby's parents have forgotten they are parents and are out to dinner with friends. They want life to be the way it was before they had their child. They want to feel their "freedom" as parents and don't want their new baby to change their lifestyle in any way. They go out to dinner without their child because it is socially unacceptable to bring infants into nice restaurants. The mother is happy because she can drink wine again and does not have to worry about how it affects her child. The baby is alone in his crib, watched by a babysitter or grandparent. He reaches out for his mother but she is not there.*

The Tragic Child Raising Method of the West

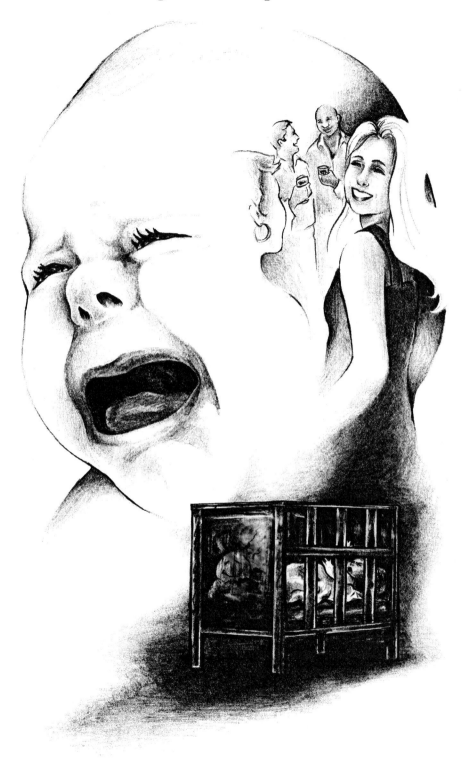

In the picture of the tragic child-rearing practice, we see an experience that is all too common today, yet this is the sanctioned pattern for most modern parents. The baby feels excruciating sadness and loneliness, and he begs for the attention of his mother; even a little bit of it will help him feel better. He is empty inside, because she, his warmth and light, is absent. His mother feels an inner struggle, and she has difficulties balancing her work life with caring for her baby. She is torn. Her heart is unhappy, and her unhappiness spreads. The only way she knows how to get out of her predicament is through avoidance. She withdraws from life, perhaps through watching television, but anything could do. She tries to buoy up her mood by engaging in activities that are considered pleasurable in the modern world, such as enjoying a fine dinner and wine with friends. The wine temporarily numbs her to her problems. Over dinner, the conversation is all about her baby. The parents are glad to boast of the joys of parenthood and their new baby. Meanwhile, he is suffering, missing the warmth of his mother and her luscious, satisfying, and nutrient-rich milk. His heart is broken. He gives up on life.

The "modern" negligent way of raising children turns the baby into an object of parental gratification. The baby is merely a status symbol, or an emblem of one of life's achievements. Or worse, the child's main purpose may be to perpetuate the parents' genetic legacy. The child is a manifestation of their blood lines, and what matters to the parents is that their memory lives on, rather than how much care and love they bring to their parenting. Even though they go out to "enjoy" themselves, modern parents ignore their own personal feelings and desires. Their life is centered on work (which usually involves making profit for a company) and stimulating leisure activities, but certainly not being parents. Their child gives them some temporary feelings of value and satisfaction as they carry out their dreary lives, much like a pet dog or cat would. The modern parent probably wonders why so many other parents have children when it is so difficult and time consuming. They have forgotten their true nature. And we, as a culture, have forgotten ours.

An Embodiment of a Mother's Love:
Breastfeeding

Many parents say they want a healthy child. Are you willing to follow through completely with the one necessary and crucial step to creating a healthy child? This one simple step is breastfeeding your infant on cue. Many children in the West are breastfed for 3-9 months, and each sitting might be short and incomplete. Today's children are not having their innate expectations of breastfeeding met.

With breastfeeding, the infant receives a pleasurable gift of life-giving, soulful connection with his warm and supple mother. He receives a biological feeling of peace and relaxation. His body becomes soft and receptive. All his troubles and worries float away as he suckles into a blissful sleep. For the mother, breastfeeding is relaxing and peaceful, rather like relaxing in a hammock in a tropical resort. All panic, tension, fear and anxiety melt away from the baby as his mother's bosom caresses his face. Many mothers may want to go on vacation, perhaps precisely because they are not giving themselves the daily vacation of breastfeeding their child.

During breastfeeding, hormones are released that stimulate the feelings of love, connection, and bonding. The typical mother does not eat foods that give her the tremendous supply of nutrients, including Activator X, needed for breastfeeding. As a result, she may find breastfeeding irritating and uncomfortable because it quickly uses her body's vital resources. Her body may no longer be able to produce the hormones associated with breastfeeding because of her imbalanced diet, which increases her discomfort. Breast milk is the baby's ideal food. The healthier the mother is and the better diet she eats, the more nourished and healthy her baby will be. Babies feel deeply at peace when their mothers eat a diet high in healthy animal fat.

Shortchanging your child when it comes to the breastfeeding session is like consciously depriving your child of the full nine months in the womb he needed to properly develop. An abbreviated breastfeeding period leaves infants weak, and with a sense of incompleteness with the world. Breastfeeding is like an extension of the umbilical cord, an integral part of the second womb. Not fully breastfeeding severs the second umbilical cord, and the developmental phase of attachment abruptly ends. These parents unconsciously do not want their children to thrive in the world and deprive their children of breastmilk. As I have said, this is a result of deeply rooted pain in the parents.

Breastfeeding on cue, the way native people do it, means that when your child is hungry you give him what he needs and wants. Many mothers are resistant to giving their son or daughter all the breastmilk that they want. Why might mothers do this to their own children? I think you know the answer.

It is normal for a baby to sometimes suckle for one hour or longer on one breast. As she feeds more on the same breast the milk becomes thicker and creamier. This is because milk with a higher fat content develops as the feeding continues. Breastfeeding is a natural biological function, and nursing 10-20 times per day or more is normal.

Babies many times get hungry at night and require nursing. This means in order to fulfill your baby's hunger for breastmilk, she needs to be sleeping in your bed or in a bed that is connected to your bed — as a matter of convenience. Giving your infant breastmilk throughout the night is a simple way to stay rested as a mother. You can lie down and even fall asleep as your infant suckles. Do not listen to people who think that breastfeeding is outmoded or to people who say breastfeeding promotes tooth decay. Tooth decay is caused by a deficiency of nutrients, not by breastmilk. In some places where infants and children have a high protection against tooth decay, they are breast fed during the night, as needed, for many years. Breastfeeding at night also has another widely important and overlooked benefit — it promotes normal physical development. At night, your baby's body is rapidly growing. Her cells are dividing and removing waste products and debris produced through normal cellular metabolism. At these periods of rapid growth, children need food that is easy to assimilate, that does not strain the body. This food is breastmilk. Your baby will sleep better, and that means you can sleep through the night or only wake up a few times for a very short period to get the feeding started. It is wrong and ignorant of doctors, dentists, and anybody else to say that breastfeeding is unhealthy or that nighttime breastfeeding is unhealthy. These comments are not based on scientific fact, but rather on a cultural delusion.

Michelle says: "It's not just the milk or the formula or sucking a pacifier that brings peace and fulfillment to a tiny person. It is the closeness with mothers. It is the direct bond of physical touch, of the lips to the nipple, which allows the baby to feel safe and have his place in this world. Our true intention is to nurture our babies so they can feel safe in the world. Mothers mistakenly think that there is something more important than breastfeeding their children. It helps when the father or friends and family are supportive of breastfeeding. It is a great act of service to the world to breastfeed your child for many years. Besides the discouraging influence of society, mothers don't want to breastfeed long enough because of the pattern of passing along an imprint of lack and unfulfillment, which is wrapped up in the negative pleasure pattern. This is a tragic mistake."

One common way that a mother disconnects from her baby is by weaning her child too soon. Reduced breastfeeding is often associated with the mother spending time away from her baby.

When a child is fully breastfed, he will be weaned at **4.5 to 7 years** of age. That figure will provoke a reaction of surprise in many because it is so incongruent with how most of us were raised. It is also contrary to the typically recommended breastfeeding length of one year.

Indigenous practices for breastfeeding vary widely. In a large survey involving dozens of indigenous groups, the average length of breastfeeding was three to four years.[450] In some indigenous Eskimo groups, weaning occurs when the child has reached about 1/3 of his adult weight. For boys this would take longer since they grow larger, around 6 and 7 years of age. Girls are weaned at around 6 years of age.[451] Eskimos exhibit some of the finest physical development on the planet. For example, the adult Eskimo man can carry one hundred pounds in each arm, and one hundred pounds in his teeth for a long distance.[452]

Based upon this model, I place the minimum age of healthy weaning at four and a half years. **The ideal length of breastfeeding is six or seven years.** As we examined in Chapter 5, a majority of our modern mothers are deficient in nutrients. And this deficiency carries to our children's earliest experience of nurturance when, as a modern society, we encourage mothers to breastfeed their babies only for a small fraction of the time required by Nature for success. On the other hand, breastfeeding beyond seven years could also become unhealthy. Children who are breastfed until completion will feel an upwelling of goodness in their heart. They will feel as though they matter.

Science also shows us that breastfeeding is superior to bottle feeding. The mortality rate for bottle-fed infants in one study was over ten times higher than breastfed infants.[453, 454] Breastfeeding also helps reduce long face syndrome, SIDS, and otitis media, or middle ear infections.[455]

If doctors and other "authorities" were looking out for your child's best health interests, then they would honor the evidence that has been presented. Breastfeeding is the best way to keep your child healthy, and needs to be carried out for the duration of several years, and be provided on cue. While on this subject, I must mention that ALL INFANT FORMULAS are modernized foods. They will set your child up for inferior health and must be avoided. If you must use a supplement under a special circumstance, you can find healthful homemade infant formula at www.westonaprice.org/children/recipes.html . Low breast milk flow can be improved with 1-4 cups per day of carrot juice, or carrot and celery juice that is freshly juiced. Please add 1-4 ounces of cream. (Excess carrot juice consumption may promote tooth cavities.)

Breastfeeding is one of the most feminine and motherly acts. The fact that our culture does not fully endorse prolonged breastfeeding is an example of how our culture does not honor the divine feminine nature that exists in all women.

Instead, we make careless claims that breastfeeding for more than 6-12 months is somehow unnecessary. The child who desires the breast is responding to the instincts with which Nature equipped him. **Your child's desire for full and complete breastfeeding is a program designed by Mother Nature, the creator herself.** In responding to this desire, you are following "Her" principles.

With frequent on-cue breastfeeding, the resumption of your normal ovulation pattern will be delayed, sometimes for a period of up to two years and usually for at least six months. This creates a natural child spacing which, as we have discussed, is important for a mother's health, as well as for the health of her next child.

Exclusive breastfeeding means providing only breastmilk for your child and nothing else. Even in the case of healthy mothers, I suggest that you observe and honor your child's reflexes to eat food. This usually means introducing some safe foods, at least in small amounts, beginning anywhere from 5-7 months of age. When Yeshe started grabbing at food we listened to her cue and knew she was ready for some food. Children who are breastfed begin to need other nutrients, like iron, at about 6 months of age. These nutrients are not readily provided in breastmilk.

Breastfeeding Adopted Children

I have read of three accounts of mothers breastfeeding children who were adopted. Dr. Price wrote that an Aborigine mother died and her mother (the baby's grandmother) stimulated her breasts to start producing milk by rubbing ground up parts of a special insect on them. (Photographs of this insect are in Dr. Price's collection.)[456]

Dr. John Christopher, an outstanding Western herbalist, was able to use the *blessed thistle* herb to help women produce breast milk. Blessed thistle can bring back dried up breastmilk, and in at least two other cases regularly drinking blessed thistle tea stimulated women who had not been pregnant to produce breast milk for babies. The successful regimen included three cups of blessed thistle tea per day, and plenty of fresh vegetable juices.[457] I share these stories in order to illustrate that a reality exists that is beyond the limited scope of what we believe is possible.

Bottle Feeding

If for some reason a child needs to be bottle fed, a traditional Indian feeding cup called a paladai may be healthier for a child to use than a bottle. The paladai promotes suckling needed for breastfeeding.[458] I had difficulty finding one of these but there are special pouring dishes and candle holders that have the same shape and can be used as an alternative to bottles. You'll have to experiment.

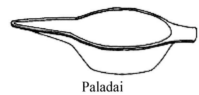

Paladai

There is also a device called the lact-aid nursing trainer system. This allows you to introduce a supplement along with regular breast-feeding, which may be needed for special cases. See **www.lact-aid.com.**

Slings, not Strollers

Occasionally, special circumstances limit the mother's ability to hold her child. Holding the child and/or using a sling is a far more intelligent way to care for your baby. Strollers are inconvenient to haul around everywhere and are completely dysfunctional in any type of natural environment. While in a sling or being held, the baby feels directly connected with her caretaker. The child's immediate experience of her environment is coherent as she sees the world in context with her mother, not separate from her. Strollers also make breastfeeding cumbersome. Clever use of slings can allow for a mother to move about and breastfeed at the same time.. Slings make it easy to perform household tasks while keeping your baby cozy and close. Michelle can cook, clean, garden, do laundry, shop, talk with friends and play with Sparkle quite easily while Yeshe is in a sling. Michelle uses a

long wrap sling and sometimes a New Natives shoulder sling, depending on the occasion. The wrap sling allows both hands to be completely free. Take time to find a sling you feel comfortable with. At first it is a bit of a struggle to use, but once you get used to it things can flow quite well.

For videos to show you how to use slings visit www.babywearing.com.

Some parents find the New Natives organic baby slings a simple sling to start with:

Father, a Loving Protector

When the soul begins to enter the infant's body at the time of birth, he is instantly aware of the energetic connections he has to both his mother and father. If they are not present for him physically or emotionally then he will feel a tremendous shock and pain. As adults, it is hard for many of us to fathom what it is like for an infant to feel the loss of one of his parents. Even if the father is physically present, the infant can perceive a loss if the father is emotionally detached, even in just a few minutes' time. The infant's perceived experience of loss of his mother or father can be likened to an atomic bomb exploding: complete and massive devastation for the newborn.

A physically present father is not sufficient for the infant, because he is expecting an emotional presence, a feeling of connection. Children look for a feeling of warmth, communion and belonging. They have an innate desire to bond with their fathers, as the father contributed to half of the genetic creation of the child. The newborn baby wants to feel an energetic "yes" from her father. She wants to feel and believe that her father loves her deeply, and that her father is truly holding her in his heart. The child yearns for a father who is joyful and happy to have this little person here, a father who supports and encourages her. Of particular importance, the baby wants to feel that she is good. That her complaining, breastfeeding, sleeping, and playing are welcome and acknowledged. One of the greatest tragedies of our culture is that so many fathers are unavailable. Abandonment of children by their fathers is a central cause of a deep underlying pain in our culture and on the planet. The withdrawn or abandoning father is a central cause (but not the only cause) of a deep rift between men and women.

While the mother's role is nurturing, the father's role is as a protector. These are not the father's, nor the mother's, only roles. However, these are essential roles which have slowly evolved over time. An indigenous woman who is carrying her child (maintaining the continuum) is quite helpless to defend herself, especially if she has more than one child. The father's primal role is then to protect her and their children. This response is a genetic encoding. There is a vast array of qualities that you might offer as a father other than protection. Our discussion now at hand, however, is about the particular quality of being a protector. The ideal father offers loving protection by holding a vibrational energy container of safety. Women can feel more vulnerable to outer forces when they are pregnant or have young babies. As a mother raises and nurtures her child, she wants to feel secure because she is maintaining a second womb for her baby. The father provides this security; he provides the outer shielding that protects the second womb. The modern distorted version of security is simply a man who makes a lot of money. And although financial abundance does provide some security, it is far from the complete picture.

Activity for fathers: creating a field of protection. This exercise can be done by both parents. The tangible feeling is quite different when a man does it, but one is not better than the other; participation from both parents is different and essential. Doing it together is a way that is most likely to encourage the father to participate. At least give it one try. If the mothers reading this book want the fathers to participate, they will need to give fathers some extra energy around it. To produce a field of safety and protection, the father feels in himself a rootedness in his being. He first connects to a deep connection to his own metaphoric mother, the Earth. A positive and present father creates a field of protection and safety for the mother, during the time of pregnancy and after, by being deeply

rooted to the earth from his tan t'ien, which is a core energetic point located 1.5-2 inches below the belly button, precisely at the center of gravity within the father's body. Feel this spot and even place one or several fingers on it. Do this standing up with legs a little wider than shoulder width apart and knees bent slightly. Holding this awareness on the tan t'ien and the Earth connection, the father creates a field of safety within which he can hold the energetic container of his family. The field is created by the clear intention of the father to protect and to create abundance in his family. You can invite in the spirit of supreme safety and peacefulness and use it as help. Safety is also a thought or intention of holding the feeling or concept of protecting children and caring for them. Much like animals marking their territory, the father's role is to protect his "territory"—his home, his family, his children. This protection is not in the form of ownership, but from the surrendered place of mutual respect, love, compassion, and understanding. Men possess genetic programming to feel this protective instinct, as perhaps thousands of years ago groups of men would help protect their village from neighboring tribes, or from large predatory animals.

When he is rooted to the earth, the father's energy field feeds the mother, and feeds the energy body of the baby during the time of pregnancy and childhood. Women also feel safe and comfortable around men who want to protect them, rather than in the presence of men who are trying to satisfy their childhood needs by being with them. The father feels more supported if he has a group or clan of men supporting him, working in harmony together for their higher good. Mutually holding this field of safety and protection for each other a small group of families will feel safe and protected. Needless to say, if all men, or even just one percent of them, were doing this then there would be an all-powerful field of protection pervading the planet. Everyone would feel safe with each other, with themselves, and with life. Violence, war, and strife, would be virtually impossible in this scenario. This is how important a healthy father is.

Men Working Together in a Positive Manner

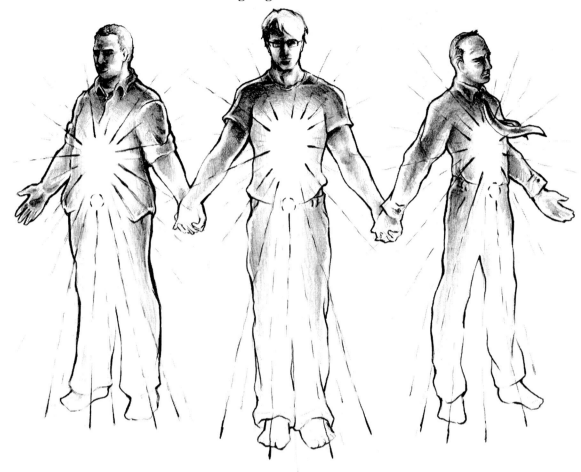

These men are working together to support their families. Their intention as fathers can be reflected in these words, spoken for their families, "We will fiercely protect you, and strive to honor you."

The Consequence of Distorted Father Energies

The outer world today is in part an active creation of men who do not embody the essential role of the loving protector. In fact, many fathers embody a distorted and dark form of this role. Many men work together to create the destruction of our planet, usually in the service of greed and profit. This is a shameful part of our culture and creates deep pain. Rather than working together to support and protect women and their children, these men inflict violence upon them. The devastation we have inflicted on our Earth is a reflection of the inner devastation that many men must feel due to their imprint from childhood, when they were devastated by a loss of love from their own mother and father. The Earth symbolically represents holding, protection, nurturing and support. The Earth supports us and helps us feel safe. The destructive, distorted father energy many times comes in the form of a father who, rather than protecting his children and his wife, hurts them and is physically or emotionally violent. This man then becomes the cause of the mother and child feeling unsafe, and the primary source of their pain.

The model of this destructive father, embodying negative masculine energy, is passed down from one generation of men to the next.

The children of abusive or absent fathers grow up to expect or even behave in a similar manner. Our culture is a living demonstration of the divine qualities of the father expressed in their distorted manifestations. The modern father is unavailable, withdrawn, and ultimately extremely disconnected from himself and his family. It takes extreme internal disconnection to be capable of violent actions against those whom he loves. Since children make an internal map of reality based on their childhood experiences, a child's map in the case of an unhealthy father will include such beliefs as, "Men are dangerous" or "Men are distant and unavailable." Or even worse, "We must obey male authority because otherwise we will be punished." This child will either grow up to be just like his father, or will expect men to behave that way in society. When male destructive energy is accepted, tolerated and expected, it perpetuates itself.

The Divine Masculine

Underneath the distorted denser layers of masculine energy (which is in both men and women to different degrees) lies the divine masculine, which we all want and need in our lives. We want to raise our boys to be healthy men and good role models for the world. To overcome the darkness of the masculine we must look at the darkness, feel it within us and how it affects us, and let this feeling stir and move us. The destruction only stops when we all work to examine our own inner destructive tendencies. Acting to protect the Earth is an important part of this work too. The Earth can represent the qualities of both our mothers and our fathers. Seeing this parallel explains how we unconsciously treat the earth the same way our mothers and fathers treated us.

On the *New Earth* (envisioned in Eckhart Tolle's book of the same name), fathers realize their true potentials as the missing heroes we so desperately long for. Men can reclaim their masculine identity, which protects and loves women, children and other men, and can become the living embodiment of the fictional heroes of today.

(To Fathers) You are the hero that your child, your wife, and your planet have been waiting for.

Women are heroines when they embrace their true divine feminine nature, which includes the qualities of strength, nurturing, safety, compassion, and joy.

(To Mothers) You are the heroine that your child, your husband, your community and your planet have been waiting for.

Both men and women have within them the distorted form of the divine masculine energy. The masculine energy is yang; it is outgoing. The distorted form can be violent and aggressive, either overtly or passively. We can only heal this imbalanced trait when each of us allows himself to feel and experience our own internal pains regarding the actions of men in our culture. Whether it is war, genocide, pollution, corruption, or violence towards women and children, we can begin to claim our right to heal and live safely on the planet when we stop numbing ourselves to the pain of these internal and external events. We must start feeling and acknowledging the depths of our emotional and psychological experiences in this culture of violence. Through feeling our fears, and dropping down into the tears, we can break out of the vicious cycle.

I have to make this point again because it is both so urgent and so often overlooked. When we see something wrong in the world, the world does not just require or ask of us to try to fix what we see wrong. We must also equally look within us to see what is wrong in the inner world. When we see outer pollution, it usually triggers an inner voice that is full of judgments and negativity. "Look at those people, living unconsciously," we might say, or "Look at all this disgusting pollution," and so forth. It can also trigger numbness: "Who cares?" or "It's their fault, it's not my responsibility," or "I have enough problems already." Yet we miss the fact that these judgments are also a form of pollution. We create psychic pollution, in which the negative parts of our self add to the psychic pollution of the planet. If you want to change the world, change yourself first. Change how you see the world. Start by paying attention to how you feel towards the bad things in the world. Notice when you feel upset, angry, negative, uncomfortable. This is the drum beat of your awakening. Too many people are trapped in the cycle of waiting and hoping for the world to fix itself. And I can tell you for certain that you can wait for eternity and the world will never be how you want it to be. When you can make inward changes by feeling or even just acknowledging those difficult, painful, and trapped feelings you become empowered to make real outer world changes. How do you think it came about that I wrote this book?

(*To Fathers*) No matter how challenging the relationship is with the mother of your child, the father's presence during pregnancy, birth, and the child's growing years is crucial. Even if the father is present but also is working and is away from home often, this affects the child. Know that even though you are not the primary care taker of your child, your child needs to feel your love and support, and is nurtured by your loving energy. Just as he feels with his mother, nothing can bring a young child greater happiness than to feel the loving presence and embrace of his father.

Regardless of whether you are a man or a woman, if you feel a deep sense of deprivation, loss, or emptiness in your life, if life seems dull, out of alignment, and with little excitement, then it is likely that you are suffering from the pain of the devastating loss of the one you loved the most. It does not matter if your parent is still alive or not, it simply has to do with how you feel about them, and how present they were for you. Feel and tune into this sensation now.

(*For Fathers* and Mothers) Being a protector is about being in contact with the sensations of your body. It is about honoring yourself as a human, and simply being. You are more than just an entity that seeks pleasure and avoids pain. When you experience yourself in your humanness, you will also transcend some imbalanced emotions and feelings towards the opposite sex. If you are a man who has a tendency not to be present, to aggression, and to avoid your innate responsibilities, then I pray for your healing.

Nothing is Like a Father's Touch

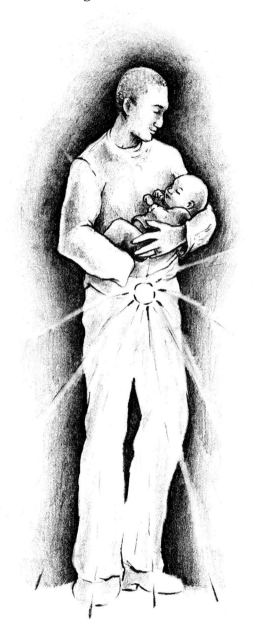

The father provides a sense of safety, love, affection and support.

Activity: father healing (or mother healing). To aid healing yourself I suggest that you create a prayer that comes from deep within, from the truth of your being. Invite in and align yourself with the divine will and the divine masculine from the highest reality. From this place ask for forgiveness and surrender. In your own words you can say, "Father, forgive me." Or you can use a prayer I mentioned earlier, "Show me, Father, the real reason for my difficulties, so that I can solve them."[459] (Of course replace "Father" with the name or image appropriate to your religion or beliefs.) You can begin to heal the separated parts of yourself that cause you to create more pain on this planet. If you are not motivated to do this for yourself, do it for your child-to-be. You are in control of whether you and your child experience the great joy and satisfaction of being together, or great sorrow with the disappointment of loss, or of aggression at your hands. It is time to end violence on our planet, to realize the importance of harmony between men and women. It is time for fathers to be responsible, to help motivate this change by being aware of their true nature as a loving protector. Fathers can open up to the power of the divine masculine, which is all-powerful, to make positive changes in the world. If you want to change the world and make it a better place, you can absolutely do it. And if WE want to make a better world, WE can do it! It begins with that first choice, that quantum moment of change when you realize that you can truly make a difference.

Other Roles of the Father

(*For fathers* and mothers) Acknowledge that you are one with your partner and child. There are an infinite number of roles that a father has. This discussion is meant to liberate your thinking to unlimited models and suggestions so that you feel more confident and supported in who you are and who you want to be for your children.

A father's role is to:
- Provide healthy nutrition.
- Provide financial support, which manifests as food, shelter and clothing.
- Protect the boundaries of the mother.
- Protect the boundaries of the children.

- Create a safe and comfortable living environment.
- Relate honestly to your spouse and children.
- Make sure your child is nurtured and taken care of.
- Protect your child and partner against unnecessary medical interventions or other negative outer world influences.
- Most important, shine like the sun. Be who you are freely; that is how you can let love enter the chambers of your being.

Gender Roles and Your Divinity

The masculine principle is outgoing and leads to action.[460] The feminine principle is of receptivity, of letting the activating forces work their lawful way toward fruition.[461]

Men do not embody only the active principle and women do not embody only receptivity. Both men and women have active and receptive principles that need to be purified, balanced, and unified. Each person is totally different. It is possible that one woman's healthy active/masculine energy may be stronger than a man's healthy active/masculine energy. The reverse is also possible.

The divine masculine and feminine principles can be distorted in each one of us. One example of the receptive principle in distortion is if "instead of surrendering to the self-activated inner powers, one surrenders to another person's authority… By the same token, a woman who surrenders her autonomy to a mate because she is too fearful and lazy to assume the consequences for her own actions makes a travesty and caricature out of femininity."[462]

One example of the active principle in distortion is this: "A man cannot dare to be fully a man and to activate the creative force in a deliberate and purposeful way when his unconscious is still steeped in hostility, rage, and anger. For, the activating principle then threatens to express these destructive impulses."[463]

Both men and women have an active and receptive side. In distortion, the receptivity is lazy and fearful and allows one to be controlled. When the active principle is in distortion, and there is too much negative current tied up with it, the individual holds its expression back to prevent destructive behaviors. As we begin to notice and accept these emotions within us, then we begin to emerge from the destructive patterns. Of course, there are many other distortions and higher qualities of the active and receptive principles that are not discussed here.

Various deities, as well as human role models, can help remind us of our own divine masculine and feminine traits. Use whomever you feel comfortable with. The role models of the divine feminine and the divine masculine can be used to help remind you of, and to help heal, these parts within you. Find the energy, spirit, or form of the divine feminine and masculine that appeals to you.

Divine Feminine– Mother of the world, beautiful and powerful, full of love and compassion.

Divine Masculine– Finding the greatness within, unconditional love and acceptance, true compassion, and revealer of the path of salvation for all who suffer.

One Common Confusion

Because of confusion surrounding the masculine and feminine principles in our modern times, men and women have become uncertain about what their roles are. While women can have a strong and healthy active current, they are not fathers. While men can have a strong and healthy receptive nature, they are not mothers. It is possible for a woman to be fatherly, and for a man to be motherly, and they can do a good job at it. But it is not the same thing as a fatherly man and a motherly woman. In an ideal situation, both men and women fulfill their true roles. These roles I am referring to are not the diluted and oppressive or culturally imposed roles. I am referring to the divine roles represented by the figures of the divine mother and father.

The father needs to be the best father he can be, rather than aspire to be a mother. The mother needs to be the best mother she can be and not try to be a father. When you do not live up to your full potential, as a mother or a father, then you have failed your child. You can never be who you are not. A man cannot breastfeed a child; he cannot get pregnant, so he cannot be a mother. Women bear children, and women nurture children with their loving breast milk. Because of this, women cannot be fathers. Because of imbalances of the inner masculine and feminine qualities of partners in relationships, and because of **mass** societal confusions and distortions, one common mistake is making fathers mothers, and mothers into fathers.

When the mother is truly the mother, and the father the father, then the child will feel at ease in the world. Nature designed the child to feel certain things. The creator designed the child to breastfeed and be nurtured by the mother. The creator designed the child to feel held, protected and safe by both the mother and father. When we honor and surrender to our humble roles, then we honor our child in a deeply loving way.

If for some reason your child is missing a mother or a father, then it is important to acknowledge your child's needs for that male or female energy. In some indigenous groups, when a mother is absent the child may be adopted by another mother so that the child will still receive her bonding stage of attachment, and receive the physical nourishment of breastmilk. If for some reason one parent is missing, try to find a surrogate, maybe a trusted friend or relative, who can fill in some of that lost energy.

Stages of Individuation

Stages of Individuation, Healthy First & Second Stage

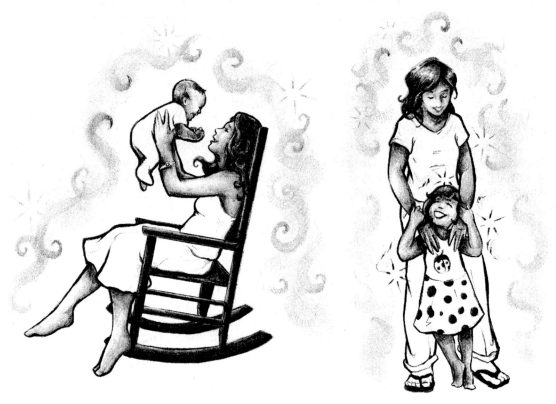

First Stage on the left: Early in her child's life, the mother keeps the continuum with her child intact. She does not leave her. She gives to her child selflessly and unconditionally. She thus fulfills her child's many needs.

Second Stage on the right: In the second stage you see that as the child receives enough of her mother's attentions, she feels fulfilled and satisfied. The mother is constantly giving to the child and filling the child up with her goodness. The aura around the child represents her budding sense of self. The role of both parents is to affirm the child's self and to affirm their unique personality, not to try to make them into an image of the parent or to conform to societal norms of what is "accepted."

The stages of individuation depicted here are an overall picture of how a healthy child can develop. Children slowly grow and there is a natural rhythm of expansion and contraction. What you see in the pictures, which includes how the child's aura might look, is how a child can slowly develop a sense of herself. This sense only becomes healthy when the child is fulfilled. This rarely happens in the Western method of child rearing.

In the first stage of infancy, the child cannot differentiate herself from the world.

She thinks that she and her environment are one and the same. She believes that she is her mother. If the child is allowed this belief and her mother gives to her unconditionally, her real needs are met and she will evolve naturally. The happy child mimics her parents and their behaviors because Nature designed the child to copy the successful patterns and approaches to life that her parents have. As the child is fulfilled, she starts to have her own energy field and her own self.

Healthy Individuation, Third & Fourth Stage

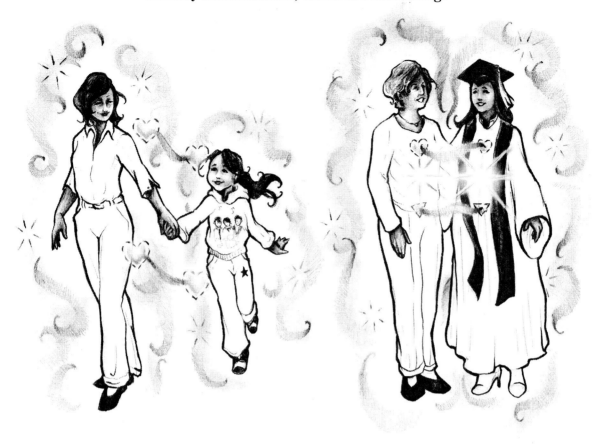

Third Stage on the left*: The young child is supported by her mother. Her mother gives her space to be, and at the same time allows the flow of energy and relation between herself and her daughter. Both are happy and satisfied by their relationship. Its framework is love and togetherness.*
Fourth Stage on the right*: This child has developed a strong bond with her mother. She trusts her mother. They stay connected through their relational cords, which are strong, robust, and filled with joy. The mother and daughter feel mutuality, honor each other, and respect each other. She has received fully from her mother, and feels assured and safe in both her active and receptive qualities.*

In the second stage of individuation the child believes that she is omnipotent, and one with the world. She wishes and believes that all her impulses should be met immediately by the mother. She is floating in a sea of life, not realizing good or bad, but having pure experience, and feeling oneness with both her father and mother. If she is frightened, she searches for and needs that safety net of her mother to hold her. There is an interplay where the child explores the world and then returns to the mother's second womb. Yet, when this child is com-

pletely fulfilled by not being abandoned physically or emotionally, she never experiences a loss of her innermost self. She will become more confident exploring the world as a feeling of her loving and present parents integrates into the cells of her body. She believes she is love; she believes she is lovable because that is how she is treated.

In the third stage of individuation this child is beginning to really feel and test her independence. She finds that what she likes is different from what her mother likes. On one hand, she seeks to imitate her parent, and on the other hand, she begins to find her own unique expression of herself. This child is both intimately sensitive and very self confident and trusts herself. It is important to understand that if you practice the continuum of care, your child might actually seem to develop in some ways more slowly than other children. This is because she actually is able to experience her childhood. The other children are forced, through painful "lessons," to skip many of their developmental stages and thus might seem older or more mature. The healthy individuation process is a deliberately slow and lengthy process. This extra period of care will produce a fine and capable adult, full of love, compassion and energy.

In the fourth stage of individuation you see the beginning of the mature individual adult. She stays in intimate communion with her mother. In healthy individuation, although the child is physically an individual, physically a self, and emotionally her own person, there is a deep and abiding connection to her parents. Through that connection, she feels connected to everything else, including the force that creates the universe. She never separates from this force too much, because her connection to her parents was never severed by force or abandonment. The parents and the life-force are synonymous to the infant, and so she experiences, in her own way, God. This child, as a young adult, will be mature and compassionate in a deep way. She will radiate positive energy, and seek to engage people in healthy relationships because her imprint was of a healthy relationship. She will experience union with a partner as a young adult because she expects that type of experience from life. Her lessons in life were not learned by her parents teaching her ideas, but by her parents embodying their love for her in their surrendered action of giving unconditionally.

Opposite page, top picture.
The First Stage on the left: In the first stage, the infant's body does not have contact with his mother's body. He rests against a car seat baby basket. He has limited contact with his mother. She stays distant from him and she does not give to him fully. As a result, his energy field does not feel fulfilled. He does not receive the mothering he needs.

The Second Stage on the right: In the second stage, the child feels constantly needy. Many times, this is a sweet and innocent neediness, and doesn't seem like such a big deal. To protect herself against these constant "demands" the mother pacifies her child. The mother continually refuses to give her child fulfillment. What is not evident is that the mother actually spends tremendous amounts of energy in not giving to her child. As a result, the mother passes along her dissatisfaction and avoidance of life to her needy child.

Opposite page, bottom picture.
The Third Stage on the left: The child learns how to manipulate his parents to get his needs met, since his up-front feelings of neediness have been almost constantly rejected, punished or ignored. Over time, this child develops strategies to satisfy his needs in a new way. It is as if his own mother is acting like a child, expecting fulfillment from him.

The Fourth Stage on the right: In the final stage, this child is grown up but he experiences a constant underlying feeling of fear and unfulfillment. He does not respect his mother and harbors anger and resentment of her, and rightfully so. He tries to avoid, manipulate, or control other people to get his needs met, because that is what was done to him. He has a superficial relationship with his parents. He cannot wait to leave home and fly to the other end of the country to go to college, and his relational cords to his mother are in tatters. The mother is happy her child is finally grown up, and she is happy to be past all those "difficult" and "needy" early years. She is proud of how quickly her child grew up and now is concerned about his rebellious nature and what she sees as an unproductive attitude.

Stages of Individuation, Thwarted Development First & Second Stages

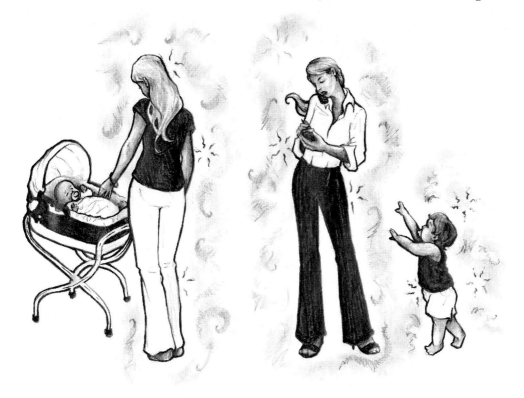

Stages of Individuation, Thwarted Development Third and Fourth Stages

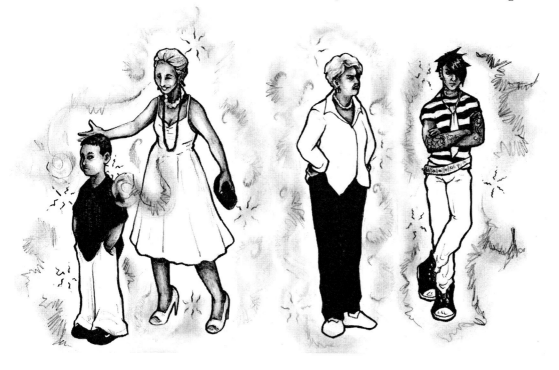

The first thwarted stage of development. Many of our childhoods involved mostly the thwarted development illustrated here. Viewing these pictures might bring up painful feelings for you. Beginning in infancy, this child's dearest, most precious loved one turned her back to him and treated him in an inhospitable way. The continuum of care was never initiated and this sweet and innocent newborn baby was alienated from his mother. He is alienated from all that matters in life. He knows something is wrong but cannot put his finger on what it is.

The second thwarted stage of development. Having never really bonded to his mother, the child's body is filled with numbness and indifference to life. The world does not care about him, so he thinks. Life is a struggle and a burden. He is often punished in different ways because he is too needy. He always wants to attract his mother's attention but only fails. His mother entertains him by buying him toys and video games. When he is needy she gets angry or irritated at him. She believes that the child needs to please her and tries to teach this boy to be a good boy and listen to his mommy.

The third thwarted stage of development. By this time, the growing boy has given up on ever getting his needs met. He has a deep sense of unhappiness. His energy is depleted and he is lethargic in some ways. He wants to learn about and explore the world, but something thwarts him from doing so. It is his latent feelings of abandonment. One cannot imagine the lonely world of this child, who grows up in emotional isolation, never feeling bonded or connected to his mother. He thus feels unloved and unconnected to the world around him. He has developed many clever strategies to manipulate his mother into giving him some energy and attention. Most of the attention he receives is negative.

The final fourth thwarted developmental stage. As a teen, this boy cannot wait to get away from his parents. He treats all his friends as objects to use for satisfying his needs. He now will focus his attention on outer world success. He wants to be rich, famous and successful so that people will pay attention to

him. When he goes to college he switches gears and devotes his energy to his school work, studying long hours. He spends his early twenties working long hours, making a fairly large amount of money, and hoping to meet a beautiful and caring woman to share his life with. But he wonders why all the women he meets are mean and cruel. He doesn't realize that it isn't the women that are the problem, but that it is his imprint. His imprint tells him that in relationships women are mean and cruel. This is because he experienced that cruelty as a child, in the form of abandonment and neglect from his own mother with whom he once longed to be. His imprint is to "love" such a woman, and he carries imprinted meanness and cruelty himself, and thus he feels attracted to women who are like him. Life for him is filled with unhappiness and the few fleeting pleasures he experiences are during his three weeks of yearly vacation. Even if he meets the woman of his dreams and gets married, his life will be filled with disappointment. He will continue to look to the world, to earn more money, buy fancier cars, bigger homes, and more prestige for the fulfillment that he can never find. Something is missing within him; it cannot be found in the world.

Note. Human development proceeds as a constantly flowing force of life. While there are stages of more complex learning, these four stages represent larger stages and approximations that are designed to illustrate how a child matures and develops a sense of himself through his bonding experience with his mother.

Additional note. It is part of our life's work to heal the distorted and darker parts of ourselves. If you have raised some of your children in unconscious ways, it is not too late to make an important difference in their lives by beginning to relate to them with more awareness. Nothing is frozen in stone. Darkness is numbness, inertia, and stagnation. Light is fluidity, movement, and a feeling of rightness. If you cannot heal mistakes you have made in the world, and cannot change how you were raised as a child, you can mourn and go through the grief and find forgiveness. I wouldn't want anyone to think that if he were raised a certain way, or has raised his own children a certain way, that he is doomed to suffer without hope. There is always hope for the truth.

When the child was not fulfilled by the selfless actions of his mother or family, he cannot individuate in a healthy way. He will view himself and the world in a separated, imbalanced and unrealistic manner, because a part of his psyche did not develop properly. Nature did not prepare the child for being raised without the continuum of care, so he becomes imbalanced psychologically in many ways and then seeks to hide his imbalances in order to fit in the world. His energy field is never full and he does not complete his process of individuation. The child is battered emotionally and psychologically from his failed attempts to have his parents attend to his natural needs.

Each time parents thwart the bonding process the child is physically and emotionally hurt. As an adult, this wounded person's actions are tainted with the pain of unfulfilled needs. Consciously or not his actions will be harmful to himself and/or to others. He is a captive in a cycle of pain, trying to have his needs met yet constantly being rebuffed. He cannot see individuals for who they really are because his parents did not see him for who he really was. If you recognize this condition in yourself or you see it in others, try not to judge it, but rather recognize it and hold it in your awareness with love and compassion. Love and compassion are the keys to healing our wounds, because it is what the hurt and vulnerable child never received.

Many of us experienced our childhood in this way, to varying degrees. Here in each of us lie the seeds of evil, which manifests itself as numbness. We learn negative patterns and behaviors in our early years. We embody these experiences and unconsciously treat others the way that we were treated since that is our imprint of how the world is. One of the key steps to healing is to observe and fully acknowledge your negative and positive behaviors in an honest way. Do not pretend that you have no problems, but at the same time do not dwell in judgment of how horrible you are. You need to find the middle ground of acceptance so that love will blossom in you once again. For now, simply notice your habits, notice your inner feelings

and impulses that you likely ignore or discard. Perhaps you will catch yourself acting in a childlike manner. Take note of it. See if it reminds you of the past. See if you can feel the deeper feelings underlying your behaviors.

Natural Infant Hygiene

Babies were not designed to wear diapers. Nature never made a diaper tree for us to use, right? Nature had a different plan in mind. In much the same way that Nature expects parents to *understand and meet* the baby's hunger signals for breastmilk, Nature intended parents to learn to anticipate their child's elimination needs. In many indigenous cultures, the parents either "know" when the child needs to eliminate, and they take him to a nearby bush, or they let the child pee at any moment all over everything, and then just laugh about the amusing design that Nature has given us.

There are advantages for children who do not wear diapers. First, there is no big white puffy thing between their legs that can cause rashes and other discomforts. There is something inhumane about allowing a child to wallow in their own urine or feces, even if only for a minute. In some cases, diapers can encourage an unnatural rotation of the legs of the child from the top of the leg bones. I am speaking here more of plastic diapers than of cloth diapers. If a baby wears a diaper all the time, he can become alienated from his own groin, the central portion of his body. Do we force our children to wear diapers to cover up their "sinful" or "bad" parts? Our genitals provide us a feeling of pleasure, of the life force, our creativity and our rootedness in the Earth. A child who is not wearing a diaper has free access to see, feel and examine his or her genitals. Children are likely to do this frequently when they reach a certain age. They see their genitals as an amusing and curious piece of flesh, another fun thing to play with in their personal world. These early explorations are a part of our natural evolutionary and developmental process. When this stage of self-exploration is allowed, babies will feel that having genitals is natural and good, like the rest of their bodies. Such natural self-exploration is of course discouraged when the infant's genitals are encased most of the time in big puffy diapers. Preventing this stage of development and discovery might have significant and subtle unforeseen consequences such as imbalanced sexual habits or feelings in adulthood.

Natural infant hygiene means allowing your child to go about diaper-less, while you learn to understand and synchronize your activities with your child's elimination communication. It is practiced in indigenous groups all over the planet.[464] Understanding a baby's elimination needs is a loving way for parents to enhance bonding and deepen their connection with their baby. It also can save quite a bit of money on wasteful disposable diapers, as well as resources and time in washing cloth diapers.[465]

Even if you do not practice natural infant hygiene, it is a good idea to let your young children be naked frequently, or be in loose, comfortable clothing without a diaper enough of the time so that they have the opportunity to get accustomed to their bodies and have access to all of their parts.

The practice of natural hygiene involves watching for cues, communicating with your baby and relying on intuition to determine when your baby needs to use the potty. When you feel it is time, you take your child either to the toilet, or to the bushes if outdoors.

In our family's personal practice of natural hygiene we at first had pee going everywhere. Michelle was very frustrated when first practicing this. But eventually, the practice became more convenient and made caring for a child easier because much less time is spent on cleaning the baby and changing diapers. In the end, Michelle had a 98%+ success rate for knowing when our daughter needed to pee. Potty training was totally effortless and natural as a result. With Yeshe, we are using cloth diapers about half of the day, and the other half she is diaper-less. For us, having two children somewhat complicates the practice, but nevertheless, with natural infant hygiene, one diaper can last most of or the entire day because it never gets peed on.

Michelle says: "Natural infant hygiene is really fun, and really pleasurable to do. Our elimination is just as important as the eating that starts the cycle. The bond that can come as a result of listening to your baby's cues makes natural infant hygiene worth the effort. It is a huge pleasure when you can communicate with your baby in such a way, before they can even talk. Practicing natural infant hygiene has deepened my bond with my daughters. It has been very challenging at the same time. Now, after overcoming the challenges, I know it was worth it."

I recommend the book, *Diaper Free!* by Ingrid Bauer. Not only does it explain natural hygiene very clearly, it is also a great support for natural heart-centered child rearing. Learn more at: **www.natural-wisdom.com** .

Why Babies Cry

Babies talk to us and tell us how they feel by crying. Many parents can mistakenly have an inner judgment of the cries of their baby. The judgment might arise from the parent thinking they themselves did something wrong (which could be true), to being angry at their child for crying and whining. I encourage you to let go of any judgment of your baby's cries and rather to do something extraordinary: *listen to the cries*. When you can override your judgments of yourself and your baby, your baby's cries become a blessing. The cries become a blessing when you acknowledge the mistake you made, or you find a way to meet the child's needs. Cries also become a blessing when the child releases pain, hurt, sadness and frustration from her experiences. I don't suggest that you should make your children cry, but if they do cry for some reason, I suggest that you really feel and hear their communication to you. You can be happy that your child is able to communicate to you how she feels. At the same time, if there is frequent and repetitive crying, this can be your child's way of responding to consistent imbalanced patterns from you as parents.

There is no time that a child cries that she is not communicating a message. There is no time a child cries when she is not experiencing some type of discomfort. Parents tend to disregard their own internal, natural responses to their crying baby. Understanding the cries of your baby means feeling your own internal responses to them. Because many parents themselves are cut off from their own delicate emotions they cannot feel what their baby is communicating, or they don't want to feel it. This sad situation began when the parents' cries, when they were children, were not heard as well, and so the pattern became imprinted.

When your baby cries, feel how their cries resonate in your physical and emotional body, and have compassion for your child. If you listen closely to your baby, you will likely have a sense of what exactly your baby is crying about. Never abandon, punish, control or threaten in any way your child because he cries. Let him cry, and encourage him to release all of his feelings, while physically holding him. Thwarting your child's crying in any way gives him the imprint that his expression of life through crying is bad. It doesn't cure his crying; it makes him hide his crying inside, which causes very uncomfortable inner turmoil. Suppressing any of a child's communication to its parents will result in the child concluding that part or all of him is bad. The child will believe that in life he is unseen and unheard. If your baby is crying give him what he needs, and if he continues to cry, or cries because he feels hurt, then listen to it. Be with them compassionately until the crying is done. In this way, the child will feel that his expressions of frustration, pain, or sadness are accepted. When you do this, you will encourage an open line of communication with your child that will remain intact as he gets older.

A baby cries because he or she feels discomfort. This discomfort requires immediate attention from the parents. A baby cries because he is hungry, he is in physical pain, he has an unresolved pain from the past, he needs holding, he is frustrated, or he feels conflict in his parents. For example, if the mother or father is angry, this can strongly upset a baby since he can feel the anger intensely even if it is not directed at him. In the early stages of his life, the baby's mood is very connected to how his parents feel.

If his parents are angry then he will feel uncomfortable.

Crying in the case of hunger, of needing to be held, or because of physical or emotional pain needs to be addressed by the parents immediately. On the other hand, crying from frustration over, say, his toy breaking, or the shoe getting lost, needs to be honored and given space by the parent. This is another type of crying, which is sort of a growing pain. Many parents, however, assume that all crying is the "growing pain" variety, and that their child must work out his feelings by himself. In such cases, these parents are subconsciously hurting their child and getting negative pleasure from their treatment of their child. This all happens, as I said before, because the parents are numb to their own feelings, and they are teaching their child to be numb. I have seen that 90-100% of crying from my daughter is not the result of her imbalances, or her learning to deal with the world, but a result of her pain from the imbalances in myself and Michelle. She responds to our collective familial imbalances. The conflicts that seem normal to adults or do not bother us can be torture to children, as they can feel them acutely. **I have seen strange, unexplained crying in my daughter that stopped when my partner changes her mood and state of being.**

Babies and children wish to constantly experience pleasure. Everything they do is designed to give them more physical enjoyment and to have more fun. When their current of pleasure is thwarted by an unloving, or not fully aware parent, this can cause a child great agony and frustration. A child sees some crayons lying on the floor and begins to color all over the walls. He experiences great pleasure and bliss as he picks up the colors and, smiling and laughing, moves toward the wall. Then suddenly, mother comes and shouts "Don't do that! Stop!" Children do not think anything they do is wrong or bad, because it is not. Children have incomplete awareness and control, so how could anything they do be wrong? And yet they get the message that they did something wrong when they feel a strong negative energy emanating from their parents.

In the case of trauma and unresolved pain, the child will repeatedly create situations when he begins to feel tense and emotionally irritated, as if everything is bothering him. An aware care-taker will be able to witness this, and give the child emotional space, usually while holding the child, to release and discharge his or her pent up emotions. A common way that parents do not give children emotional space is by trying to "fix" the feeling. Parents typically distract their children from discomfort, for example. Or they thwart expressions of pain by shushing the baby, or by trying to make the baby laugh. **This thwarts the useful purpose of crying. The parent's job is not to stop the crying, but to address the cause of crying.** The parent also might give up, or withdraw because he does not understand his child's behavior. It may seem to be unreasonable behavior, but really the child is trying to heal an imbalance, and trying to make sense of the world. His actions come from innocence and are harmless. If your child's feelings are hurt, he or she needs to have the experience of feeling these hurt feelings (this does not mean abandoning the child to "learn" from the growing experience, as I have said). If you distract him from feeling his hurt by giving him cookies or making him laugh, he won't have the opportunity to discharge his emotions. He will also become a cookie addict. Another mistake parents make is to abandon their child by letting him "cry it out." This is a cruel thing to do and is a passive aggressive form of punishment. It gives your child the message that getting upset is unreasonable, and he will be punished for it through emotional abandonment by his parents. As you saw in the drawings, when a child "cries it out" alone he becomes disassociated from his body because the feelings are too intense to experience without the grounding support of a parent. If you notice yourself feeling uncomfortable when your baby is crying, be alert and present. Do not try to fix your uncomfortable feeling. Allow your child to have his feelings and at the same time, take necessary action if something physical needs to be taken care of. If it is not a physical concern and your child is sad, or feeling some type of emotional hurt, just be present with him, holding him compassionately, tolerat-

ing his pain, and allowing the feeling to be completely released. When a child has a hurt and he is not allowed to fully cry and release the hurt, then his body will slowly become frozen, as it is part of our biology to fully release our emotions. Children are often upset about some behavior related to their parents not being aligned with their higher selves. In this circumstance the parents will need to tolerate their own distorted emotions in order to be able to hold a safe space to witness and honor their child's feelings.

Michelle says: "We live in a divine universe and we are all divine creations from love. The challenge is that an aspect of ourselves has forgotten the experience of this reality. When our children and babies cry, it is because they do not feel love pouring from us. We do not believe anymore that we are living in a pure and loving universe, and it is our responsibility as adults to challenge this belief. It's perfectly normal for babies and children to cry. Understand that their cries are for perfection in the world and for contact with the divine, the more perfect world they came from. It is important for us adults to remember that it is possible for this world to be peaceful and harmonious. Our children can tell us exactly when we are off the mark, not being our true selves. Any time they cry or make us feel frustrated or agitated it is really our problem, not theirs. Our love for them is blocked, and our agitation is a sign of our own imbalance. This gives us a perfect opportunity to look deeply into those imbalances and bring compassion and love for those parts of ourselves. When we can allow our feelings through acceptance, we can learn to love our children in deeper ways."

Children Want to Participate and Be Treated As Equals

Babies, toddlers, and all children want to mimic and copy what adults do. Children have an innate ability to learn what their parents do, and your child will copy your various behaviors, even how you pick up a spoon, or how you move your lips to make words, because he intimately knows you and feels a part of you. Nature designed the child to copy the parents' pattern of survival, which works well when the parents know how to function well, emotionally and actively, in the world. Keep this thought in mind in Chapter 12 on schooling; because when children cannot mimic their parents' or adults' patterns of success, then they miss out on an important developmental stage.

To educate a child, we need to allow him to copy what he perceives as our patterns of survival. We do not have to force children to participate in what we do, but we need to allow them to participate in reasonable ways in adult activities. For example, if a mother is washing dishes, the child naturally wants to copy the mother and wash dishes. Now, the child may only want to wash the dishes for five minutes and then do something else. A space can be set up for the child with a small sponge and water so she can play and pretend to wash dishes. The dishes may not actually get clean, and the child's version of washing dishes might be spilling water everywhere, but the child has fun because she has a sense of <u>participation and belonging</u>. When the child is older, she will want to help out by washing the dishes, and by then she will be an expert at it. It is a child's longing, and Nature's intent, that a child feels a part of her clan (family) through participation in the normal activities of the adults. Normal adult activities are caring for other children, food preparation, food gathering (usually done at the grocery store), and income producing activities.

This idea is contrary to the notion of forcibly training your child. If you command and order your child around, you will inhibit this natural process and usurp his own budding sense of will and independence. Never force a child to do any activity, unless there is an emergency. When a child is forced to do something, he equates working with being forced and usually does not feel happy with the activity since he did not choose it. The child is then split between his desire to do what the parent wants, and the desire to act spontaneously in the moment. When I use a computer, I let my daughter have time to use it as well. She just hits the keyboard, but she is still learning my patterns of success. (She is very bored with the computer and doesn't last too long here, and it's probably not her path.) It is important to know that children do not always have long attention spans (neither do many adults). Naturally, they want to play and do many things. So make a space for your child to participate in the family, and allow your child to exercise her free will to decide to participate or not. Healthy parents trust their child's inner will to determine what activity the child wants to do. If the child is given space and allowed to express her own volition and will, then the child will equate working with playing. In the long run, if given her personal freedom your child will automatically feel full enthusiasm for everything you do. She will find happiness in cooking, cleaning, talking on the phone, shopping, or whatever it is you feel is important.. Parents need to be supportive of their child's instincts and developing will. Children need to be allowed to be children. Children are unable to follow many of the unrealistic expectations parents have for them because they are not in the stage of development when they can meet those demands. When children begin the transition to adulthood, around age 14, they will be able to be responsible in those specific ways we want. But we can't expect this from them at age 2.

In *The Magical Child*, Joseph Pierce writes of the different stages of the child's development. To support your child's development, the environment must acknowledge the developmental period the child is in. In other words, you cannot teach a two-year-old to read, or to cook his own food. But you can teach that to a twelve-year-old. It is common for parents who are not in touch with their child's developmental stage to rush through the early phases of their children's development. They try to get their child to take on the productive capacities of later stages when the children are still the most needy. Or the opposite happens, and they spoil the child by giving him too much of what the child does not need (lots of toys, for example).When a child is spoiled like this, he never has the space to develop his own sense of self and uniqueness in the world, and remains unhealthily needy. So there are two extremes: the child is forced to grow up too rapidly by unreasonable expectations and demands, or he is not given space to grow up, and is forced to remain child-like. Most parents oscillate along the entire spectrum, depending on the situation. How do you know if you have imbalanced parenting practices? You can only know to the degree that you are aware of your own internal habits and patterns. By noticing the sensations in your body as you live in the present moment, you can get a sense of how harmonious your parenting is. If you feel good about yourself and life and if parenting seems conflict-free then you are in some degree of harmony. If you don't know how you feel, or wish that you felt good and are many times struggling with your child, then you are out of harmony (and remember, it is not their fault; it is your responsibility to change).

Children's Pleasure Principle and Taboos

Perhaps you can feel yourself holding your breath from just reading the title of this section. I know I can feel myself straining as I hold my own breath. Pleasure is the natural expansion into life that allows the free flow of our full energy currents. It is accurate to state that in our culture we have taboos attached to the pleasure principle, and especially when speaking of children. We must speak about our experience, and acknowledge our feelings about our children's expression of their pleasure principle so that we can create a safe and nurturing space for them to explore their self expression. If they are allowed this, they will open up to feeling more love and enjoyment for everything. Wanting your child to feel good and enjoy life is an aspect of your

higher parenting self—the divine parent that can blossom within and through you.

Embrace, accept, and honor your child's pleasurable feelings. The Pathwork suggests that we cannot separate our pleasure stream from our feelings of love. [466] Further:

The truth is that infants experience physical pleasure more strongly than the average adult human being. The infant is not burdened with guilts, shames and misconceptions... Thus, in the child's early years, its pleasure is directed to its immediate environment — to the parents. [467]

The child's currents of pleasure are an inherent part of Nature's design for the human being. Parents need to witness, and emotionally honor their child's pleasure currents. When the child's natural pleasure principle is not thwarted but allowed to develop normally, the child progresses towards healthy adult sexuality and thus to healthy adult relationships and feelings of love.

When the baby is caressed, fed, loved, it experiences acute physical pleasure in contact with its surroundings. [468]

As I mentioned before, the child experiences intense pleasure in contact with his or her parents. Whether or not of the same sex, each parent stands in the foreground at certain periods of the child's development. This is normal and healthy for these limited periods. But such feelings are labeled sinful and perverse. The child soon absorbs these ideas, even when they are not expressed directly, because they permeate the atmosphere and the adults' conscious and unconscious thinking. [469]

The basic struggle of the infant is to attain the pleasure and eliminate that which stands in the way. This simple, primitive struggle still exists within each individual. [470]

As parents, we strive to maximize our pleasure and minimize the pain we experience in parenting and in life in general. For example, we take more vacations, make more money so we can have fun, and do less work so we have more time for recreation. That is exactly what our children do as well. We do not want to experience pain, and we do not want our children to experience pain. Many times, however, we mistakenly create taboos or express our squeamishness in regard to our children's pleasure impulses. Children's pleasure impulses can include physically caressing their parents, breastfeeding, playing with their bodies, including touching their genitals, and running around naked and spreading their legs in ways that adults normally do not do. Children also love to make huge messes, yell, scream, and otherwise dive in to explore the world in a big way. Children's pleasure-seeking activities are natural, playful, fully-engaged leaps of exploration.

I encourage you to honor your flow of life, and the flow of natural feelings in your children. Be aware of your boundaries, and maintain a safe space for your children to feel their full and pleasure-filled selves, so that they may mature into healthy adults who can easily create fulfilling relationships. Our pleasure currents are an instinctual drive towards wholeness. When you honor these strong and healthy impulses, you have gone a long way to helping your child grow and mature.

Circumcision

Please do not circumcise your infant boy. If you could ask your child for permission to perform the procedure, he would tell you that he does not want to be circumcised.

Circumcision as it is practiced today is much different from how it used to be practiced. As a religious rite of passage, it was done approximately at age 13. In **ancient Jewish circumcision, the entire foreskin was not cut off, but just a tiny bit of the tip**, and only as a token. There are many writings that describe how ancient Jews could conceal their circumcision by placing a small tie or other holder on their

remaining foreskin, which was already a custom in Greek culture, where nudity was normal in public baths and other social interactions. While the traditional age of ancient circumcision is unclear it is likely that this tradition mimicked the custom of many other native groups, and occurred close to the age of 13. It is possible that later religious traditions have changed to insist that circumcision occur during the infant stage when the boy is not able to protest.

Routine medical circumcision as practiced today is not the same procedure as the small token of foreskin taken as a rite of passage for adolescent boys. It is male genital mutilation. In the modern procedure, the entire foreskin is removed completely. How we progressed to removing the entire foreskin of infants just a few days old I do not know. I believe it is a very cruel mistake that we continue to circumcise newborn infants, no matter what the claimed reason. There is no biblical commandment that states, "Circumcise your newborn infant." If there were good religious or ceremonial reasons to circumcise boys in the United States, then we would need to use more traditional standards, and wait for the child to reach age thirteen. At that age, it is then possible to use local anesthesia for pain, and the child understands what is happening, and has developed physically, emotionally and sexually while remaining completely intact. The advantage to holding off circumcision until this age is that the boy will develop a relationship to his genitals as Nature intended. Nature intended for boys to have a foreskin during their very early formative years. The foreskin is a guardian, and through childhood it protects and allows your son to experience a natural form of self-exploration. When an infant is circumcised, the erotic tip of his penis is prematurely exposed to his awareness. The process is excruciatingly painful. The imprint of the circumcised male is that life is painful, that having a penis is a cause of pain, and that one is punished for his masculinity. He may also believe that it is normal for men to be sexually and physically abused. In about 80% of the world males are left as Nature intended. Circumcision does not prevent any type of disease in any way, as popular propaganda and myths would have you believe. Infants go into traumatic shock or scream violently when the flesh on the most sensitive part of their body is cut off. Circumcision can disrupt the child's bonding with his mother and cause the infant to act irritated. Side effects include hemorrhage, infection, and even in rare cases, death. [471]

When examined more closely, circumcision even conflicts with many traditional Jewish laws and values, such as doing no harm. [472]

The American Academy of Pediatrics came out against routine circumcision over 30 years ago, citing "limited scientific evidence to support or repudiate the routine practice of male circumcision." [473] Cutting a young baby's skin with a knife without anesthesia is a malicious form of cruelty, and it should be made illegal.

In a greater sense, we need to ask ourselves why we need to cut our little boys' penises when they are born. Have we gone mad? This is an assault on manhood. Are we saying the male penis is wrong and bad, so we must deform it after birth? When you wonder why the distorted male consciousness is running amuck on this planet, then look no further than this painful imprint given to many infant boys.

What many women and men don't know aout circumcision is that the foreskin plays an important role in adult sexual intercourse. A circumcised penis functions differently from an uncircumcised penis in the sexual act. The foreskin provides an extra layer which reduces friction and in important ways changes the experience of the sexual act. The foreskin also protects the male's sensitive glands, leaving them softer, more lubricated and more sensitive than the uncircumcised male. As couples have reported, when the male has restored his foreskin through "foreskin restoration," intercourse is much more fun and enjoyable. Foreskin restoration is a long but relatively painless process involving various methods and devices to safely stretch the foreskin, over a period of one to several years.

For further information visit:
www.circumcision.org, and
www.jewishcircumcision.org.

Car Seats

Car seats are made for babies, but babies are not made for car seats.

Certain common aspects of modern society quickly become obstacles for mothers who wish to keep the continuum of care of their infant intact. One such obstacle is the car seat. Though laws vary from state to state, my understanding of the law in California is that a child is required to be locked into a car seat while the vehicle is moving or is in the flow of traffic. Now as you well know, babies and young children want to be held by their mothers and want to breastfeed, so they don't want to be locked in a car seat. Some mothers might claim that the right to breastfeed one's child overrides the legal requirement to have a child in a car seat. I am not a legal expert, so I cannot say if this is the case. Still, many mothers resort to abandoning their children in the back seat while the child cries and screams for their attention and struggles against the restraints.

We have dealt with this predicament in the following way. Until Sparkle was older, I always drove with Michelle and Sparkle in the back seat. Michelle could breastfeed and remain connected to Sparkle. Breastfeeding in a car seat is uncomfortable for the mother and baby. If Sparkle complained too much then we would pull over, go for a walk, and then put her back in. When Sparkle was younger she hated car seats. As a result, we rarely drove her anywhere. When we did drive, we waited for her to take a nap, and then off we went. Sometimes we would wake up very early to run our errands and she would sleep in the car. When Sparkle was older, around the age of three, Michelle made short driving trips with her in the back seat. Sparkle had a blast.

You may have a car-seat-happy-baby, but in general babies don't like car seats. They scream when confined and kept away from their mommies. There are no legal alternatives that I know of to allow the baby to stay on the mother's lap. Of course, there are transportation alternatives: riding a bike with a front-mounted car seat facing the parent, walking, using horse and buggy, or taking public transportation are just a few ways in which the mother can hold her child. In most states, if your car or truck only has front seats you can legally have the baby in the front, so at least they can see you and you can touch them while you drive. Managing a car seat can be very difficult and we still have frequent difficulties with this issue.

There are many ways to maintain the continuum of care while driving. Some are legal, some not so legal; some are safe and others not so safe. It's not the baby's fault that he wants to be connected to his mommy, but our fault for disrupting that process through restraint systems that separate the bond. Really take time to consider ways to foster the bond between mother and child during transportation, and invite in your creativity and the deva spirit of driving babies safely, to help you find healthy ways to transport your children.

With the problem of driving in mind, we tried to choose our living location with adequate activities to do without driving. For you, this might mean living near a playground or a park. For four years we lived within walking distance of the beach, so Michelle went to the beach every day for her activity. Now we live in a forest, so there are places right at hand for walks and a stream to visit. All of these require no driving at all.

Conclusion

The infant was designed by Nature's ineffable laws. The infant has certain expectations of life and of her parents that were programmed into her by the Creator. These expectations are easy to summarize. Your child expects to be fully loved and cared for and to have all of her needs met. Your son or daughter expects to be held, nurtured, and to be kept by your side. Your child expects to be fed nurturing breast milk.

The result of keeping the continuum in place for Sparkle for four and a half years now, is that we experience her as being with us as a family, as if we are one entity or unit. She has been included in almost every activity we do, which gives me a feeling of peace and contentment. Michelle and I feel we are deeply connected to her. I am intimately aware of her needs and

wants, and I desire to fulfill them. Now when I do things without her, which is not very often, I feel a sense of loss. I wish she were with me so that we can experience the joy of living together.

The supposed "freedom" parents enjoy by abandoning their children are desires of a numbed mind. The selfish "little me" in us, the childish inner part, would rather go traveling, spend the day out, or go out to a nice restaurant, club, or party instead of being with the children. If there is an activity that Michelle and I are interested in attending which does not include children, we simply do not go. If others cannot honor our children then they do not honor us as parents. Since most parents give in to their selfish desires at one time or another, fulfilling our selfish desires at the cost of being present parents has become acceptable and the encouraged norm for our culture. Having fought through those negative desires, I can assuredly tell you that it is not children who are wrong for wanting to be with their parents. **It is our society and our culture and parents who are wrong for not wanting to be with their children**. We are wrong for not establishing societal norms and social settings where children are an included part of life.

As I am thinking and feeling about my connection with my daughter, she is calling for me in the other room. She says, "Hug you," which means that she wants me to give her a hug. And like the hundreds or thousands of times before, I stop what I am doing, leave my desk to go pay attention to my daughter and give her a hug.

When we deeply honor ourselves, we deeply honor our children. Your child is designed to feel this honoring and to elicit it from you. Your child is designed by Nature to be loved and to be acknowledged. Ultimately, your child is a child of God, and on a spiritual level he is designed to be treated as an individual and at the soul level, as an equal.

The choice is yours: take up the challenge to honor the innate needs of your true self, and thus honor the innate needs of your child, and receive the creative fulfillment of honoring your destiny in the world. Or, create vast amounts of suffering. As we proceed to the next chapter, I will

help remind you of the wise choice arising from
deep within.

10

Parenting: The Center of Your Longing

Parenting is a fundamental part of the experience of being human. To become a parent may be the one life experience which changes your whole life's purpose. Committing fully to your role as a parent is a fulfillment of your longing to understand your purpose for being in this world.

Intention: To help you realize part of your real purpose in life — to be a nurturing parent. To do this we must look at what makes us good parents, and what inhibits us from being good parents.

The sooner you understand that negative thoughts and feelings are obstacles to your ability to parent, the easier parenting will be. Wise parents know that when there is difficulty with their child, whatever it may be, the difficulty is an opportunity for their own awakening. Wise parents know that their young child has no self; that is, no negative aggrandized self, and so their child expects the same selflessness from his parents. When you maintain a rigid and frozen belief system about who you are and how you live life, you will tend to use your defensive mechanisms of control, avoidance, and blame in your approach to parenting. However, when you have an expanded sense of self, then you are able to engage the higher qualities of love, devotion, patience and clarity to aid you in your parenting. The negative self resists change and hinders expansion. So as a parent, you are constantly negotiating between this *higher self* and the *lower self.*

As a parent it is important to be completely honest with yourself. Acknowledge when you feel tired, hurt, or incapable. Through experiencing your inner truths and through feeling hidden fears (which will emerge in your role as a parent), you can find your steadfastness and inner strength. In Chapter 2, we learned of the Loetschental Valley Swiss who paid homage to the kind *Father*, and his divine presence in the special summer butter. It is time for us to pay homage to this same kind *Father* in us, and in our children. It is time we pay homage to the evidence of his divine presence in ourselves, in our children, and in our spouses. Without the presence of the divine, how could we even exist? How was it that you met your spouse, chose a life together, and through your union now rejoice in your newborn child?

Loving Your Child Means Serving Your Child

Have I spent fourteen months of the last two and a half years of my life devoted to writing this book for personal gain or attention? No. While I will be grateful for any remuneration for my effort, and I do feel a sense of satisfaction from sharing with you, those are not my primary purposes in writing. I wrote this book as an act of selfless service. We should not continue to allow ourselves and our children to suffer. Through this book I wish to share with others what I know to be truthful, in the most honest way I can, and in the hope that I may help empower people to find their strength as parents.

I wrote this book in service to the goodness that is in you — that *is* you — which comes from the goodness in me. I write in service to the *higher self*, the divine spark in each of us that unites us all. I wish to honor you, and my connection to you, by writing what I hope will help you and your family to grow and to become healthy and prosperous in as many ways as possible.

For quite some time I didn't know what to do in my life and my constant prayer went something like this: "I know I can do something good for the world; I want to help people, but I don't know what to do. Please, show me, help me, let me be a vehicle for You. Let me be a vehicle for the highest goodness and truth to enter into this world. However it looks, I want it; help me open to it." And a few months later, I started writing. Then, without having much of a goal or plan in mind, I wrote a short version of this book to share with people. Wanting to expand on it, I wrote the full version, which you are now holding.

My intention to act selflessly was, and continues to be, inspired by the teachings of Amma (www.amma.org) who is known in the West as *The Hugging Saint*. A woman of Indian birth, Amma began her ministry in 1981, with the principal goals of aiding the disenfranchised, charity to the poor, and advocating peace among all religions. Her primary means of communication is through expressing her motherly compassion by hugging the many people who visit her. Amma is a vehicle for love to flourish in the world, and is a wonderful role model for us as parents, as she embodies the qualities of the infinitely compassionate, understanding, and patient divine mother. I am always moved to tears when I see her selflessly serve other people. When I visited her ashram, I experienced firsthand her unconditional love, which radiated a feeling of intense peace and joy that some have labeled as bliss, or a river of love. Her message is simple, and also similar to that of other spiritual teachers:

Love is our true essence. Love has no limitations of caste, religion, race or na-

tionality. We are all beads strung together on the same thread of love.[474]

I learned from her that if I truly believe in the higher qualities of love, compassion, truth, and justice, then my actions must reflect that truth. I interpret the core of her message to be something like: "Why waste your life in mundane pursuits? Why not take a leap of faith and do something extraordinary? Place your *selfish* goals and desires behind you and begin to embrace the attitude of compassion towards others." This awareness motivates us to behave differently, and is a gateway to a more fulfilling existence whose purpose is to be a servant to the divine.

One way you can experience or express love is through selfless service. Selfless service does not mean to give yourself away or to starve while you feed others. Selfless service is a practice that comes from the part of you that has no self. The self is the created identity you think you are. The self that says, "I am this." Or it says, "Life is this way." Selfless service demands service to the life force, in service of the purpose of life in order to experience peace, joy, and unity. When you let go of expectations of what you should be, of how life is, you can transcend your limited thinking mind and experience an ocean of love. For most people, this experience isn't a sudden great opening; it comes slowly through consistent practice. That feeling is in this book, to the degree that I can embody it. The more you read these words and breathe them in, the more you can expand and connect yourself with this timeless energy that has the power to change you in positive ways, and to point you in the right direction.

When you truly feel love and compassion in your heart, other people may not notice, since our culture does not value these emotions as highly as other social skills and ambitions. Dr. Weston Price, however, noted that the Australian Aborigines, who exhibited a high degree of alignment with Nature's laws, based their religion on the golden rule: "that life consists in serving others as one would wish to be served."[475] And when I see Amma devote herself to serving others, including serving and embracing me, I cannot help but want to do the same, in my own way. Amma gives freely to everyone; in her eyes all are equal and all deserve to be loved and cared for. She embodies the spirit of the Divine Mother, the ideal love that all children need. We needed it as children, and our own children need it now. Divine love is a total surrender to feelings, regardless of whether we think those feelings are positive or negative, in support of our children. The Divine Mother loves all of us unconditionally. You are loved by her.

Activity: divine love. Invite in the deva, the spirit of the Divine Mother (however you imagine her). Allow her to embrace you. Feel her love inside of you. When you feel loved within, this love is contagious and radiates to everyone.

I often feel tender compassion for all parents, and particularly for all children. I really understand and relate to children's challenging experiences of growing up. This book is intended to reduce or eliminate some suffering by offering you a truthful perspective on life, and by providing insights into the causes and effects of illness on all levels of your being. I find it incomprehensible and wrong that vital health information has been hidden from view. And so this book is my humble gift to you.

Right Action

Sometimes as a parent you are not going to know what to do. You might find yourself in a dilemma where you do not know what is right or wrong. There is a spiritual and yogic practice of right action that can help you to align your will power. While in many cases the right action is difficult to know, I will give you some pointers to help you discern the right action.

Right action will sometimes be a part of your parenting practice. If your child wakes up needing attention at 4:00 am and you have an appointment to make at 7:00 am, you may not be happy, and you may be so tired that you do not want to take care of your child. It may seem to you that your meeting is more important. But even when you feel totally miserable and unhappy, and resent your life as a parent, that precious being, your child, is still there by your side, still expecting you to be the perfect, attentive parent. Right action entails a philosophy similar to the concept discussed in the section on painless birth: "not my will, but Thy will" be done. Your child's needs are not designed to accommodate your schedule. Right action means understanding that you are greater than any petty doubts, fears and frustrations; it means serving your child unconditionally, while acknowledging the challenges and difficulties such a choice brings.

Parenting is a Part of Your Path Homeward

If you begin to experience chaos and craziness as a parent, you might start to wonder, "Why am I doing this?" You might ask yourself, "Who am I?"

Parenting is your opportunity to fulfill part of your spiritual purpose on Earth because it is an opportunity for you to become more aware of the moment and more open to love. It is an opportunity which you have the choice to embrace, or resist. Every moment there is a precious little being with you and her every thought and action brings your attention to the here and now. Your son, or daughter, is not lost in thought or distracted by the thousand things that typically make up the days and fill the heads of adults. Children can be beacons to the present moment, and help us understand our own inner child, as well as how to be free. The Pathwork says:

> *Every human being senses an inner longing that goes deeper than longings for emotional and creative fulfillment... If we would try to put the meaning of this longing into concise words, perhaps the most accurate "translation" would be that it is a feeling or sensing that another, more fulfilling state of consciousness and a larger capacity to experience life must exist... The longing is realistic when you start from the premise that the clue must lie in you; when you wish to find the attitudes in you that prevent you from experiencing life in a fulfilled and meaningful way; when you interpret the*

longing as a message from the core of your inner being, sending you on a path that helps you to find your real self. [476]

When you experience disharmony in your relationship with your children or your spouse, and you begin to look within for the answers of why is this happening to you, then you have embarked on your spiritual journey. Knowing that there is much to gain from understanding and acknowledging your hidden inner parts can be a positive motivation to face the difficult times of your life. This journey helps you grow as a person, and thus helps you fulfill the spiritual aspect of being incarnated in a body.

Allowing Your Child's Emotions through Accepting Your Own

You will no doubt have reactions to something that your child, spouse, or other family member does. In Chapter 7 on fertility, I discussed how our defensive postures can negatively affect our physical health. These defense mechanisms can and will affect your children when you become a parent.

Children will respond to and react to the hidden agendas and feelings that are within their parents, even if they don't do this consciously. A child will, for example, automatically react to your impatience, and act in ways that will make you feel more impatient. The child's response is an energetic mirror of your emotional state. No matter what you do to change the external environment, your child will still feel uncomfortable and perhaps provoke you, because he is reacting to something that is alive in you. Children can help magnify the internal distortions and conflicts that we harbor.

Thus, it is important and helpful to be very truthful and honest with ourselves, and to give our inner condition proper attention and acknowledgement. Take time or space to observe what you are experiencing and the sensations you notice in your body. You might say to yourself, "I feel impatient with my child." Or better yet, say this to someone else. Once you acknowledge the feeling, explore it. What is its purpose? Why is it there? I hope you will have

someone who can listen to you without reacting to you and without trying to "fix" your impatience. In that way, you will have some help to decipher the meaning of your hidden thoughts and feelings which have created your impatience.

People tend to become completely caught up with their emotions. In the moment, they "become" the emotion that they are experiencing. When you believe you are an emotion it seems that the only way to "fix" or alter the emotion is to create some change in the outer world. But this will only effect a superficial change. Let's say a mother cannot tolerate her feeling of impatience. This mother is having sensations of irritation and feels strain in her body. She loses sight of herself, forgets that she is an embodiment of love, and that her child needs her to care for her. Lost in the experience of impatience, she believes that she is the very embodiment of the discomfort that she is resisting. At that moment, the mother believes this feeling will never end, and so she is impatient, the impatience continues to build, and she does not want to tolerate the feeling anymore. Once she cannot tolerate the feeling, she will react to her child in a variety of ways, trying to make her impatience go away. She might snap at her child, yell, leave, or just shut herself down.

Sometimes outer world change is exactly what is needed. But often it is most important to simply feel one's feelings. Remember, you can take action and also feel your feelings at the same time. Every time you feel an uncomfortable emotion, try to be the awareness or space *around* the emotion. Fully feel the sensations of the life energy moving through your body in that moment. Emotion is energy in motion. If you can feel your emotional current fully, it will dissolve itself and disappear. When you don't feel it fully and avoid or resist it as most people do, it continues to return in a vicious cycle. Rather than shun or repress their feelings when their baby makes them upset, parents should embrace this as an opportunity for inner learning about the rough edges in their personalities. This is how the kind *Father* shows us where we are not aligned with life. He created your child and your partner to remind you of all your imperfections so that ultimately they can be healed. And make no mistake about it, <u>anything</u> can be healed and accepted. Without strong guidance most of us are not able to accept everything, and ultimately it is our own laziness, numbness and fear that keep us from releasing these emotions in a healthy way.

When a child is responding to an emotional hurt or pain you cannot fix the hurt, and you should not try to make your child stop crying. You need to hold a space of awareness, while in deep empathetic contact with your child, and give him the message that yes; it is okay to feel upset with life, even to be angry at your parents. Your child wants to know that if he is in pain he will still be honestly loved and accepted for who he is. If he is not given the space to be upset, the imprint he receives is, "When I am hurt, I am not loved." The conclusion about life the child might then make is, "I should not be hurt, or show my hurt, or I won't be loved." From this conclusion many of the child's feelings go into a dark closet and are forgotten until one day he becomes a father and the cycle begins again. Young children experience many frustrations and pains in their daily lives. They need supportive parents who give them the assurance that it is okay to be loud and to express their feelings about life, whether these feelings are happy or sad, bright or dark. They want to know that they are fully accepted for being that way. The Pathwork explains that when a childhood pain is naturally gone through and endured, it ceases and does not create numbing defenses.

Feeling pain directly and fully strengthens resilience and the ability to live fruitfully and productively, and it certainly increases the capacity for experiencing pleasure and deep feelings. It is only where pain has not been experienced that defensive numbness occurs -- and hence neurosis, destructiveness, deadness.[477]

In other words, it will be helpful for your child's emotional health if you adopt the attitude that it is acceptable for him to experience his feelings, no matter how loud, obnoxious, or angry your child becomes. Now, the feelings

might need some directing: if your child is angry and throwing rocks at your car or, even worse, the neighbor's car, you won't want that to continue. But you could allow him to throw stuffed animals, or other softer objects. Allowing the expression of your baby's or child's feelings is different from the modern parenting strategy, which is to fix, distract, derail, ridicule, ignore, or avoid the child's painful feelings.

Witnessing and experiencing is a tool used to help us engage more with life. To witness is to benignly watch and observe ourselves compassionately from a loving and patient perspective. The witness is the observer underneath your thoughts that simply witnesses without reacting. Witnessing helps us detach ourselves from our emotional reactions and to see them through fully. To be clear, the objective is not to avoid your emotions, but to witness them and let them be felt. Each of us has many different aspects of our personality. We have many different sub-personalities and moods. These parts are often in conflict with each other, and produce uncomfortable feelings. Witnessing your feelings gives you the space to feel the full range of emotions that come with being a mother or a father. When you make mistakes, rather than judge yourself look at the origins of your judgments, and how they create and enforce a negative self identity. Take a moment now and witness your thoughts. What are you thinking? Witness your feelings; how do you feel? Witness your body; what are the sensations right now? How are you breathing? Witness your spirit; what does your soul long for? Witness the world around you; what do you perceive through your senses? Practice being your own witness and notice when and how you take stock of your life.

Daily review, as previously discussed in Chapter 7, is a process that supports your healthy growth as a parent. It allows you to observe your disharmonies in a way that creates a positive energy current towards healthy change. Please attempt to practice the review (or to write in your journal about your difficulties and frustrations as a parent) at least twice a week, and ideally once a day. Practicing the daily review can be quite pleasurable, which should help motivate you to do it regularly. The daily review will help you feel better about yourself and your situation, and bring clarity to your problem solving. From the daily review that I practiced for myself, I was able to make the next leap and now share some of my conflicts with Michelle. When she simply listens without offering critical comments, usually a solution pops into my head. The daily review, done by yourself or with a friend or partner, in the end will help you be more empowered in life by enhancing your ability to make good decisions and to use your time more wisely.

Embrace your Dark Side

Our shadow aspects—our unconscious darker sides—represent a denser, lower-vibration energy in our being. These aspects are sort of like the bad part of town, but it's inside of us. There is litter everywhere and the buildings are falling apart. In this internal dilapidated slum anger, rage, pain, greed and other negative feelings lurk. The lower self arises as a defense against our pain, our numbness to our feelings, and it is a way we disconnect ourselves from others. Our dark side is the negativity we act out with ourselves and others.[178] Your child can see, feel, experience, and even bring out your dark side. The dark side remains in darkness because we secretively choose to keep it hidden, and therefore also keep it alive. Our dark aspects remain strong and powerful when we deny that we have negative impulses, thoughts, and feelings. That denial of the inner darkness contains within it negative pleasure. Whenever you have a negative experience that results in uncomfortable feelings of envy, greed, spite, hatred, anger, maliciousness and so forth, welcome it. This is not to say that you should act out these feelings unconsciously, but welcome and observe these dark emotions in the light of your objective awareness. I know it doesn't feel good; it creates tension, and is uncomfortable, but those discomforts must be gone through, like growing pains. By embracing these dark emotions and being thankful that you can find or see them, they slowly begin to dissolve and lose their power. We can therefore illuminate our darkness by

going through it. A significant portion of our darkness arose from our imprint in childhood, from the day we were born when we were not loved the way we longed to be. Within many of our adult bodies is a hurt, abandoned and mistreated child. When the inner child acts up, try to understand her experience, so that she can get the love and care that will help transform her negative feelings.

Practice Core Energetics or Bio-Energetics

Negative feelings arise in everyone, and it is not uncommon for a parent to feel frustrated half of the day. So, you need some techniques to help you deal with these feelings. Ignoring our feelings—including hunger or thirst—will eventually lead to a sour mood. Sour moods can negatively affect and even unconsciously harm your precious child. One good solution for this dilemma comes from the work of Alexander Lowen and John Pierrakos, who were both students of the famous psychologist Wilhelm Reich. Originally the work was called Bio-energetics. When the two creators separated, John Pierrakos formed Core-energetics, which is similar in many ways to Bio-energetics.

According to Bio-energetics, feelings become stored in our physical bodies, particularly in our musculature. New feelings may be stored on top of older emotions. Through various emoting types of movements you can help release these trapped feelings. A typical emotion that many of us embody is anger or rage. Rather than hold in the rage and keep it bottled up, you can release it by hitting pillows (or via other creative forms of safe acting out). In this way you do not direct the anger or hostility toward your child or spouse, but direct it away from them, into a neutral source such as the pillow.

If you do not understand what it is like to release your feelings, then you can look towards your children as examples. When they are angry they might jump up and down. Or they might hit people or throw things. These are just their natural unbiased impulses. If Sparkle gets angry and starts hitting things, rather than try to punish her I encourage her. I stick out my hands and let her hit or kick me. I let her be angry at me. Michelle does the same. Needless to say, her anger is short lived and in fact she is rarely angry. Remember, never punish your child for his expression, or the resulting repression will feed his negativity and hurt. Try to understand and heal the experience that caused the behavior.

If you frequently experience feelings of laziness, stagnation, dissatisfaction, lack of aggression, then this is a good sign that you have repressed your anger and hostility. As a practice, just hit some pillows or the mattress every morning. Making sounds as you do so also helps. When you perform these exercises, make sure your child feels safe or that you are in another room. The aim is to consciously acknowledge your anger or rage. Usually a child will copy his parent; so if a child has tantrums, then you might also be having your own version of tantrums that you are not totally aware of.

Michelle says: "Part of the job of the child is to provoke the parent; some will do this more than others. It is normal for children to have tantrums. Be a role model and show them how to use that energy in a healthy and positive way. To respond in supportive ways requires creativity and spontaneity. It is not always the same every time. We shouldn't smother our children's feelings and tell them not to cry or have tantrums. We should help guide their energy to positive outlets of expression."

Alexander Lowen's *The Way to Vibrant Health: a Manual of Bioenergetic Exercises*, is full of these demonstrative exercises with illustrations and descriptions of how to perform them.

Feeling Irritable and Irrational?

Your mood, or your spouse's or children's mood, is <u>substantially</u> affected by both the type of food you eat and the overall health of your body. When you have a short fuse, or act or feel irrational and impatient, you are probably just really hungry. I have noticed this in myself, and I assume it is very common that people ignore their hunger needs. This comes from the early childhood imprint of being ignored. When you

are hungry, you usually do not have much time before you will go over the edge emotionally. I believe that as our hunger increases our body actually starts to shut down, like the sleep mode on your computer. Your blood sugar declines rapidly when hunger sets in. Following the dietary guidelines suggested in this book helps to reduce these stressful periods, as your blood sugar levels will be much more stable.

Have You Forgotten?

Many parents-to-be and even adults who are already parents have lost touch with one of the deepest of our soul's longings — to have a child. Even if you do not feel this longing, or only feel it at times, search for it. You can observe this in your children because their longing is only to be with you. Your longing, therefore, is to be with them. Do not doubt it. In fact, nothing will bring you more fulfillment than bringing your full and attentive presence to being with your young son or daughter. This truth is encoded in our DNA. Who put it there?

The creator Herself.

In allowing this truth to manifest itself, you allow one of the divine purposes of creation to unfold. There cannot be a higher, more spiritual, or more worthy task than to be with, and experience life in close communion with your children. And a crucial part of being with your children is being engaged positively in relationship with your spouse. Your children need both of you united in love and mutual support.

The Call of Life

Real change begins when you acknowledge deeply and honestly to yourself that you have the dangerous potential to create pain for the one person whom you love the most, your child. When you walk with the knowledge that you are imperfect (in a non-judgmental way), that you are fragile, and that your life is temporary and impermanent, then that knowledge allows the dimension of timelessness to be here in you. You want to walk in the world acknowledging that you are human and fallible. It is through your deepest humility and truthfulness that you can find your faith, your trust, and your divine self. The ego can thrive upon suffering and negativity; that is why popular cinema and the news are filled with just that. The Pathwork explains:

> *The actual — not theoretical — activation of the real self with its vibrating life, limitless abundance, infinite possibilities for good, and its supreme wisdom and joy happens to the exact degree that you dare take a look at the temporary truth of yourself. This means feeling what you feel; having the courage to transform yourself into a better human being for no other reason than a desire to contribute to life, rather than to make an impression and grasp for approval. When the immediate barriers to transformation for its own sake are overcome, then the real self with all its treasures will clearly manifest.[479]*

Noticing Your Defense

When we were children, many of us did not receive everything that we needed and wanted from our parents. As children we learned how to constrain and censor the life force flowing into our bodies, and the result is that we hold back, control, attack and avoid many life experiences. The partial cutting off of the life force means that we do not often feel bliss and pleasure. Our children constantly need and long for us to hold and love them. In order to begin to free ourselves from the shackles of separation, we must notice our defensive behaviors so that we can understand and feel the real emotions that motivate and fuel them.

Pride

The prideful part of us is the distorted aspect that thinks, "I am better than you." This is not the proud parent who feels a glow at her child's every success. Rather, pride is a defensive mechanism we use to protect ourselves from pain. For example, the young child in the image wants to "Play, play, play!" His mother has had enough playing; she is above that. She is above her child's needs. She wants to "relax" and not do anything. She feels unhappy and overly tired but doesn't know why. Rather than play with her child, she ignores him. He notices his mother is ignoring him and tries harder to get her attention, until she finally snaps at him in anger.

Michelle says: "We all have defensive postures. It is important to accept that they are there. This is a human flaw and you do not have to take it personally that you have them. We typically hide the negative aspects of ourselves and pretend they are not there. We can really start working on the long process of changing them only when we first own up to them. Otherwise we will always be wondering why things are wrong and never find the source of the problem."

Self Will

Self will is the overuse of will in an attempt to control the outer world. This is a real mistake since we can control so few of the things that we wish we could. Control is actually an attempt to censor our real feelings, rather than take rightful action in the world. Self will is disconnected from wisdom and from emotion, and so thwarts fulfillment and creates negativity. Self will is imposing and tyrannical, and other people can feel it. Tyrants can be passive as well; be aware of the lazy tyrant who gets his way through manipulation.

Mother in Pride Defense

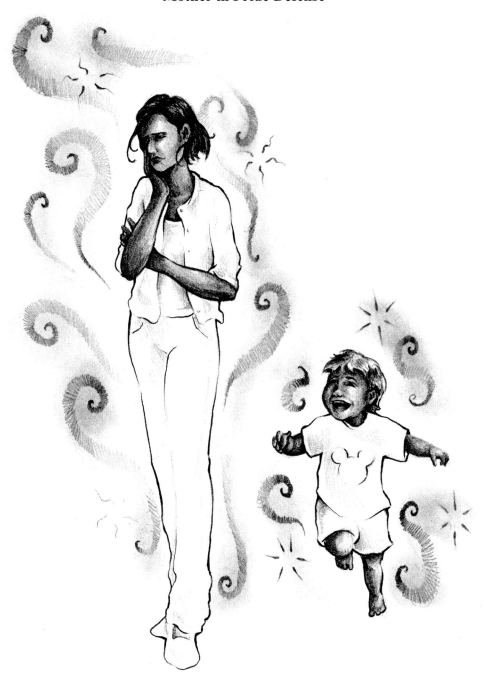

In this picture, you see the child being his normal innocent self. This child wants and needs attention from his mother. The mother in the picture feels scornful, irritated or upset at her child. She also thinks that these feelings are "bad" or "wrong" to have. Rather than project them at her child, she lifts her energy up and away. Soon this child will feel upset and rejected because his mother was not present for him. The pride defense can also be manifested as passive-aggressive behavior.

Father in Self Will Defense

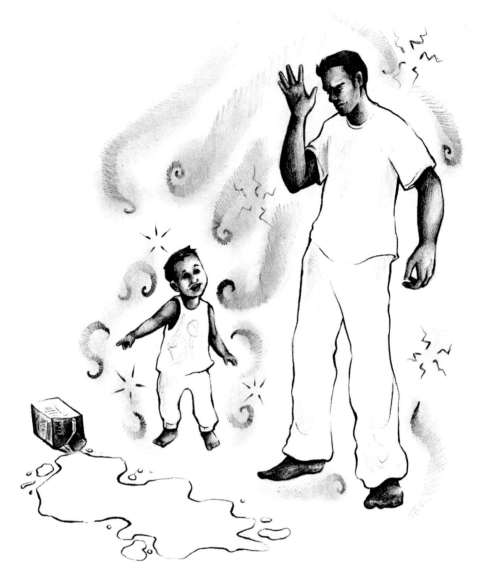

In this picture the child is so happy to have discovered how much fun it is to spill milk all over the floor. He wants his father to be proud of his joyful creation of milk artwork. His father is tired, and has been working on household repairs all day; the last thing he wants to do is clean up the child's mess. He is wondering when his son will grow up and be a good boy. The father sends out controlling and forceful energy to try to "teach" his child not to spill the milk and not to inconvenience his father anymore. The father is trying to teach his child, "This is how life is." And, "Do not have fun if it bothers me." In the picture the child is still happy after he spills the milk. "How exciting," he thinks. His father is angry, "Don't do that! Bad!" Once the child receives this huge dose of negative, forceful energy he will feel humiliated, as if he were bad. The child wants his father to honor his excitement and mirror it back to him. Now the child may feel so ashamed of himself *that he stops drinking milk, or stops playing with toys in certain ways. The shame comes from somewhere deep down, feeling that his father does not love him. And at that moment it is true that his father did not act from his heart. Because the child is still not individuated, he will reflect his father's withholding of love on his own self image. He will grow up to not love himself in certain ways and the pattern will continue.*

Mother in Defense of Fear

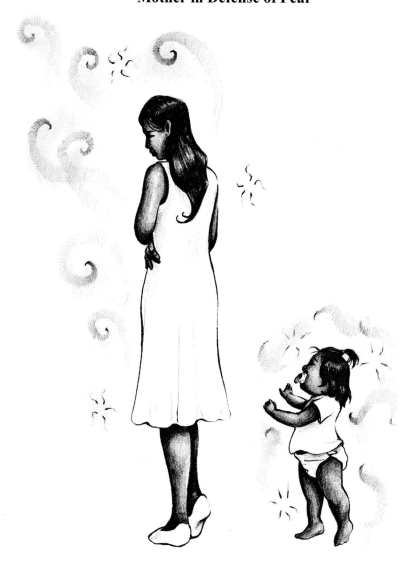

This mother is pulling her energy away from her child because she experiences her child's innate needs as too much for her to deal with. As a result, she has pacified her daughter with a pacifier. But her daughter's neediness will not go away; in fact, the more she tries to teach her daughter how not to be needy, the needier her daughter becomes. In the mother's mind, there is something else she needs to do. She does not know what it is. She thinks that if she gets what she needs then finally she will be able to give her daughter what her daughter needs. But until the mother figures it out, she

finds her daughter's needs annoying. This mother is disconnected from her feelings. She wishes her child would learn to be less needy and learn to take care of herself. Her strategy is to ignore her child until her child gives up being needy. In essence, this mother is defending her feelings of not wanting to be a mother. She is missing out on the joy, and fulfillment of giving to her daughter. Grief separates the mother from the experience of communion with her daughter. This mother's real need is to feel her grief and sadness so that she can be present for her child. What the mother feels is missing is really a part of herself. The daughter will feel miserable about herself and eventually become enraged and despondent because she is never mothered and her mother always avoids being present for her.

Undefended Mother*: This mother uses a balance of her reason, will and emotion in a positive way. She is not perfect; however, she accepts when she is imperfect and looks for the deeper truth underlying her errors. She lives in communion with her daughter. She sees, knows, and feels that her daughter's needs are also her own needs. Her daughter's needs speak to a part of herself that wants to fulfill those needs. This mother experiences a real feeling of joy and love for her daughter. Although her daughter does not consciously understand the reasons, she feels so happy and joyful to be alive, and she feels almost constantly safe and fulfilled. That cord and stream of mothering, the continuum of contact, of love and affection is nearly always there for her. This mother can tolerate her child's demands: the impatience, and the frustrations that her daughter will feel at times. This is because this mother can tolerate those feelings in herself. As a result, this mother does not punish, does not avoid and does not withdraw from her daughter's needs. This healthy mother is grounded within herself, and feels patient, loving and present. She has become a healthy adult, and is therefore devotional. She constantly seeks and embodies her inspiration for motherhood. She realizes that NOTHING can be more important than embracing her true self in the role of mother. She lives in deep surrender to what is, and accepts with both power and humbleness her feminine role as a nurturing mother.*

Fear, pride and self will all work together depending on the circumstances; one is not isolated from the other, and many people have a tendency to use one defense mechanism more often than others. In childhood we developed these defense patterns in response to pain, in-cluding the early imprints of not being loved as we longed to be. It was our way of surviving the pain. Giving up our defense postures can feel like dying, because we are letting go of parts of ourselves that we believed were necessary for our very survival. When you drop your defensive postures, you usually will experience some pain, sadness, and grief. Any time you can feel even the slightest bit of those feelings, they can create a gateway for your more peaceful and vital self to emerge.

Most of us use all of the defensive postures, depending on the specific situation and how we are feeling. We cycle between fear, pride, self-will and being undefended and joyful. Those parents in the images are examples of different states we will experience daily as parents. Our goal is to spend more time in the undefended zone, in the realm of play, joy, love and compassion, and less time in the painful zones of fear, pride, and self-will. To do this, you must not avoid your feelings. Do seek out the root cause of your discomforts.

These defensive postures can also be seen in our children and in other people. People defend themselves against us, and we then out of habit adopt a defensive posture towards them. When people are defending themselves, they are hiding feelings that you trigger in them; but these will be emotions that they are ashamed of and are doing their best to resist. The solution to this sort of standoff is to hold a caring and compassionate outlook while remaining unprovoked by the defensive behaviors of other person. This is easier said than done, as the defensive postures change rapidly from moment to moment. For now, just aim to recognize them, and if you recognize that you or someone else is in a defensive posture, then seek the deeper truth in that moment.

Mother who is Undefended

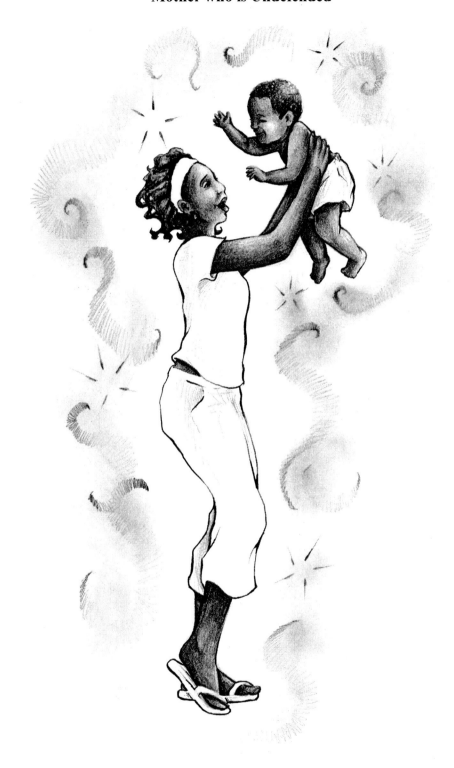

Moving Away from Blame in Relationships

I know; it's so much fun to blame your partner that you probably won't want to give it up! However, with the ongoing high rate of divorce, and children being born to single mothers, it is important to make every effort to encourage good relations between the mother and father in the interest of the newborn. The steady rock of two loving parents helps the child experience a safe, secure and happy childhood. A child will experience anguish, pain, and fear if his parents do not act as a harmonious unit. The child will feel divided inwardly since his happiness is dependent upon a healthy, united family structure. Nature designed children to expect peace and harmony from their parents; a family life full of discord can be a painful shock to the young child. If parents spend their energy arguing over their child, then their child might come to believe that something is wrong with him and he must be the cause of the disharmony. The child will then respond to this sadness and pain by withdrawing.

For this reason it is a good idea to air any problems, hidden attitudes or resentments you hold towards your partner. Keeping these sentiments bottled up just increases their potency, and will eventually lead to moodiness, arguments and outbursts. Typical resentments include "You don't give me what I need," "You never listen to me," "You're mean and stupid," "I hate you." We hold these feelings towards our partners inside without articulating them because of our own immature and fearful consciousness. We are waiting for our partner to reach out to us and soothe our feelings. Our partner never reaches out, and the issue is never addressed. The Pathwork examines the connection between blame and unhappiness:

Therefore I say to all of you, my friends: whenever you are unhappy, look first for that side of you that says no, for whatever reason. Then look for the side that blames others even if only subtly, indirectly and secretly. Look at your emotions where you make a case against someone or something -- against life at large, perhaps.

Because no matter how wrong others may be, they can never be responsible for your suffering, no matter what the appearances are. If you do not blame anyone, but overly blame yourself in a very destructive attitude that does not find a way out, then you are doing exactly the same. For this kind of self-blame is only a disguise for violent hate and blame of others.

If you wish to connect yourself with the causes of your suffering and truly remove these causes, this must be the process: really wanting to see where you say no to what you want most – no matter how impossible this may seem offhand. Question your emotions extremely carefully, and look at them when it comes to practical reality. Notice how you act contrary to what you imagine you want so much.[480]

Activity: nurture your relationship. To nurture your relationship, give to your partner as you expect to be given to. Your spouse has likely arrived at adulthood with some amount of emotional pain and neediness that he has naturally brought with him to your relationship. To work through this emotional "baggage" requires a surrendered action. Take extra time to communicate compassionately with your partner. Set aside even five minutes and really let him know how you feel, and what is going on with you. This works best if you first tell your partner something like, "I would really like to communicate my experiences with you and have you listen to me with your heart without judgment. Do you have a few minutes?" Hopefully your partner will meet you half way and listen. Be sure to give to your partner freely from your heart, as well. Make the extra efforts to do things that he likes — cooking special meals, giving a massage, or any other kind of special attention. Be sure to be patient as most of our piggy banks of love are pretty low. And it takes a lot of deposits to fill it up to the point where you can unconditionally give and receive. So nurture your relationship, not in a way that is self-sacrificing, but by offering genuine and heartfelt communication and interaction. When mothers and fathers work together this way, each freely giving and receiving from the other, they will have plenty of energy and love to give to their children.

Work, Careers and Keeping the Bond Intact

In our modern life, we have convinced ourselves that personal success is directly linked to material gain and with our position in society — especially with our careers. It is important to understand the difference between doing work and pursuing success in the world in order to support a false and fragile self image, and doing work because it serves a higher or more meaningful purpose, such as motherhood. Many mothers decide to work or go to school when their children are very young. These mothers leave their children at daycare or with relatives. However, I believe that motherhood is a meaningful job, a meaningful position in society. It is far more important than being a secretary, graphic designer, lawyer or doctor. If you don't believe this, it is time to take a look into what you value most in the world.

Many of us have unfortunately been raised to believe that we are only valuable and important when we go out into the world of work and pursue a career. In other words, your value as a person is based upon what you do in the world. Who you are becomes a mere label: I am a "vice president," a "consultant," a "manager," a "real estate agent," and so forth. Many people choose to work for a big company, and thus their energy is spent making money for someone else. While I am not opposed to pursuing a career or to working, I do believe it must be done while keeping the mother-child bond intact. This means that if you have to go to work, then your baby goes with you. Work in the world must be secondary to your real job, which comes with real and lasting rewards — the rewards of being a mother.

Being a mother is a worthy task and has value. While these days motherhood may be a cultural status symbol with only sentimental significance, in truth nothing is more important than being a mother.

If a woman has a career, but its pursuit comes at the sacrifice of her children, that career should have no value in our society. Many mothers with young babies take **pride** in being away from their youngsters and being unhindered to do other things in the world. Such values are sadly misplaced. We must begin to respect and value the roles of motherhood and fatherhood as absolutely central to the healthy functioning of our society. If you feel pride from leaving your child, from "having your life back," transform this feeling into the genuine pride of being a sensitive, loving, and present parent for your child. Even if society, your spouse, co-workers, or friends do not value your actions, your son or daughter will, and so will I. A proud parent is one who allows respect and joy to flow into her through her mutual relationship with her child. True pride is an inner feeling of satisfaction that only comes when you utilize wisely your life's task—your heart's longing—as a parent. When you answer this inward call, you will feel successful because you have devoted yourself to something that truly matters, both for the sake of your own family, and for the family of humanity.

Michelle says: "Your children need a real mother. A lot of intense feelings can come with being a mother and maintaining the bond with your children, because we were not raised to do this. We need to work together with our family to support this bond. Women who leave their children with someone else in order to work believe that they are an important asset to the business they belong to. But they leave behind those to whom they are the most important: their children. The workplace can always find a replacement for you. But your children will not be able to replace you. Being a mother means being with your children. When you are pregnant and thinking about leaving your child, then you have already begun to abandon him. If my child was in a day care, I would not feel fulfilled as a mother. We have the innate longing to feel connected with our children as mothers. We need to be with our children. There is no rush for them to grow up; there is plenty of time."

In indigenous cultures, the mother is always with her baby whether she has work requirements or not. If a modern mother feels she must go to work or to school, she can set up a schedule so that she does not work excessive hours and can have her child with her. This arrangement might present difficulties depending on the child's age and the particular work or school demands and limitations, but there is no reason it cannot be done. If a baby comes to work with her mother, what do you think her favorite activity in life will be? It will be going to work. When the child is fulfilled and happy with her mother, she will remember the experience and will want to recreate it later in life. When I was around the age of eight my mother took me to work with her. She owned a small typesetting shop, and made graphic designs, typed up letters, and printed out documents. I would sit nearby and draw, color, and play games on an old computer, and sometimes help her with some of her work. And now look at me. I am doing similar work: designing, writing and laying out books and websites.

Money often controls parents' choices about how they raise their children. It seems like part of "harsh" reality, but many families choose lifestyles that require two incomes to support. If a mother chooses to destroy the continuum of care in order to go to work without her baby, her decision is not in harmony with the divine. In indigenous groups, mothers worked with their children in a sling. Choosing to break the mother-child bond comes out of deep-seated negativity that is hardly perceivable at the conscious level because it is so painful. We have a well of pain within us that covers up our natural responses to life. Many of us have a difficult time fathoming how our child really feels when she cries, because of this cover. This well of pain whispers to us in our own dark solitude. If we enter and explore the well, however, the experience can renew us.

THE WELL OF GRIEF

Those who will not slip beneath
    the still surface on the well of grief

turning downward through its black water
    to the place we cannot breathe

will never know the source from which we drink,
    the secret water, cold and clear,

nor find in the darkness glimmering
    the small round coins
        thrown by those who wished for something else.

I feel the sadness in our culture. The higher self — the true self — of every mother does not want to leave her children. And we know that children love to be with their mothers, and suffer greatly when pulled away from them while they work. I feel our profound collective suffering surrounding this issue; it is a deep well of sadness.

Modern mothers don't realize that gold coins—our true wealth and prosperity—lie at the bottom of this metaphorical well. The gold lies beneath our grief and pain; we can find it by penetrating those feelings. If only we knew the vastness of this treasure, everything else would fall away as we devoted ourselves to uncovering this precious soul substance. Parenting can be our gateway into the well, and thus it can bring us gold: salvation, happiness, and real freedom. But those who do not descend to the darkness will never know the secret of the water which nurtures us. This is the parent's calling and challenge in life; it is speaking to you.

Activity: honor yourself for being a mother. Our society does not do a good enough job in honoring mothers. And as a mother or father yourself, you might have downplayed the importance of your parenting "job." Ideally, there ought to be enough financial abundance in our society that mothers would not have to even think about working. Mothers should not have to worry about having enough to feed, clothe, and house their children. You're doing well as a mother, so keep taking care of your precious baby. Put what's important first!

Perhaps you are faced with the difficult question of choosing work or staying home with your child. If you choose to work, are you aware that you are putting a dollar value on the precious time you spend with your child? You will trade your income per hour for time spent with your baby. Have you considered that the added income will be coming at the emotional expense of your child? Is such an exchange really worth the few thousand dollars a month?

Mothers who pretend that they are not mothers by becoming wage slaves are a symptom of the *disease called modernization*. Mothers who go to work sever the psychic umbilical cord established between them and their children in the "second womb" stage of development. It is both shocking and frightening that we regularly abandon our children in this way in western culture.

When a mother leaves home to work, it is important to examine what happens to her income. Consider first, taxes. The state and federal government can easily take away 25-35% of your income for taxes. So, while you are away from your child working, 25-35% of this time goes to support the government and its activities, rather than to you or your children, for whom you are supposedly making this sacrifice. This is like working two to three months of the year for nothing.

While you are away at work, someone must watch your child. If you have two or more children your childcare costs will be much higher. This is part of why our society created the public school system. With their children attending public schools mothers can work, without directly paying for childcare. Without a public school system—which I think would be a good thing — most parents wouldn't be able to "afford" to sever the mother-child bond by sending the mother off to work. What we have today is an uncomfortable and disturbing vicious circle. Part of a working mother's income goes to taxes, which helps pay the salaries of public school teachers, who entertain the mother's children all day in the name of *public education,* which allows the mother to leave home and work. Schools and day care centers become surrogate mothers. Nearly all of them offer only a fraction of the love, nurturance and support a real mother can give her child. In these settings the child is also deprived of the most precious source of physical and emotional nurturance: breastmilk.

In our culture it is common for mothers to wean their children before the age of one, thus depriving their children of nature's super food imbued with mother's warm love and compassion. If the mother's intention is to breastfeed for a longer period, as Nature designed our children to expect, then it is much more difficult to interrupt the continuum of care. Yet it is our culture's destructive and perverse goal to support the mother in physically and emotionally abandoning her children so that her labor in the workforce can be exchanged for cash.

One reason a mother might choose to go to work is the enticement of good health insurance benefits. But have you considered being able to avoid doctor visits because your child never gets sick? Your child is much more likely to stay healthy when you care for him and feed him good food at home than when you leave his nutrition up to school meal programs.

When you examine how much of your salary goes into taxes, increased transportation costs, gas and insurance for the extra car, child-care expenses, along with the other expenses associated with a typical job, such as emotional stress, physical strain, and more money spent on pre-made foods because of no time to cook, it seems that even a moderate to well-paying job just isn't worth the effort.

Grandparents sometimes make working more feasible by offering to watch your children while you work. Is it worth it? Why don't the grandparents just help out a little financially so the mother does not have to work at all? If grandparents chipped in for groceries, gas, and even small contributions to rent or mortgage, then that sum would probably come close to what would be left over, after taxes and expenses, from mother's income.

Thoroughly investigate how much money you would actually take home from a job, and consider what you are getting in exchange for sacrificing that time with your child. Companies that want to retain their professional employees who are new mothers can often be creative in arranging reduced, work-at-home hours. Also, mothers and fathers should make sure to file with the state after their children are born; many states and companies provide some paid family leave. While not as generous as in some European countries, where mothers are paid for a full year's leave, it does provide some extra financial help. Mothers who have to work can choose to work at daycares (with their children) or start their own daycares or other jobs that include their children.

Our society should honor motherhood on its highest altar. We know that strong, vibrant, healthy, productive, and loving boys and girls can be created through the continuum of contact with their mothers. Our wished-for future society, in which there is no war, no violence, no poverty, and no fear, begins with our hope for the future: our children. We do not have to continue letting our children suffer because mothers have misplaced their true longing for the fulfillment of their life's most important task.

Parenting, the Olympic Sport

Parenting is a physically active undertaking. Holding your baby or young child requires strength, grace and dexterity. Protecting your children from danger, or making sure they don't destroy a friend's house during a visit is just a part of the job. It takes more energy to clean up messes, make extra food, do extra laundry, and juggle your day-to-day tasks while keeping your child attached to you. Think of parenting as a physical work out, rather like going to the gym. Everyone knows that we should exercise regularly. Now is your chance to get in good shape; embrace the extra physical demands of parenting!

Living on a Small Income

For about a year, Michelle, Sparkle and I lived on an income of about $750 per month in a very pricey part of California. I earned that income working a few hours on the weekends teaching three or four yoga classes. Michelle didn't work at all. We lived in a studio apartment that was about 200 square feet; we had to roll up the futon every day so that there was space to sit or eat. A small shelf contained our full wardrobe, which probably could have fit into a single suitcase for all three of us. We didn't even have a full kitchen, and only a little fridge. Sparkle was just a few months old and neither Michelle nor I knew what to do with ourselves or our lives. With that low income and a family of three we qualified for food stamps, which added over $350 a month to our food budget. We spent almost nothing on anything other than food or rent. We rarely bought clothes or toys, and rather than buy a new computer, we used the old one given to Michelle a long time ago. Baby clothes came as gifts from friends. Our few occasional large expenses were paid through credit cards. We lived in government-subsidized housing in which our rent was proportional to our income. We hardly drove anywhere accept for the five minute trip to the store. This wasn't an ideal situation, of course; I was going to school, and the expense of that far exceeded our income. We also lived next to an amusement park, so in the summer it was noisy and crowded. But it also had great rewards: we could walk to the beach, and I could surf. With our small income, however, we continually endured stress and constraint in how we could live.

Michelle was frequently upset over our cramped living conditions even though I was quite satisfied with them. She finally called the manager one more time to ask for an upgrade. "Well," he said, and explained that normally you are not allowed to move. But they needed an assistant manager, so Michelle took the job and we were upgraded to the best unit in the complex. It had two bedrooms (it was still small), a quieter location away from the street, and even our own small garden.

I continued to go to school and began working part time for my parents, and was now making $2000 per month. While still not a comfortable income, it covered our expenses enough to keep us going for a few years. I kept my old car, a Honda which I still have, and we sold Michelle's car. Our small duplex was spacious because we had no furniture except a roll up futon. Our friends gave us a few chairs. Most of my income was spent on food, rent and credit card bills. We lived this way for two years.

A few months after we moved to our larger apartment we started having problems with our new neighbor. It was very difficult to live where we were, but we were stuck. My income was too small to move to nonsubsidized housing. In Santa Cruz, our subsidized rent was $600 per month. In some parts of this country, that could pay for a mortgage on a much larger house. Michelle and I longed for a change. But we didn't just sit there and do nothing; we talked about the issue seriously almost every day. We sought to change our inner world, not the outer world. Eventually we freed ourselves inwardly from the constrained situation and began to feel more spaciousness and peace where we lived. However, when the local government decided to spray pesticides over our home, I listened to an inner urging and immediately moved our family into my parents' home. My parents were not

thrilled with this move, and they were even less thrilled when we ended our subsidized housing without having anywhere else to live. Although our condition was very stressful for a long time, a series of unforeseen events made our decision to stay at my parents' house extremely fortunate for them. Unexpected family circumstances required that I attend to many affairs that I would not have been able to had we not moved. Never-before-imagined resources came to us, and today we live comfortably in a spacious cabin in the forest in a very peaceful and serene setting.

I am sharing our story with you because even though it was often difficult and stressful, Michelle and I were able to live comfortably, eat well (all organic foods), and have shelter and transportation with income from only one of us. Many situations and energies threatened to break the bond between Michelle and Sparkle, yet I would have nothing of it. If we had had to move to another country, live on a farm, or do anything else to ensure that Sparkle and Michelle could stay together, we would have done it.

If we could survive comfortably on such a small income, without any savings and very little resources, most people reading this book can do much better. Before I engaged in personal growth and real change, I was very unhappy. In this unhappy frame of mind, I felt very strongly that I deserved to go out to dinner, live in an expensive place, and have a nice car (I never had those things, but I desired them). My unhappiness was leading me towards a wasteful lifestyle, towards being miserable working for lots of money and then spending the money on luxuries. These thoughts incapacitated me such that I was not motivated to get a job, and nobody would hire me either. I kept thinking of the outcome of my actions. It all seemed so pointless. The typical career lifestyle creates a vicious cycle, requiring a lot of work to afford the nice apartment, car, vacations and so forth, and then perpetuating the unhappiness through an unfulfilling job. The modern paradigm is no different: parents expect to pay for a big house, lots of stuff to fill the house, and two new cars, all requiring huge amounts of cash. I don't want to suggest that deprivation is the solution to this dilemma, but rather, simplification. An acquaintance visited us today, and he lives in his van. He says he's never felt so free, and that he never has to drive anywhere to get home. You might expect that someone who lives this way would be unhappy and uncomfortable, but for this fellow, living in his van has made his life a grand adventure.

If money is the issue that keeps you away from your children, then try to think outside the box. Build a house on a friend's property. Live in a tent or with your parents or other relatives, convert a garage or other property, rent a small studio or live outside of town where the rent is cheaper. Or live in the center of town where you won't need a car. Become a farmer, get a goat or chickens and have your own eggs and fresh milk. It is our ideas and beliefs of how we want to live that cost us so much money. You might also try to develop passive sources of income. Find ways to make money when you are not working, such as any form of internet or local business, real estate, and inventions or products. Finally, make sure you spend your money on what's important. Shop in resale or consignment stores instead of buying everything new—this is good for your bank account and the environment. Many people lose money paying for policies and insurance that are overpriced or that they do not need. Read up on taxes and find ways to save there.

Activity: manifest your dream of an abundant life. How you live in the world is a reflection of your beliefs about how life should be, which is very much affected by your imprints from childhood. Michelle and I now have almost exactly the life that we dreamed of. Michelle and I talked about what we wanted and needed, drew pictures, and called in the deva spirits to help make it happen. It took us about two years to really bring our dream to reality. Many times, we would fail at things and wonder what went wrong. We only understood later that what failed us in the outer world were things that really didn't serve our best interests. I see many people trying to create the life they want, and the only thing preventing their success is their lack of focus and limited imagination. You truly can create your dream

life. Align your intentions with it, pray for it, and then *act* to make it happen. There are many opportunities in the world out there. Life is only as good as how we feel about ourselves, so examine closely your internal world. If you want to change how you live, invite in the infinite possibilities for abundance.

I know someone who works over 40 hours a week at a high paying engineering job. He would really like to spend more time with his children. Meanwhile, it has always been his hobby to photograph weddings, and he really enjoys it. He is now starting a wedding photography business, and if everything works well he can replace working five days a week as an engineer with one or two days on the weekend while earning the same income. Most important, this father will realize his wish to spend much more time with his children.

Change takes work. I have worked very hard over the last year writing books and articles and creating websites to earn my income. Working hard is not a struggle when there is a positive goal at the end of the tunnel.

Unrealistic Boundaries

Many parents refuse to accept the fact that their young child's nervous system is immature and that the brain continues to develop over many years. The young child only begins to have some grasp of the adult work world at about 6 years of age. It can take up until they are 23 years old for young people to have some handle on life. That is why, for example, there are age restrictions for driver's licenses. It is unrealistic to confer certain responsibilities on your children when they are not yet able to understand them and their biology prevents them from fulfilling them.

This is especially true for children under the age of 6. They are floating in a sea of consciousness and don't yet understand the logic of the adult world. A one- or two-year-old might hear your words as a jumble of noises, and see your expressions on your face and be amused that you are looking at them.

While attending a play and singing group for children near our home I recently observed a mother who had a certain unrealistic boundary with her sixteen-month-old child. The toddler wanted to climb on some folding chairs. Her mother placed her hands on her daughter's hands and said, "No, we do not play on these chairs. You can play on your play structure at home, but not on these chairs." The child had a huge smile on her face and was happily running around all over the place. To a young child, a chair and a play structure are the same; they are both things to climb on. Being at home or in a classroom does not matter to a toddler. If she sees something, she wants to play on it. So when this mother tells her child "No," the child will be confused, since earlier that day she did the same thing at home and it was okay. Why is it wrong now? There does not seem to be any reason from the point of view of the child; the "no" seems completely arbitrary. This same mother told her child to "Share, share, share," her toys with another child. And the one-year-old just ran around and pretended to give the toy to the other child. Again, this woman's child does not understand the concept of sharing. A toddler can easily think everything she touches is hers. How could she share? Even if this child did understand the abstraction of sharing, she is at a stage of development in which sharing is not as much fun as playing with the toy herself.

Pay attention to the areas where you micro-manage your child. Ask yourself, is it really necessary? Absolutely protect your children from harm. At the same time, this protection can go too far and become a separated form of parenting. Generally, micro-managing thwarts the child's expression of life, and ends up being a waste of time for the parent, so nobody is having fun. If you are a micro-manager then you imprint that on your child. Your child will look to you first, rather than to himself, to see if what he is doing is right or wrong. This child will learn not to trust his own authority and impulses, and to only trust the outer world authority. Or conversely, the child will grow up to become hyper rebellious, in passive or overt ways, and always do the opposite of what is instructed.

To stay out of this trap, I recommend that you try to really understand and appreciate your child's level of awareness and intelligence about life

Setting realistic boundaries for your children means that you are aware of possible hazards in the environment. For example, a sharp object lying on the floor are dangerous if a child is running and playing near by. Streets and moving vehicles are dangerous for children. Again, the young child's intelligence wasn't designed to expect the danger of the car.

The way Michelle and I created realistic boundaries for our child was to create spaces where our daughter could play freely. We did not want to micro-manage what she does and jeopardize the fun of her childhood. We also did not make just a play room that was safe. Our whole house is her play room, because she is a part of our family, and we wanted our home environment to be united and harmonious with her needs. Also, we didn't have to obsessively watch everything she did. We would be mindful in public places because we understood that since she was able to climb on a chair at home, she would expect to be able to climb on the chairs wherever we went. We also took her to the beach often, where she could run around and do whatever she wanted, and we did not have to limit her behavior too much, except for grabbing her when she tried to run into the ocean. Playing in the ocean water and splashing around is one of her most favorite beach activities. Understanding Sparkle's perspective as an infant led to unexpected results. For example, when she was a baby she loved stuffed animals and would become very attached to the ones we had. But then we would go to the clothing store, or to a friend's house, or to this or that appointment, and people would all have stuffed animals for her to play with. Just as at home, Sparkle assumed that those toys were hers to keep and play with. Needless to say, when we explained to the person that she was now very attached to this toy, they would just give it to her. Sometimes we would return the toy a few days later after she got bored. The point is that we all found a congenial way to indulge Sparkle's enjoyment in hugging stuffed animals both at home and while out in the world.

We also make it a practice to not impose our will on our daughter. Many indigenous groups function this way as well. We rarely make her do anything with the expectation that she will want to participate. We do our best to honor her and let her be as she is. If she is angry with me, or if she makes a mess, then I am okay with that. I honor her for the pleasure and enjoyment she wants to have as a child. This includes never instructing her to say things like "thank you" and never making her say "hello" or "goodbye" to anybody. This is an example of giving her space to be as she is. Why should we try to control her as if she were a puppet? Why not let her have her own natural response to life and to others? As a result of our parenting, it is really funny when people talk to her, or try to tell her something. For example, sometimes people will try to make her say something. I usually start laughing when they do this; since we never imposed our will on Sparkle she feels no need or desire to do what other people tell her to do. If they try to elicit a response from her, she usually just ignores them. Just the other day my brother was trying to teach her how to play the card game Memory. At first she played along. Then she became bored. My brother tried to explain the rules to her, but she ended up kicking the cards everywhere. Again I thought it was so funny; she is doing what she enjoys as a child. Children aren't meant to follow adults' boring mental lifestyles. These are the subtle joys of a parent practicing alternative principles. Sometimes Sparkle won't answer us either and we are her parents. When she does this I understand that she is exercising her power. I pay attention to her behavior, and let it be as it is. In general, children will copy their parents; that is how they learn. Don't waste your time or energy controlling your children or telling them to do anything unless it is absolutely necessary.

Being aware of the space and of the boundaries your child needs is a way to support him, to create a safe and grounded space for him to grow and thrive in. The examples I've shared carry a message for you to look for ways to really honor the stage of development your child is in. It causes children pain and stress to be expected to do more, or to act in ways that they are incapable of because their biology is undeveloped and incapable of meeting the demand. Practicing realistic and respectful boundaries means deeply listening, honoring and accepting your child for who she is, including her physical and emotional needs. **Rather than trying to mold your child into who you want her to be, you want to support and nurture the vibrant being your child already is.**

Health and Safety Boundaries

After being in several types of therapy groups, I have discovered some things that are difficult to hear. Many adults were sexually invaded in some way as young children (this is perhaps somewhat less common for boys but it still happens frequently). Even if the invasion seemed relatively minor, it is the intention and the circumstances of the invasion that can cause great harm. Typically the perpetrator is not a stranger, but a trusted authority such as a doctor or a teacher, or often a family member from the extended family. The violator can also be from the immediate family, such as the father, or the brother. A person whom you do not deeply and unconditionally trust should not be left alone with your child, even for a few minutes. Even if this person is an important family member, or someone whom you think you should trust but just don't, then listen to your intuition and don't allow your child to be alone in that person's company. Don't allow yourself to be swayed by the thought that, "It's okay, it's just for a short break, everything will be fine." If anybody attempts to separate you from your child in such a way that you won't be able to see what is happening to your child, even for just a few minutes, then that's a red flag of warning. You can feel a sense of unease in yourself if you are thinking about taking a short break away from your little one and the person you're going to leave him with isn't exactly on your wavelength. What if your child needs to go potty? Have a diaper changed? Has an itch? Also be careful with older children watching young children unsupervised. If the older child was abused or violated in some way, he may try to do the same to someone else, not even necessarily consciously; it just happens.

While the babysitter may seem like a nice innocent young woman to care for your child, what if she invites some friends over? Who are those friends? While your sister or cousin may be wonderful to watch your child, what about their husband's friends who may be over while you are away?

Medical procedures and exams can also be invasive from your child's perspective. The amount of physical touching that your child undergoes during an exam should be minimally invasive. Don't leave your child alone with people whom you don't know, even for two minutes. Children usually cannot protect their physical boundaries because that is their parents' job. It is your job all the time; you don't get a break from it. Don't make the foolish mistake of expecting another adult to protect your child's boundaries unless that person has your unconditional trust.

I wish we lived in a mutually trusting culture where everyone has each other's best interests at heart and children would be safe in all settings. But that's not how the world is today. The message here is to place extra attention and energy on planning that your child's boundaries are protected. Don't remain unconscious or oblivious to ways your child could be harmed without your knowing; think ahead and always use your best judgment.

Being a Positive Role Model

One of your baby's innate expectations is that you have the ability to respond to life's circumstances and to make decisions. As your baby grows into a toddler and then to a little person, he will at times have difficulties in making decisions. There are two extremes here in how parents will respond to this. There is the parent who constantly controls his child and makes decisions for him: "Do this, don't do that." And then there is the absent parent who says, "I'll do whatever you want." The problem with the controlling parent is that the child is never able to develop his sense of self. The problem with the laissez-faire parent is that the child can feel lost

and uncared for. Children don't necessarily need to have everything that pops into their mind, and parents can help them to learn discernment.

Being a responsible parent means you will attend to your children's real needs. For example, your child expects that you will feed him, but sometimes he may not know what he wants to eat. You will provide good food for your child and hope that he will eat it. If asked, your child might wish to eat his favorite foods: cookies, fruits, and other sweets. If you always give your child the sweets he wants, he will be unhealthy. Your child also won't respect you because he wants you to be an active and guiding presence in his life. A wise parent knows what her child needs and provides it for him, without the child needing to ask or make decisions. As the parent models good decision making, the child imprints these healthy patterns for making decisions. None of this is to be taken as a suggestion that you should deny your child his true needs or force your child to do something he doesn't want to do. You need to be an authoritative guide, but also make wise and balanced decisions. Do not merge your consciousness into the world of your child, but rather, understand, respect and honor his world from your adult awareness of his real needs for food, attention, caring, play and safety. Sparkle likes to play and make messes. This is natural, so I support her playing and making a mess. Sparkle also likes to eat fruit often. We give her fruit only sometimes after she's first eaten nourishing foods. Sparkle likes to play with friends, and go to the beach and the river, so we do our best to do these things with her. Some days we are limited in doing everything she wants, so we don't do all of them. For much of her childhood, we have done one of these fun activities every day. Sparkle likes hugs, and when she needs a hug we always hug her. When she wants to be held, we always hold her. Sometimes she wants all the space on Michelle's lap. We cannot always give her all the space at that exact moment because Yeshe needs space. We do our best to make sure she has all of the space a few times per day until she feels satisfied, but she cannot have it all day, whenever she wants, because sometimes Yeshe needs extra attention.

Tantrums

A tantrum is just your child moving their energy. That is all. Your child is expressing the laws of physics and the physical world. Loud stomping, screaming, throwing things, and hitting are simply expressions of moving energy. These activities are not "bad" in the case of a child. A child has no control of his or her feelings, other than to let them flow, or to try to repress them. From a child's perspective, that huge expression of rushing energy seems to come out of nowhere. A tantrum is a natural response to their environment; it comes from their frustration with how they have been treated and raised. Your child's tantrum might disturb your neighbors, and disturb your own sense of how you think your child should behave. And that is the purpose, to get you to change and to look at something you are not seeing. The disturbing energy caused by a tantrum is absolutely no reason to either stop your child, or to punish them. (I would only redirect a child if he were in danger of being hurt, but I would not stop him.)

If your child does have tantrums I would take this as a sign that, as a parent, you are not hearing your child, not understanding his feelings, and not holding a space for your child to just be a child. Because you do not understand him, he needs to express himself louder so you can hear. He is so desperate for you to be there and hear him that he goes wild and has a tantrum. **Tantrums usually occur because the parent is unwilling to understand or meet the child's needs.**

A tantrum is a high volume expression of a need or a disappointment. This is a time to be thankful that your child is sharing with you passionately what really matters to him. The only exception to this is an autistic or otherwise mentally disabled child whose natural perceptions of life are incoherent. In this case, the child is expressing something more than just a frustration. A mother told me that her autistic son had tantrums lasting several hours every day. Needless to say, they eventually got the message across. So terrible and painful were the tantrums that the mother took every effort possible to cure her son's autism, and she succeeded. As part of her success, the tantrums stopped.

I can only tell you what I do when my daughter gets angry, or starts yelling. I listen to her. I acknowledge her. I have absolutely never tried to obstruct her energy movement. If she is angry, then I accept it. I won't leave her just because she has a displeasing mood. I want to understand her mood, what caused it, and where we can go from here. Every time Sparkle has had a tantrum it has been from feeling unloved and uncared for. Yes, on the outer level there is a need going unmet; but on a deeper level, she is affected by her perception of not being fully loved and cared for.

Wise parents listen to their children's tantrums and use it as a wake-up call, a message that something needs to drastically change — in the parent.

Sometimes when Sparkle gets angry it is due to pain that has gotten trapped within her. And she may say things like, "I don't want you," or just run away and hide. I want to honor her in that state and I let her be. I can do this because I know that children's moods change. Ten seconds later, my daughter wants to play with me.

Any time your child expresses an emotion or physical movement, it is an impulse that they are not fully in control of. They are exploring the infinite possibilities of the expression of life in the physical world. If you thwart or punish your child's expression, the expression doesn't go away. If your child is angry and starts throwing things or hitting you, yelling or punishing them may make the behavior stop. But their natural life impulse goes underground. So even if you stop your child's anger response on the surface, deeper down he is controlling himself. Conversely, if you really give your child loving and present attention, he will become happy and agreeable. Parents wrongly think that punishing children will make them obedient. This is really a form of emotional abuse. On the surface, the punished child is well behaved; underground he is a ball of pain and anger. His life force is stagnant within him, making his entire life uncomfortable, less pleasurable, and filled with unhappiness.

Physical abuse. Striking a child, or spanking, is physical abuse. Spanking disconnects your child from the root of his being. That is why parents spank the butt, because that is near the child's root and pleasure center. As a result, spanking disconnects the child's rootedness with the Earth. Spanking is extremely painful to the child even if he does not admit it. Parents who want to ruin their child and transform him from a happy compassionate person into a fearful and loathing tyrant are the ones who spank their children. The parent's role is to protect and nurture the child, and spanking or pinching, hitting, jabbing or slapping to punish a child is a form of deep betrayal. The child's hidden thoughts will be, "I am going to get you back one day," because they are powerless against a big adult, and "I hate you," and "I will never trust anyone again." Children trust their parents deeply; that is their innate design. When the parent breaks this trust through physical or emotional violence, a deep thorn of pain is thrust into their child's heart. This is reparable to some degree, but it is better to never do it in the first place.

The So Called Terrible 2's

The main thing terrible about the two's is how parents treat their little children. As the two-year mark rolls around, your child starts to become more of an individual. He wants to do his own thing. At the same time, your child is very bonded with you and has a difficult time separating himself—who he is—from you. So while he sometimes wants to do his own thing, he also wants his parents to do it for him or with him because he does not yet recognize that he is an individual. If your child has thwarted needs then this can result in very expressive responses in the two's. Parents then judge this child's individuation and expression as "terrible."

It is hard to imagine what can be more cruel and disheartening than for a parent to consider his child as terrible.

The terrible two's are not inevitable. Yes, children are self-centered; yes, they can be loud, yell and cry, and make lots of mess. But this does not make the two-year-old phase terrible. Little children can become tyrants, and they want everything their way. This is how they learn about what it is like to be an individual and to be grounded in the world. When the continuum of care is kept intact, when your child has never been abandoned by you, and when she is still getting the nurturance of breastmilk, this developmental stage can be not too difficult and not terrible at all. In fact, it is enjoyable to see your little person become so versatile and proud of her abilities in the world. At the same time, both the parent and child feel the small growing pains of letting go of infancy.

I have also noticed that during the two-year-old phase the child needs a wide-open energy container. Your child needs space and freedom to be herself. If she doesn't get it she will complain. The mother or both parents are like the honey pot to the two-year-old. Sometimes your child will want honey from the pot (attention, affection), and sometimes she won't. She can go back and forth rather rapidly. Your job is to keep the pot full of honey and available at all times. This can be very challenging. Your child will say she wants something, and two seconds later say she doesn't want it! Part of the child's individuation happens through the energy center in the solar plexus. The solar plexus energy center and the cord connecting you and your child remain open. When your child wants something from you, she is connecting to your relational cord—that honey pot in the solar plexus. Any time Michelle protested about Sparkle changing her mind all the time, I reminded Michelle that she also changes her mind often. A healthy parent stays open and allows the coming and going of her child without withdrawing or trying to control or deny this form of love. This back and forth dance is a part of your child growing up. Support this dance; do not fight it, and do not control it. Notice what your defensive reaction is when you have difficulty with your child as she goes through this phase of individuation.

Saying Yes to No

When your child says one of his favorite words to you — "No!" — it is important for you to understand how to respond. "No!" is one of the most pleasing sounds to the wise parent. When your child says "No!" to you, he says an inward "Yes!" to himself. "No!" is how your child begins to find himself. "No!" is something your child says to feel powerful, even if he changes his mind a few minutes later. So when your child says "No!" understand that it comes from the inner "Yes!" that he gives to himself and to life.

Final Words on Emotions and Accepting Life

This brief discussion of self observation and self awareness is just the beginning of the long road of personal awareness. Both the *Bioenergetic Manual*, and the *Undefended Self* can be a good place to start with a more detailed roadmap of how to expand your awareness. People who want to grow emotionally usually find ways to make it happen that are appropriate for them. Whether through a group of friends, a therapist, a religious group or other practice, there are many ways to grow and mature. None of the things I mentioned doing are necessarily simple. They require patience, compassion and understanding, not just for your child, but for yourself. It may be difficult, and life may be difficult, but that is no reason to give up striving for the highest expression of yourself as a parent. Have faith, pray and align your energy for the highest good for yourself, your children and your family.

I have outlined many principles for helping you love your child more, by primarily witnessing when you are not present for him. You are able to choose love in any moment and to choose to maintain that heartfelt connection with your child.

It is your choice to be present from moment to moment. For the practice of mindfulness, and yielding to rather than opposing the flow of life, the works by Eckhart Tolle, *The Power of Now*, and/or *The New Earth* can be helpful. Both are available in mother-friendly audio CDs.

Parents can also find dozens of excellent examples and practical tools for heart centered parenting in the book *Raising Our Children, Raising Ourselves* by psychologist and parent Naomi Aldort.

There is Good and Evil

Now it is time to really dig into a difficult concept. We are going to enter the heart of darkness in the world. People tend to judge things as either good or bad. Even worse, some people are unable to discern good from evil and continually find themselves ambivalent. It is common in our culture, especially in politics, for a compromise to mediate a conflict of seeming opposites. This is also seen in journalism, when both sides of a story are told from a supposedly neutral perspective. Both sides have their conviction and perhaps are even right, or so the common belief goes. Our society does not believe that we can find absolute truth or absolute right and wrong. Sometimes we don't know what is right or wrong for the other person; our short-sighted vision limits our knowing what is best in the world. When people are locked in a battle of opinions, you might resign yourself to the idea that both sides have value. Both are right and both are a little wrong, you believe. Perhaps behaviors which you see as wrong are serving some as yet unforeseen higher good, you might say to yourself. You might wonder how you can judge what another human being is doing; perhaps their mistake will actually help them in the bigger picture. And if you don't know what is right or wrong, then you cannot do much about anything wrong in the world.

People believe that many things are relative, and that there is nothing that is inherently good, or inherently bad. Good or evil exists only "in the eye of the beholder." The media attempt to display this perspective by "neutral" reporting of facts. But this is not the truth. There are things that are inherently good, and there are things that are inherently bad. This is not merely an opinion; there are facts and truths that can be found and experienced.

The existence of evil is watered down in our culture. Painful truths are whitewashed, or they are exaggerated to the point where we miss the truth. Our viewpoint has become so fractioned that we cannot trust mainstream media for the bigger picture. And not seeing the entire picture is part of the evil principle. It is a limited and constrained consciousness. We are falsely taught to believe that right and wrong is in the eye of the observer, and that there are not many ultimate truths to rest our weary souls upon. If there is a truth, then, so we believe, "scientists" would have discovered it. The classic example is, "If there was a cure for cancer it would be front page news." Well, I wish it were that way. The news does not actually offer an unbiased opinion as they claim, but rather false neutrality where their real position is hidden. They set the agenda, putting in and leaving out what they please. Even when science finds the equivalent of "a cure for cancer," it doesn't get reported. Many real cures have already been found by real doctors and health researchers But the mainstream does not consider it news; it is censored.

We are directing our energy, consciousness and intention towards these outer world forces as if they were arbiters of truth. They continue to perpetuate a belief system that offers problems but no solutions.

You need to understand that **there is good and there is evil** on this planet. I hope I have demonstrated to you goodness and evil in relation to the modern plague. The modern plague represents evil, darkness, separation, pain and suffering. We are sometimes wrong in our interpretation of right and wrong, but that does not negate the fact that some things in the world are right, and some things are wrong (and some things do exist in a grey area). Knowing what is right — truth, justice, love, compassion — is a part of goodness. Where each one of us is numb, the resulting laziness and lack of clear vision about the truth makes us easily affected by evil and negative influences from both within us, and outside of us, because those forces live upon lies.

Evil is, and results from, numbness in the soul.[481] We learned to be numb because we experienced so much pain when our continuum of care was broken as infants. Numbness was the only survival solution.

Three stages of evil

1. Numbness towards the self as a defensive mechanism.
2. Numbness towards others: we can watch people suffer and not feel any discomfort.
3. Numbness to the point where we can inflict cruelty on others. [482]

Many times we see evil in the world but we look the other way. Perhaps we think that someone else will take care of it, or that it isn't our business. We know something is wrong, or it does not feel right with us, but we do not say or do anything about it. We are stuck in fear, or believe we are incapable. This is because we are inauthentic with our own feelings and attitudes. By not speaking out against evil we are allowing it to continue. If you will not speak out against it, then who will? If everybody expects his neighbor to do something, then everybody will just be waiting and not acting. As a result, the evil actions will continue. A powerful but hidden reason why you might not speak up against evil actions is the *negative pleasure* you get from being a bystander. You can participate in the evil action without having to face the consequences because you can tell yourself that you did not actively cause the wrong action, so you are not responsible for it.

There are good and evil ways to raise children. There are no grey areas. There isn't a yet-to-be discovered truth. The truth has always been here, and is recognizable through observing our feelings, and watching the examples in Nature. We can raise our children in truth, with a spirit of love, communion, and clarity, or in the spirit of evil, in separation, materialism, and confusion. When you are aware and understand how your day to day living habits affect your children, it will be much harder to stay separated from them. The earmark of separation is insensitivity to other people's feelings, including your children's. When this numbness is thawed, the separated behavior becomes so intolerable (because it is painful) it collapses and cannot be continued.

While you may say a clear "no" to evil actions in the world, do not fight the evil with more evil. Fighting and negativity strengthens the energy forms that create evil. For example, if you protest against violence or injustice by inciting a riot, on the energetic and physical plane the violent action adds to the violence that was already there, even if it appears that the protest is working. Consider the concept, "Do not resist evil." "All the negativity in the world stems from something one believes in that is not according to reality."[483] "Do not resist evil in you. By that I mean give up the appearance, the pretense that evil does not exist in you. Give in; go with the movement of life." [484] Evil must be faced and overcome primarily within the self. Only then can evil be dealt with outside the self.[485] That doesn't mean to say and do nothing about evil in the world. But you will be much more effective at stopping evil in the world when you understand what is numb in you.

Do not go through your life, through your pregnancy, and through your years as a parent ignoring how your unconscious attitudes, and the unconscious energy you have, may result in evil deeds or actions towards your children. Do not ignore how your attitudes or your numbness affect the dear ones around you: your children and your spouse, your friends and your relatives. Say yes to life, and pray for divine help.

11

Vaccines
Kill Innocent Babies

You cannot deal with an enemy whose existence you ignore, whose weapons you do not know and recognize.[486]

Intention: To learn about the harm caused by vaccines so that you will not allow them to be administered to your children under any pretenses. To motivate you to spread truthful information about vaccines to others.

Numbed by our social collective unconsciousness we have given away to supposed authorities our personal power in matters that concern our health. As a culture, we have allowed these "authorities" to maliciously abuse this stolen power and thereby endanger our health. The result is that we have today such routine and accepted medical protocols as vaccines for numerous disease states. As long as we choose to ignore the truth about the pernicious effects of vaccines, we will remain powerless to avoid their dangers.

The truth is that vaccines, are not safe.[487] In fact, **vaccines do not work**. It is a real crime and an abomination for anyone in our country to promote vaccinations or to vaccinate children. I will be unequivocal: I do not advocate for parents' rights to choose whether or not to vaccinate their children. There is no grey area in this discussion as far as I am concerned. I do not believe that parents should have the choice of whether or not to poison their children; I believe that vaccinating children should be illegal. Vaccines are toxic, even deadly, and should be avoided at all costs!

A Pain-filled Truth

I mentioned in the introduction of this book that some of what I say might cause uncomfortable and even painful reactions in the reader. This chapter might bring up these emotions, and much more. Our modern medical system, which includes the mass vaccination of children, literally makes us sick and even kills us. It is part of the global illness that I have called *modernization*. As disturbing as much of this information may be, I nevertheless urge you to be open to the truth as you read, for your sake, the sake of your children, and all children.

Why Vaccines Cannot Work

With the advent of modern civilization came widespread diseases that were once non-existent among indigenous peoples. Disease arises as a response to the environment. It occurs when the body tries to remove toxic material through alternative means when the main avenues of cleansing and purification, such as the liver, have been damaged. How can one be vaccinated against such a disease? When we remove the toxic influence, or improve our health through a nutrient-rich diet, the chance of contracting disease decreases or disappears.

How, therefore, can an attenuated virus injected into your infant's bloodstream prevent a toxic accumulation, or a nutrient deficiency? Quite simply, it cannot.

Would it surprise you to learn that the entire premise of vaccination is a complete fallacy? It is a hoax. In fact, it is a crime cloaked in the guise of public welfare policy.

The concept of vaccination is based upon the germ theory of Louis Pasteur, which he himself repudiated upon his deathbed. Vaccine science postulates that we are victims to diseases that enter our bodies from the outside world. The typical theory of how vaccines work is:

Your body makes antibodies for the disabled virus it is exposed to via the vaccine. These antibodies help protect you against similar live viruses you contact later. The antibodies destroy the vaccine virus, and thus the child suffers a mild form of the disease, and his "immune system" is built up against the disease. The similarity between the injected virus in the vaccine and the virus said to be responsible for causing the particular disease is the key to the efficacy of vaccination.

It all sounds quite logical doesn't it? Give your child a small, non-harmful disease to prevent the supposed devastating effects of the real disease.

The following diseases are said to be caused by viruses: measles, polio, smallpox, hepatitis, rubella, mumps, chicken pox, influenza, meningitis, Varicella-zoster (shingles), human papillomavirus (HPV), and rotavirus. Immunization is either suggested or required for all of these. Immunization is also suggested for some bacteria-caused diseases, such as diphtheria, pertussis (whooping cough), and tetanus.

Have you heard of such a thing as gaining immunity to bacteria? Is that even possible? I am not aware of any science which supports the premise that our bodies can become immune to bacteria through injections of foreign substances. That means you can forget about getting a diphtheria, pertussis or tetanus vaccine, because you cannot build immunity to bacteria. **The majority of diseases we vaccinate against are viruses**. Or are they? A more careful look at viruses shows that the diseases associated with a virus in fact are not caused by a virus. In fact, there is no such thing as an infectious disease virus.

Around1890, German physician Robert Koch and bacteriologist Friedrich Loeffler hypothesized that if diseases are caused by a virus, it should be possible to isolate the virus organism, and then use that isolated organism to create the same disease in another otherwise healthy animal. These criteria are known as Koch's postulates.[488]

As technology has steadily improved since Koch's time, science should have been able to conclusively prove the existence of viruses under Koch's postulates, and to have isolated a virus under the microscope. However, no one has been able to isolate any viruses to prove that they exist. Naturally one would expect that the medical establishment would announce this astonishing scientific discovery that disease-causing viruses do not exist. But instead they did something far more sinister: they pretended to have isolated the virus by following the acceptable protocols under Koch's postulates. In other words, *there is no such thing as a virus*.

When scientists claim to have isolated a virus, what they really have isolated is a mass of cellular material in which they believe a virus exists. If this material is filtered from sick animals believed to have a disease, and the material will kill cells in a Petri dish, then it is believed that the deadly virus has been discovered. Researchers then take some of these blended and partially filtered animal parts and look for RNA strands. If they find an RNA strand they report to the world that they have "mapped" the virus.

As German virologist and molecular biologist Dr. Stephan Lanka asserts (translated from German):

Viruses which are claimed to be very dangerous -- in fact do not exist at all.

The pictures of influenza, herpes, HIV, measles, hepatitis B, smallpox and other diseases are not pictures of viruses, but pictures of damaged cells with typical particles or other cellular material. In Lanka's words,

It must be said that these photos are an attempt of fraud committed by the researchers and medical scientists involved, as far as they assert that these structures are viruses or even isolated viruses.[489]

The proof of an infectious virus like hepatitis or rotavirus rides on the existence of some entity that can enter into and damage a healthy cell, then replicate itself and exit that cell in order to pass the infection to the surrounding cells. Yet in animal and human biology no such disease-causing entity has ever been found to exist. In any case where viruses have been proven to exist, as in algae, for example, they do not cause disease, but function as a helpful and supportive part of the ecosystem of the organism. Dr. Lanka continues:

*Actually in diseases, neither in the diseased organism nor in a body fluid, one has never seen or isolated a structure which one could characterize as a virus. **The allegation of the existence of any disease-inducing virus is a transparent fraud, a deadly lie with dramatic consequences.**[490] (Emphasis added.)*

The existence of disease-causing viruses is taught in school, reported in the media and then supported by mainstream doctors, the government and the pharmaceutical industries. The use of half truths and outright lies continues to obscure the truth of the matter. The term virus comes from the Latin word for poison or venom, which is probably related to the Sanskrit word *visha*, meaning toxin or poison.[491] The cells of our body swell and become mangled when exposed to poisonous substances (such as heavy metals, toxic foods, pesticides, chemicals and so forth) and then modern "scientists" mislabel these symptoms of environmental poisoning as specific diseases caused by viruses.

Remember the assertion of the wise western physician Dr. Henry Bieler:

The first is that the primary cause of disease is not germs.

And Dr. Thomas Sydenham:

Disease is nothing else but an attempt on the part of the body to rid itself of morbific (diseased, toxic) matter.[492]

And the modern physician, J.H. Tilden, MD, after years of wandering in the jungles of misdiagnosis:

There is no hope that medical science will ever be a science; *for the whole structure is built around the idea that there is an object disease — that can be cured when the right drug — remedy, cure — is found.[493] (Emphasis added.)*

Viruses and vaccines are both part of a devastating lie.

The awareness of this contradiction is why so many great physicians do not claim that viruses cause disease, but rather associate disease with a pernicious condition in the environment, such as poison or pollution, or malnutrition. By upholding the paradigm of the disease-causing virus which randomly attacks helpless victims, most modern doctors help hide the truth of what really makes us sick: toxins and nutrient deficiencies.

If vaccines cannot work, because the viruses they are supposed immunize us against have never really been isolated, then what are they really doing when they are injected into our children?

These large dosages of poisons are meant to cause neurological damage, learning disabilities, lowered intelligence, and diseases such as cancer in the long term.

I know that at this point that some people's illusions are crumbling. Even if you already know that vaccines are to be avoided, you may still have entertained illusions about the benign intentions of the medical establishment. Every parent who truly recognizes and feels the truth about vaccinations will help open a portal for real and effective change.

If vaccinations were truly effective and performed as advertised, we would not need laws and propaganda to enforce their use. If they worked to prevent disease, everyone would want to use them. But parents, who have a natural concern and caution regarding their children's welfare, must be coerced, manipulated, and betrayed into poisoning their own children.

Show me the Evidence!

There is no evidence that vaccines work. Vaccine promoters like to point their fingers at critics and say, "Prove to me vaccines do not work." But I have something to say to all the vaccine promoters: "Show me some evidence that they do work!"

Go to your local doctor and ask for a copy of a comparable study of vaccinated and unvaccinated populations for each vaccine the doctor is offering. Your doctor might scoff at you or dismiss your concerns as over-reactive. But press him to show you the long term studies that prove vaccines are effective in preventing disease. You will find that no such study exists. Be sure also to ask to see the disclosure label that comes with the vaccine. You will be shocked at the documented "side effects" listed for each vaccine.

Dr. Harold Buttram wrote a letter published in the British Medical Journal:

> There have never been any studies of this nature, and apparently none have been attempted. Based on personal observation, it appears that before-and-after testing has been studiously avoided by government health agencies for fear that the results would discourage public confidence in vaccine programs… [I]n my opinion the NIH, CDC, FDA can justifiably be accused of negligence in protecting the health and welfare of the American public, especially the children.[494]

Dr. Philip Incao's testimony for the Ohio State House of Representatives:

> Take a group of vaccinated children and compare them with a matched group of unvaccinated children. If the groups are well-matched and large enough and the length of time the children are observed following vaccination long enough, then such a study is deemed the 'gold standard' of vaccine research because its data is as accurate a reflection as medical research is capable of achieving of how vaccinations are actually affecting our nation's children.
>
> Incredible as it sounds, **such a common-sense controlled study comparing vaccinated to unvaccinated children has never been done in America for any vaccination.** This means that mass vaccination is essentially a large-scale experiment on our nation's children.[495] (Emphasis added.)

According to one vaccine industry whistleblower, a bad reaction to a vaccine is defined only by what occurs immediately after the vaccine is administered so that no long term consequences can be exposed. This approach virtually ignores the effectiveness period of the vaccine, which is supposed to continue for years and years. Monitoring and reporting of adverse reactions, then, should be followed for years and years.[496]

Because we are **not victims of disease** we cannot "catch a virus." However, if you do fall for the propaganda of the vaccine promoters, you will go to get a shot to protect yourself against a virus. You will then get sick, because you have mistakenly exposed yourself to disease-causing toxins in the form of the "vaccine."

To my understanding, the creation of a vaccine starts with the initial cells being grown or cultured in a nutrient-rich medium. This medium usually uses animal organs or animal parts. Many times these nutrient-rich media can be contaminated with toxins such as amoebas and enzyme inhibitors.[497]

After the cells are cultured and mixed with animal parts, they are purified in order to filter out the so-called virus that the pharmaceutical company wants to use in the vaccine. Of course, they don't filter out just the virus because the virus has never been identified for each disease, so the filter allows much more to pass through — material believed to contain some type of virus. One vaccine whistleblower, reporting under the pseudonym of Dr. Randall, reminds us that many vaccines are made with aborted human fetal tissue. He's also found foreign proteins contaminating many batches of vaccines.[498]

It is unknown whether every dose of vaccine is contaminated or not since the FDA abandoned testing vaccines over 15 years ago. Vaccine ingredients commonly include preservatives, stabilizers and other adjuvants such as ethylene glycol (antifreeze), phenol (carbolic acid), formaldehyde, aluminum, thimerosal (mercury), neomycin (anti-biotic), streptomycin (anti-bacterial), squalene (fish, or plant oil), gelatin, MSG, and phenol (a caustic, poisonous acidic compound present in coal tar and wood tar).

You can learn more about vaccine ingredients on Dr. Viera Scheibner's website.
www.vaccination.inoz.com
An infant is a pure being untouched by life. When we administer a vaccine to an infant we puncture his skin, which is a form of surgery, and pump materials into his bloodstream that are supposed to prevent disease. It has been widely reported that an infant injected with the hepatitis B vaccine is given a dosage of mercury that can only be safe for a person who weighs 275 pounds or more.

Don't be mistaken; the pharmaceutical companies know exactly how these chemicals affect children from tests they do on animals and people. They throw out large groups of test data to make it appear that vaccines reduce rates of disease. These ingredients are not added to the vaccine by accident, and they each have a specific purpose. Their purpose is to debilitate your child and to make him subject to disease.

Some vaccines are created with African green monkey kidney tissue, chicken and guinea pig embryonic tissue, calf serum, and even human diploid cells (the dissected organs of aborted human fetuses).

If fetal tissue is not used then chicken embryos and monkey kidney cells may be used. These cells enter your child's body through injection and directly alter and contaminate your child's bloodstream. How does any of this prevent diseases? Show me the evidence!

Keep in mind that when children are born they are designed to be able to drink raw human milk and they are able to digest little or nothing else. If a child cannot digest chicken eggs, or monkey kidney, then imagine what happens when small amounts of these substances are directly injected into the infant's blood.

The tests used to approve a vaccination for public use do not examine whether the vaccination prevents diseases in the future. Vaccines are considered effective if certain "antibodies" are temporarily present in the bloodstream after a few days of vaccination. There is no evidence of efficacy based on scientific double-blind experiments. And even those antibodies do not have to always be present for a vaccine to be approved.

No vaccine exists that has actually been tested and proven to work against the disease for which it is supposed to protect your child.

That is why evidence that supports the efficacy of vaccination is only found in graphs with skewed figures indicating declines in disease rates after the administration of mass vaccinations. These graphs don't show you the all-important remainder of the chart, however. If they did, you would see that the rates of the disease were plummeting *before* the vaccine was introduced as shown in the graphs on the next page.

Decline in Measles Death Rate Prior to Vaccine Introduction

Decline in Pertussis Death Rate prior to Vaccine Introduction

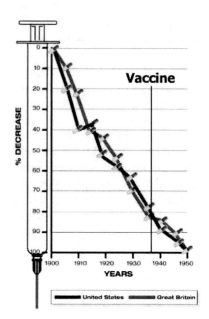

Reprinted with permission from Vaccines: Are They Really Safe and Effective? by Neil Z. Miller. All Rights Reserved. For more information, visit: www.thinktwice.com

Decline in Death Rates Prior to Vaccine Introduction

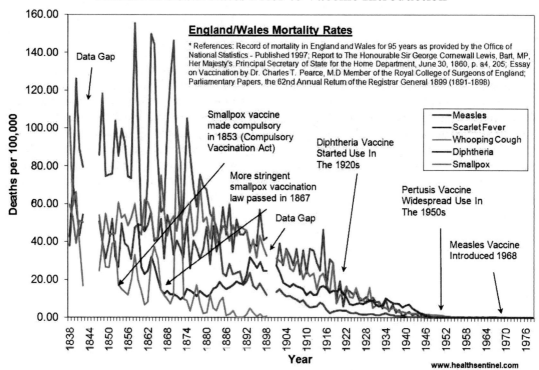

The Vaccination Lie is a Crime Against Our Children

You have probably been led to believe that vaccination is not only a good way to prevent disease, but that study after study has shown that it works. You have been lied to.

Dr. Viera Schreibner, a world authority on immunizations, reviewed 60,000 scientific articles and came to the following conclusion:

One hundred years of orthodox research shows that vaccines represent a medical assault on the immune system.

A growing number of researchers are linking vaccines to epidemics of childhood leukemia and other forms of cancer, asthma, autoimmune disease, cerebral palsy, infantile convulsions, and **sudden infant death** syndrome.[499]

A 1926 article from the Journal of the American Medical Association states the following:

In regions in which there is no organized vaccination of the population, general paralysis is rare. It is impossible to deny a connection between vaccination and the encephalitis (brain damage) which follows it.[500]

In October 2000, at the annual meeting of the Association of American Physicians and Surgeons (AAPS), a resolution was called for to end government-mandated vaccines, claiming:

Mass vaccination is equivalent to human experimentation and subject to the Nuremberg Code, which requires voluntary informed consent.

You can read the resolution at www.aapsonline.org/testimony/vacresol.htm

Vaccines are Government Sponsored Medical Bioterrorism & Institutionalized Murder

A definition of murder: The unlawful killing of one human by another, especially with <u>premeditated malice</u>. The malice is expressed or implied.

We would consider a person who murders a child to be one of the most deplorable and evil persons we could imagine. Yet when the government sponsors corporations that kill and disable our children, we call it health-promoting public policy. Our government and related establishments then threaten, coerce, intimidate, lie to and terrorize people who oppose this vaccination policy of murder.

The suffering: Below are a few documented cases of the adverse results of vaccination. These are based on publicized US Government Statistics from the vaccine reporting system.

Hepatitis B: "Since July 1990, **17,497 cases of hospitalizations, injuries and deaths** following hepatitis B vaccination have been reported to the Vaccine Adverse Event Reporting System (VAERS) of the U.S. government. This figure includes *146 deaths* in individuals after receiving only hepatitis B vaccine, without any other vaccines, including *73 deaths* in children under 14 years old."[501]

MMR: From July 1990 through April 1994, 5,799 adverse events following MMR vaccination were reported to US VAERS; this included 3,063 cases requiring emergency medical treatment, 616 hospitalizations, and 309 who did not recover. **54 children left disabled** and **30 deaths**.[502]

DPT: "A total of 54,072 reports of adverse events following vaccination were listed in a 39-month period from July 1990 to November 1993 with 12,504 reports being associated with DPT vaccine, including **471 deaths**."[503]

These are reported figures. One murder is a deplorable crime; here we have over 500 documented murders. The chilling reality, however, is that a majority of adverse vaccine responses are <u>not reported</u>. The FDA commissioner acknowledged that only 10% of adverse reactions are reported,[504] and other more realistic studies suggest that as few as 1.5% of all adverse reactions (vaccine and otherwise) are reported.[505] This means that the actual figures of vaccine injury and death are, in a conservative analysis, at least 10 times higher than the statistics I just presented, and they very well are more likely around 66 times higher. In 1993, FDA Commissioner David Kessler, MD reported that doctors failed to report up to 99% of serious adverse medication reactions.[506] This failure stems from doctors not seeing what appears before their eyes. The possibility of injury caused by vaccination directly contradicts their beliefs about vaccination. Doctors who promote vaccination — the vast majority — constantly see children being injured by vaccines. The cornerstone of Western medicine is vaccination, so doctors have the choice of admitting that their entire medical knowledge is false or continuing to deny that vaccines cause illness. Which choice do you think most doctors make?

What these figures mean is quite incomprehensible. Let's take DPT vaccines, for example. 471 deaths were reported in a three year period by doctors or hospital staff. If this figure represents only 10% of the actual number of deaths, then it is likely that **4,710 children were murdered** as a result of exposure to vaccine toxin DPT. Yes, it is shocking. And what is more shocking is to consider Dr. Kessler's assertion that 99% of serious events are NOT reported. Even if we are generous here and say that 2% of adverse reactions are reported (assuming 98% serious events not reported), this means that in a three year period, **23,550 children were extinguished from planet Earth** in the U.S. from just one vaccine. Not all children die from vaccination. Consider the additional figures of the numbers of children who showed at least a serious reaction from DPT vaccine over a three year period. If we consider how conservative the reported numbers are, this would actually be from 125,040 (assuming only 10% of reactions reported) to a staggering 625,200 (assuming 2% of reactions are reported).

While these numbers may sound astronomical or unbelievable, the data I am drawing from is published as part of the US Government Vac-

cine Adverse Event Reporting system. It can be searched at **www.medalarts.org**. When I did a recent search for the number of all people who have been reported to have died as a result of vaccines, I received the following result: "Found 3052 events with Patient Died." Of these, 2070 death reports are for toddlers and infants two years old and under. These records began in 1990, so they represent 18 years to date. For example, the first listing states, "Hypotonic, Hyporesponsive episode, Infant died:" six days after vaccination. Another, "child found dead in bed" that is a two-year-old who died two days after the DPT and HIB injection. Many reports are only for children who have died within one week of the vaccine, even though vaccines may have long term adverse effects. Because the effects of vaccines are supposed to last many years it would be less likely for the parent or doctor to consider filing a report if the death did not occur close to the vaccination date. It is highly likely that these statistics are extremely underreported. Let's assume the grossly understated 10% of adverse events reported for the past 18 years. This means that 20,070 infants have been murdered by vaccines. Using the more likely figure of 2%, the number is 103,500 infants. You can search the reported records yourself, and see the moderate to severe side effects, including death, documented by the U.S. government.

We are talking about debilitation and death on the scale of hundreds and thousands.

A very sarcastic person once wrote me that if you check the data on the VAERS site you will find a disclaimer to the effect of "these reports are just reports and have not been confirmed." First, many reports are filed by doctors, and a doctor would not file a report unless he was strongly suspicious that the vaccine indeed had caused the injury. Second, and more important, no reports are investigated because the published findings would bring the entire system to a screeching halt, with angry parents tearing down the doors of the pharmaceutical offices and dragging the criminals (including public officials who promote vaccines) to court. I sincerely hope that these vaccine criminals will be put on trial one day soon. They will be when you help spread the truth about vaccines.

Vaccine Induced Diseases (VID)

When parents allow their children to be vaccinated they are actually giving their children a disease. And this is not a hidden fact; this is part of so-called vaccine "science." To give the child a disease in order to prevent the potential for an even worse disease is the logic behind how vaccine works.

The sickness that develops after vaccination, however, does not confer immunity to the disease as it is supposed to. It is actually a new disease and illness itself, brought about by the act of vaccination — a vaccination that confers immunity to nothing.

The illness that arises is a response to poisons in the vaccine, poisons like aluminum, MSG or formaldehyde. Your child does not build up any immunity to the disease the vaccine is for. The only immunity your child builds, through cellular mutation, is immunity towards the toxins in the vaccinations. The body defends and even primes itself after repeated attacks by vaccines.

In 2001 for example, The VAERS reported 14,752[507] adverse reactions from vaccines. These included 224 deaths, and 594 cases that resulted in permanent disability.[508] Because adverse reactions are reported between 2% to 10% of the time, we can surmise an approximate yearly disease and death rate caused by all vaccinations. The real number of annual vaccine-induced illness is anywhere from 147,520 cases to as high as 737,600. The real number of **annual vaccine-induced deaths,** based on the 2001 statistics, is anywhere from **2,240** to **11,200** deaths in just one year, and the real number of annual vaccine-induced permanent disabilities in the United States is anywhere from 5,940 cases to as high as 29,700 cases.

The following is from the Centers for Disease Control (CDC.gov):

Even though most infants and toddlers have received all recommended vaccines by age 2, many under-immunized children remain, leaving the potential for outbreaks of disease. Many adolescents and adults are under-immunized as well, missing opportunities to protect themselves against diseases such as Hepatitis B, influenza, and pneumoccal disease.[509]

These scare-tactics flout the truth but are commonly used in propaganda to coerce compliance with vaccination programs. The CDC should really be called the *Centers of Disease Causation* — since they promote infanticide. Learn to see through these lies so that you will become *immune* to their noxious influence!

Part of the mass confusion and misinformation campaign involves blaming people who are unvaccinated for causing disease outbreaks. Remember, there is no reputable evidence to support these claims of the CDC. Call them and ask for the evidence in writing if you do not believe me. Here is their toll free number: 800-232-4636. How do under-immunized children create outbreaks? Someone who is "properly" vaccinated should be immune to disease carried by an under-immunized person, shouldn't he?

Pharmaceutical companies, state and federal government health agencies, the American Medical Association, the Centers for Disease Control, National Institutes of Health and the Food and Drug Administration, as well as other related institutions, clearly must be held accountable for the crimes that they are perpetrating. These are "white collar" crimes, and "institutional crimes." It will be difficult for our court system to prosecute the real perpetrators of this violence because of the long history these agencies and corporations have in colluding in their crimes in secrecy and with protection from the highest offices in the land. Information about the murder and purposeful disabling of our children through medical experimentation has been kept well covered.[510] These organizations lie to people to frighten them into believing the vaccine fallacy, while they have no scientific evidence to support their claims. I declare that these organizations and their directors will not be immune to prosecution much longer. They will face their penalties; whether it is today or in their day of reckoning. The system of lies and disillusion will dissolve, and it will dissolve first through you when the light of truth inspires you.

Vaccinations Do Not Protect Against Disease

In case you are not yet convinced of the deception and horrors of vaccinations, I have compiled more evidence for you to examine. Mass vaccinating is a relatively new practice and began in the 1800s with the smallpox vaccine. Today, a normal vaccine schedule has a young child receiving up to 24 vaccinations by the age of two. Let's examine briefly the diseases we vaccinate for most commonly, and look at the supposed risk of the disease, as well as the risks attendant with the vaccination. You will find that in many cases, it appears that the vaccination is more deadly, and has far more dangerous effects than the disease it is meant to prevent. The truth is, if we did not vaccinate at all, disease rates would further decrease, or at least would not increase.

Chickenpox (varicella)

Varicella always runs a favorable course. It has no sequlae.... PROGNOSIS.—This is always favorable. - Dictionary of Medicine (1894)

> *Dr. Ogle, the chief in the Registrar-General's Department, told the Royal Commission as a witness before it, that he had never known chicken-pox kill a child in his life. -Dr Hadwen (1896)[511]*

We can see that chickenpox is a fairly harmless disease. How about the vaccine? According to the CDC, "During March 1995-July 1998, a total of 9.7 million doses of varicella vaccine were distributed in the United States. During this time, VAERS received 6,580 reports of adverse events, 4% of them serious."[512] This included 14 deaths. One death, one adverse effect,

is too many. Not one more child should be sacrificed to this devious and unscientific procedure.

Diphtheria

Only four cases of diphtheria were reported in 1992 in the United States. What about in other countries? After the introduction of a compulsory diphtheria vaccine in Germany and France, incidence of the disease skyrocketed.[513] It should be clear now what happens when you inject toxic disease-causing agents into people.

Vaccine Adverse Event Reporting System between 1995 and 1998 reports: "During the study, there were 285 reports involving death, 971 nonfatal serious reports, and 4,514 less serious reports after immunization with any pertussis-containing vaccine."

Large scale research on over 3.3 million children in the US found 33,006 cases of acute neurological reactions (encephalitic screaming, convulsions, collapse) within 48 hours of receiving the DPT shot.[514]

Flu (influenza)

Hugh Fudenberg, MD, is the world's leading immunogeneticist and the 13th most quoted biologist of our times, with nearly 850 peer-reviewed published papers to his credit. According to Dr. Fudenberg, if someone had five consecutive flu shots between 1970 and 1980, their chances of developing Alzheimer's disease is ten times higher than if they had one or no shots. This increased likelihood is due to the dose of mercury and aluminum in every flu shot, which accumulates in the body over time.[515]

Dr. Bieler helps us understand what really causes influenza and other supposedly contagious illnesses that we vaccinate for:

> *The several forms of these intestinal crises, or drunks, follow holidays or feast-days. The lightest drunks are named colds, flu, tonsillitis; the heaviest, diphtheria. In those who eliminate through the skin (the eruptive fevers), the lightest form is called measles; the heavier, scarlet fever; the heaviest, black smallpox.[516]*

In other words, after seasonal celebratory meals, when people indulge in too many sweet foods, especially processed sugar and other modern foods (including cheap alcohols), they get sick. This is exacerbated when people do not exercise due to inclement weather. The symptoms called colds, flu, scarlet fever and so forth, are exertions of the body trying to expel the toxic substances ingested—rather like a food hangover from Dr. Bieler's perspective.

A study in the Lancet found that in over 100,000 employees, flu shots did not confer any protection to the flu. Outbreaks of deadly Legionnaires' disease immediately followed flu vaccination campaigns.[517]

In 2001, according to the CDC, 257 people died of the flu.[518] Flu deaths are grouped together with pneumonia deaths, so one has to look carefully at the statistics to see that most people, over 61,000, in fact died from pneumonia and not the flu. In 2002, 42 people died exclusively from the flu vaccine as reported by VAERS.[519] The actual number of deaths from the flu vaccine, based on error reporting statistics, is likely 420 - 2,100, far more deaths than caused by the flu itself.

Measles

Measles generally resolves itself in the patient in ten days, and is therefore often called "ten-day" measles.[520]

Measles deaths in the U.S. had declined by 99.4% before the inculcation of a vaccination program against it, so there is no evidence that vaccination played any part in its decline. (This can be seen in the vaccine chart on page 268.) Parents, however, are deluded when told that vaccination was the only factor in the decline and therefore is the only defense against the disease.[521]

An unpublished study by the World Health Organization (WHO) looked at the rate of measles in malnourished children who had and hadn't been immunized. The group who hadn't been vaccinated contracted measles at the normal contract rate of 2.4%. In the group that *had* received the measles vaccine (MMR), 33.5% contracted measles.[522]

Dr. Bieler writes:

> *It is my belief that measles heads the list of the diseases of childhood which are the result of starch and sugar toxemia. Whooping cough, croup, pneumonia, meningitis, influenza, sinusitis accompanied by a heavy nasal discharge, pink eye, bronchitis and asthma are members of the same group. The natural antidote consists of diluted fruit juices, such as apple, orange, grapefruit, pineapple, papaya and guava.[523]*

I believe that the starches referred to here are products made with flour, particularly white flour.

Hepatitis B

Hepatitis means liver inflammation. Hepatitis B is an adult disease and mostly affects I.V. drug addicts. In 1991 the Centers of Disease Causation (CDC) recommended that infants be given hepatitis B poison after birth.[524] Hepatitis B is rare to non-existent in childhood and is not contagious.[525] Hepatitis B is caused through intravenous drug use and through sexual relationships. 95% of hepatitis B patients do not need hospital care and recover naturally.[526]

There have been more than 16,000 reports of hospitalization from serious hepatitis B vaccines reported since 1990.[527]

Meningitis (Hib)

Meningitis means inflammation of the meninges membranes surrounding the brain and spinal cord.

One study in the *Journal of the American Medical Association* found that the incidence of meningitis in children vaccinated against it was five times higher than in unvaccinated children.[528]

Referring to meningitis Dr. Bieler writes,

> *These diseases are all inflammations and are due to a forced elimination of toxins. I have found the only method of curing or alleviating them is to neutralize the tox-*

ins by diet in order to relieve the congested and disturbed liver by rest and to facilitate the elimination of poison through the natural channels chosen by nature for that kind of work, such as the kidneys, liver, lungs, skin and bowel.[529]

In other words, if you want to prevent meningitis then you'll need to keep your child's blood clean and healthy, i.e., no vaccines.

1,454 adverse reactions were reported on VAERS in 2005 from the Hib vaccine.[530] This means the actual number of adverse reactions is 14,540 to 72,700 in one year.

Mumps

Mumps is considered a mild disease in childhood, with complications being uncommon.[531] In 2006, a mumps outbreak occurred in the Midwest, affecting primarily college students who had two doses of the MMR vaccine.

Polio

Dr. Bieler explains polio:

Polio, although really a comparatively rare disease, with mild symptoms such as fever, head cold and stiff neck, causes a pitiful muscular paralysis in about 2 percent of those afflicted... I also believe that the <u>most common source</u> of the particular acid the polio virus seems to prefer comes from the putrefaction of ice cream in the bowel. Polio strikes most viciously at children who eat large quantities of ice cream. One indication of this is that the majority of cases occur during the peak of the summer ice-cream season.[532] (Emphasis added.)

Dr. Bieler's assertion that polio can be caused by ice cream makes perfect sense considering independent polio researcher Jim West's proof that polio is a result of poisoning from pesticides, especially DDT, which can be transmitted through cow's milk when the cows eat pesticide-tainted feed. Milk can transmit pesticides easily because the mammary glands store and collect certain types of toxins. Chemicals like DDT are known to cause paralysis, the very same symptoms of severe cases of polio, which are falsely blamed on the virus.

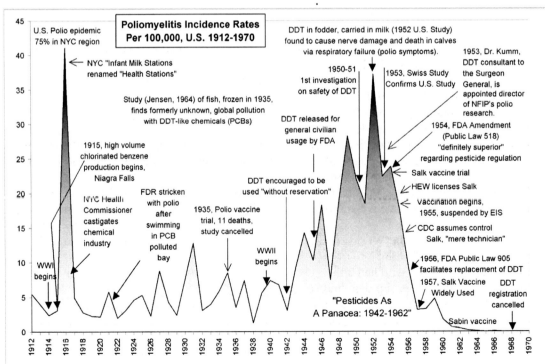

Opposite Page: *The chart shows the incidence of cases of polio in the US from 1912 – 1970. The fluctuations in the rate of children afflicted with polio, can be directly correlated to the presence of DDT and DDT like chemicals that children were exposed to primarily through milk products. While polio is claimed to have been eradicated by vaccines, in the chart you can see that Mr. West's research clearly shows that it was outlawing the use of DDT that caused polio to stop. (More recent polio outbreaks in other countries may be caused by the use of DDT like chemicals as pesticides. Those chemicals are outlawed in the US, but not in other countries.)*

It is officially accepted that since 1979, the only cases of polio in the United States have been caused by the polio vaccine.[534] However, a new disease called "post polio syndrome" has affected hundreds of thousands due to DDT pesticide blends.

The oral polio vaccine was given to children in Uganda. Greater African Radio founder Kihura Nkuba has commented that in Uganda polio is extremely rare. (This could be due to freedom from of DDT contaminated milk and milk products.) Nkuba noted that a $5 medicine is very helpful for people suffering with malaria, and yet the government of Uganda instead spent its money on the useless polio vaccine, which has been attributed to causing at least 600 deaths in that country. One can conclude that the vaccine was used for genocidal purposes.[535]

Rubella

Typically, childhood rubella has no symptoms and often goes unnoticed.[536] In 1994 for example, there were just over 200 cases of rubella in the entire country, and 75% of those cases occurred in adults over twenty.[537] In essence, this disease won't affect your toddler.

The main danger with rubella is called rubella embryopathy. In a six year period in Switzerland there were only four cases total, two from women fully vaccinated.[538]

In Australia in 1972, virologist Dr. Beverly Allen gave stunning evidence that the rubella vaccine didn't work, and that the entire concept of "herd immunization" didn't work.[539]

In an Australian study, a group of recruits was immunized for rubella, and all produced the expected antibodies. When later exposed to the disease, 80% of the recruits contracted it.[540]

In 2005, 3,193 adverse vaccine reactions to the MMR vaccine were reported.[541] The actual figure for adverse reactions is then 31,930 to 159,650 in just one year in the U.S.

Smallpox

In 1973, Professor George Dick reported that 75% of those who contracted smallpox in Great Britain were vaccinated against it. Considering how few people were vaccinated at the time, the odds of getting smallpox were significantly higher if you were vaccinated.[542]

The first vaccine ever created was for smallpox. But it wasn't created from a human disease source; the agent came from cowpox. The so called cowpox "virus"— vaccinia "virus"—takes its name from milkmaids who contracted the "virus" from handling the udders of infected cows—*vacca* is the Latin root for cow, and is the origin of the word vaccination. By transferring fluid from cowpox lesions to scratches on the skin of healthy persons, these individuals purportedly became immune to the related Variola "virus," or smallpox. Between 1870 and 1872, however, there was a widespread smallpox outbreak in Germany with more than one million people affected. 96% of them had received the new vaccination.[543] This ought to prove that the vaccine was not effective. But instead this instance is cited as proof of the success of vaccine theories.

Tetanus

Tetanus is a very rare disease. During a three year period in the 1980s, there were only six reported cases in the entire U.S. in children, with no fatalities.[544] The odds of being struck by lightning are probably much higher than of contracting tetanus.

Tetanus, like diphtheria and Hib illness, are caused by bacteria rather than viruses. Vaccines for tetanus therefore contain a toxin containing the bacterium, in the hopes it will confer immunity. The body cannot build immunity to toxins. In Germany, about 66% of those who contract tetanus have been vaccinated against it, and in Switzerland about 50% of people who contract tetanus have been vaccinated, again proving that the vaccine is useless.[545]

In a vaccine debacle, the tetanus vaccine was given to pregnant women in the Philippines. Many of those who were injected had spontaneous abortions. Further investigation showed that the vaccine deliberately contained human chorionic gonadotrophin, a chemical known to end pregnancy.[546] In other words, the tetanus vaccine was used as a disguised tool to cause miscarriage in Filipina women.

Tuberculosis

In a rare instance, a study comparing vaccinated and unvaccinated groups was carried out by the World Health Organization in the 1960s. The experiment, conducted in India with a group of 375,000 people, was ended after seven years for ethical reasons because it was shown that the vaccine had a 0% effectiveness rate.[547] It is undisputed that tuberculosis vaccines do not confer immunity to the disease.[548]

We have seen earlier that tuberculosis is a degenerative disease caused by the body's response to toxins and nutritional deficiencies caused by a modernized diet. Tuberculosis only appeared in native groups with the introduction of modern foods. Again, injecting chemicals into the body cannot provide any sort of immunity to toxic and unhealthy diets.

Whooping Cough or Pertussis

Pertussis is a disease that causes discomfort but is usually of little risk in healthy children.[549] In a 1976 report in the *British Medical Journal,* of 8,092 cases of whooping cough, 2,940 (36%) were fully immunized, while only 2,424 (30%) were not immunized.[550] These numbers indicate that those who received the whooping cough vaccine were more likely to contract the disease.

Acknowledged side effects for the pertussis vaccine include fever, local skin effects such as swelling, redness, and pain, as well as crying

bouts, a shock-like state, and sudden infant death (SIDS). [551]

Sample of Diseases Caused by Vaccines

Known diseases ("side effects") caused by vaccine introduction include irreversible brain damage, involuntary muscle movements, mental retardation, inflammation of the membranes of spinal cord or brain (something the vaccine is supposed to prevent not cause), seizure disorders, half-body paralysis, blindness, hyperactivity, high pitched screaming and prolonged crying, learning disorders, hay fever, asthma, sudden infant death (SIDS), and abdominal pain. Longer term effects can include juvenile-onset diabetes, Reye's syndrome and multiple sclerosis.[552]

According to the Centers for Disease Control, which participates in the National Immunization Program, vaccines can cause death.

[V]accines are capable of causing serious problems, even death.

After this sobering admission, however, their propaganda vigorously promotes vaccination in the next sentence:

However, a decision not to immunize a child also involves risk. It is a decision to put a child at risk for contracting serious, and potentially deadly, diseases. Getting vaccinated is much safer than getting the disease vaccines prevent.[553]

Authorities will acknowledge partial truths in order to lend credence to their reputations as authorities. This ploy allows them to lie with confidence when stating that vaccines prevent death. Keep in mind, no evidence exists that vaccines do in fact prevent death. And nearly all studies published in peer-reviewed medical journals reveal that vaccines can and do cause death.

Even according to the CDC's campaign of half truths, the choice to vaccinate remains in your hands. Risk your child being exposed to *potentially deadly* diseases, which in many cases rarely or never result in fatality or disability as I have illustrated, or expose your child to vaccinations which are definitely capable of causing death. Between 1991 and 2008 the VAERS documented 1,897 vaccine-induced murders of infants age one and younger.[554] The cold-blooded murder of over two thousand children is more than enough. Remember that the actual figures of children murdered by vaccinations are at least 10 times higher. We are killing our children at a rate of at least 1,897 infants per year. It may be far worse that that—as high as 7,439 infants per year in the U.S. alone.

I have provided you with ample evidence that the risk of serious injuries or death from most diseases that we vaccinate for is extremely low. The rates of major infectious diseases have declined over time without the help of vaccinations. A majority of the diseases that we are taught to fear don't have symptoms at all, or are caused by an onslaught of toxic foods during the holiday seasons. I conclude that the vaccines discussed here were developed for diseases that people were induced to fear the most, and the diseases for which immunity could be claimed via vaccination. In other words, the diseases chosen for vaccination programs are rare so that it is less obvious to the observer that the vaccines in fact do not work. Most people were convinced to be vaccinated and medical authorities then pronounced the success of the vaccination program in eradicating the disease. Of course, the disease in question was already disappearing. Nowadays, with the flu and HPV vaccines, it is more obvious to see that the vaccines are not effective, and in fact cause harm. When the flu vaccine doesn't work during a particular "flu season," the usual excuse is that another mutation of the flu virus is responsible for the outbreak.

The system has gone mad. Children are dying every day. We have reached the apotheosis of the plague of modernization. We poison our children, causing debilitation and death, in the name of promoting health. Dr. Mark Randall, medical whistleblower, poignantly expresses a parent's healthy response to vaccination:

If I had a child now, the last thing I would allow is vaccination. I would move out of the state if I had to. I would change the family name. I would disappear. With my family.[555]

Let's take this advice to heart, and end vaccinations. Let us invite in the spirit of revolutionary change, the spirit of hope, of freedom and of the death of vaccination. Call a friend, spread the truth, share the information, file the lawsuits, change the laws. Let's stop this inhumane madness. If you do not take action, then who will?

Numbers are cold and remote, they don't convey the feelings of emotional devastation experienced by parents and family members who have been damaged by vaccination. I believe not one more child should suffer this tragic fate. Not one more mother should have to bear the loss of her child, or have to live with a disabled child when the very thing that she believed would protect her child's health caused the damage. Vaccine injury is so common that I personally know several mothers whose children are sick due to vaccines. These mothers can easily correlate the vaccine with their child's autism or severe skin problems.

Parents regularly experience the suffering of their infants who have been poisoned by vaccination, including shrieking from pain, fever, listlessness and seizure. Here is a small sampling from actual accounts: The once healthy three-month-old, after the DPT vaccine, had swollen legs, high-pitched screaming and fever. A few days later his body became limp, and he collapsed and died. Another mother woke in the middle of the night to hear her baby screaming and shrieking within 48 hours of a vaccine. This baby died in the hospital one hour later.[556]

Based on the conservative 10% figure of adverse events reported, close to seven infants die every single day in ways similar to the babies just described from this _serial killer_ called vaccination. I cannot think of anything more horrifying than for a parent to have to watch her new baby die from acute poisoning.

We have on our hands a medical catastrophe.

Negative Pleasure and Vaccinations

Why do parents still allow their children to be vaccinated? Isn't it obvious that vaccines don't work? Why don't parents do more research before they allow vaccination? Why do parents who believe vaccines are harmful still vaccinate their children? We have discussed the motivation for this behavior earlier in the infant's perspective chapter: it is the *negative pleasure* current.

Most of us have distorted inner convictions, largely because of an unhealthy imprint during childhood. If parents are brutally honest with how they feel they will discover that some part of them might take pleasure in hurting their child. This is because the pleasure current was associated negatively with the pain that the parent experienced when a child. Vaccinating a baby is a way to inflict pain while the parent remains unfeeling and numb. If you did not feel pleasure moving through your body you would not be able to perform the action; there would be no motivation for it. You would not call the doctor to make that vaccination appointment, you would not drive there with your child, and you would not pay for it without a current of energy that had pleasure fuelling your actions. This twisted negative pleasure shows your child that it is normal and acceptable for parents and society to poison children. It imprints upon your child the way life is here in the United States: that we do not take good care of one another and in fact hurt one another willingly.

I remember being little and going to the doctor to get my regular dosage of poison (vaccine). I felt dreadfully sick, not after the vaccine but before it. I could feel what a horrible thing was about to happen to me. I had a lump in my throat and went to the appointment in complete dread. When writing this chapter on vaccines, I developed a cough and felt ill. My arm still feels uncomfortable at the site of injection of the last vaccine I had, a tetanus shot when I was about sixteen. I received a large dose of the vaccine poison and collapsed after the shot. A few months later I developed eczema, severe fatigue, and hair loss. It has been a long term struggle to heal from the illnesses caused by that last assault on my body. No child should have to suffer such insults any longer.

Negative pleasure will arise in several ways in relation to vaccination:

1. The distorted pleasure of being totally oblivious to the effects of your vaccinating actions.
2. The distorted pleasure of hurting your child.
3. The distorted pleasure of following the crowd, being a sheep, and doing what the "authority" dictates is right. The authority in this case might be family, doctors, friends, or the media.

In reality, the only authority is the Creator. Other purported authorities are false authorities—fakes and pretenders—unless they are totally aligned with the Unassailable One. Since most people possess this distorted pleasure current, many parents actually feel justified by their immutable position that they are "doing the right thing" in poisoning (vaccinating) their children. Even today I can still occasionally feel this fear in me regarding vaccination. "What if I am doing something wrong?" It is the fear of disobeying the dictates of an outside authority. But if you examine carefully who is telling you to vaccinate your child, you will find that it is merely a voice or idea in your head. In the outer world, nobody is forcing you to do anything.

How Poisons from Vaccinations Can Affect Our Bodies

Before beginning mandated mass immunizations, the following questions should have been answered by careful studies. After the vaccine is injected, what happens in the body? What happens after multiple vaccines are injected over time? What happens when vaccines that have several different "viruses" are injected at the same time? To my knowledge this evidence is not available to the public and has not been clearly researched. Whatever evidence does exist is likely locked in safes and in secret computer databases in pharmaceutical company headquarters.

To answer these questions so that you can understand vaccine-induced diseases more completely I have created a rough chain of events to describe what might happen to a child's body when it is injected with a vaccine and is not able to defend itself from the resulting vaccine-induced disease. This outline is based on my interpretation of the work of Dr. Henry Bieler.

We will assume the child's state of health and well being are good before vaccination. At the point of vaccination, the contents of the vaccine dose directly enter the child's blood and therefore travel through the body unfiltered until reaching the liver. Normally, toxins enter the body through the eyes, ears, broken skin, nose and mouth. The body has filters in all of these organs to protect against disease. The young child's body has several lines of defense against poisoning. Before the foreign matter reaches the liver, the nervous system has already sent emergency signals to the adrenal and other glands. The body immediately paralyzes many of its functions and prepares for the battle against the enemy that might cause death. The enemy, the poison inserted deeply into the body, is formaldehyde, cells of chicken embryos, live or dead cells purported to contain some type of virus, mercury, possible contaminants, preservatives, MSG, aluminum, fluoride and perhaps other heavy metals and other industrial chemicals and stabilizers not mentioned. Within just a second and a half, these highly toxic substances enter the liver. The infant's liver may already be weak or depleted because of the ill health of the mother during pregnancy, or from exposure to environmental toxins, or because of some karmic reason. The liver cannot adequately neutralize the onslaught of poisons. The infant's liver is so undeveloped that it cannot even process most normal food. But now it is waging a war against industrial chemicals and heavy metals. The liver absorbs as much as it can and starts dumping the chemicals into the highly acidic intestines to be dissolved. There, the toxin overload is too much for the body to handle, and remains stagnant, creating a diseased state in the body over the long run. The adrenal glands go into overdrive

trying to help the liver purify the blood. They raise the body temperature to help the liver try to burn the poisons. If the poisons enter the wrong channel, in the wrong part of the body for even a moment, it could mean death. The liver cannot handle the poisons and cells begin to erupt. After a few hours, the body is becoming fatigued; it can no longer neutralize the toxic elements, and the liver begins to fail. Chemicals rush into the cerebral spinal fluid and penetrate the blood brain barrier, causing an emergency shock response in the system. The infant begins convulsing, and high pitched screaming erupts. The infant's delicate internal chemical balance is now destroyed. Massive cellular death occurs as healthy cells are sacrificed in a desperate attempt to contain the poison. The kidneys go into overdrive as a backup blood purifier and the heart begins beating faster to rapidly pump more and more blood. The heart rate doubles and then triples. The poisons, too abundant to be neutralized and unknown to the infant's biology, continue to pulse through the spinal fluid and cause swelling in the brain and spine. Seizures occur as the nervous system malfunctions. If the poisons are not removed rapidly by the body's lines of defense, the heart rate continues to rise to force more filtration through the liver and kidneys. The skin erupts in rashes and blisters, the lungs fill with mucus; the swelling and the bruises are the body's attempt to contain the poisons and push them out through the skin. These are the body's last lines of defense. The baby blisters all over his body as the poisons sear his skin. If the toxins are not contained the heart muscle tires and weakens because it cannot pump the blood fast enough through the liver and kidneys to cleanse them. The toxins overwhelm the body and the child goes into shock, enters a coma state in the body's last effort to try to shut down all functions in hope that it can survive. If the baby's body can neutralize enough of the toxins then he will survive. But the ordeal may leave him with neurological or other damage, and a high potential for chronic disease. Many times the body cannot manage the poisons, as is the case for at least seven infants every day. The promise of a world of love, compassion and comfort is shattered for these children, and they die a painful death, with just a brief taste of the life they were longing to live.

Why Vaccinations Cannot Ever Work

What we call a disease, the swelling, the bumps, the fever and irritation, are the body's response to a toxic material. These symptoms, which we mistakenly label as disease, are not the disease itself; in fact, these symptoms help to protect us against the real problem. Vaccines directly target our body's responses to an imbalance, and not the actual disease itself. They are not effective because they target the symptoms. The real purpose of vaccinations is to disable the body's own natural healing and cleansing mechanisms. Thus, if vaccines really worked, and succeeded in eliminating symptoms, everyone would immediately die, because the body's ability to respond to illness would be destroyed. The results of vaccination experiments are always hidden, because if and when experiments are carried out, the results prove unequivocally that vaccines do not stop disease.

Vaccinations cannot work because the key to immunity to disease is created by a healthy lifestyle, by breastfeeding, by holding and loving your baby, and by eating whole foods. Health comes from living in abidance of Nature's principles. Let's look at proof of this.

Natural Immunity and Safety from Disease with Nutrition

A proper diet, high in activator X and other fat-soluble vitamins and activators, whole grass fed and wild animal fats (land and sea), bone broths, grass fed raw milk and raw grass fed butter, as well as complete avoidance of all modernized foods, will create a high degree of safety from illness.

Consuming a good diet does not mean that your child will never fall ill with any of these diseases. However, the good diet will decrease your child's likelihood of falling ill, and will enhance your child's full recovery. By avoiding poisons from vaccines and western drugs you will significantly increase your child's immunity to disease.

Weston Price found a correlation between death from childhood diseases and the amount of vitamins available in dairy products in the diet.[558]

When the vitamins are high the defenses are high; when the vitamins are low, the defenses are low.[559]

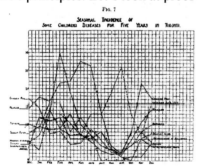

The average monthly incidences of seven children's diseases are shown in solid lines for five years for the city of Toronto, and reveal a very marked seasonal cycle. The vitamin curve as determined from samples of dairy products is shown in broken line, and is high when the morbidity incidence is low. [557]

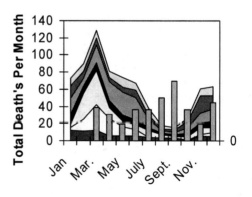

The graph on the right is a re-creation of the one on the left using the same statistics. The bars on the right represent the vitamin content of the butter. The lines represent the total number of deaths from disease per month. As the vitamin content of the butter increases, death from many diseases decreases.

Between August and September the grassfed butter contained the highest amounts of vitamins. At that time, you can see that all of the curves representing children's diseases drop dramatically.

What are the vitamins found in summer grassfed butter? Activator X, which is a hormone or hormone like substance, vitamin E, vitamin A, vitamin D, conjugated linoleic acid, and other known and unknown nutrients. This is nature's form of immunization against disease.

The best "immunization" that you can give yourself is eating a diet with whole, unrefined foods in alignment with Nature's principles.

Sacrificing Your Child on the Alter of "Public Safety"

Thousands of parents lose children each year due to vaccine traumas. Even if they don't die, many children are often left permanently disabled. The federal government created the Vaccine Injury Act to prevent lawsuits directed at pharmaceutical companies; without such protection the vaccine industry would crumble under an overwhelming avalanche of lawsuits. Filing lawsuits is very expensive, and lawyers representing the pharmaceutical industry fight back with massive force. Gag orders, supported by highly unconstitutional laws, limit what information reaches the courtroom, and the real truth remains hidden from the public eye. The laws that limit pharmaceutical accountability surely violate our constitutional rights, as they eliminate the checks and balances of the government. Rather than protect us from disease, the government allows companies to continue selling poison in the form of vaccines to our children at huge profits. The government thus significantly contributes to the suffering and death of many of our children. That being said, there are still ways to sue the pharmaceutical companies regarding vaccines and win big. The National Childhood Vaccine Injury Act states that in order to qualify for a reward, the adverse event must occur within four hours of administration of the vaccine. Only one in four claimants receives monetary compensation. Yet despite this tight restriction, in a thirteen year period the Injury Act has awarded $871,800,000 to parents of vaccine-injured children.[560]

How To Protect Your Children From Vaccine Diseases

White hat techniques (clean).

1. Do not give any vaccine to your child.
2. If you plan a hospital birth, be prepared to sign waiver forms so the hospital is not held accountable for any complications. The correct phrase is, "I do not consent to the treatment."
3. If hassled, or if there is an emergency, explain that your child is allergic to MSG or formaldehyde (everyone is), and that if injected he might die. Ask the "injector" if he wants to take a life and defend himself in court.
4. Ask for the waiver or release form. If it is not offered, continue to insist that you want to sign the waiver. There always seems to be a waiver, they just don't want you to know about it.
5. Make sure you appropriately file exemptions for your state, or join whatever religious organization you need to join to be exempt (even when you don't belong to the religion). More information can be found at: **www.vaccinetruth.net** I have found that playing by the rules of the system usually can work to our advantage when you totally understand the rules. You are the authority, and nobody can tell you what is right or wrong.
6. Leave the situation, take your child, and run! Once you get outside of the hospital, they cannot make you come back; they are not a police force. Out of sight, out of mind.

Grey hat techniques (less clean and less encouraged).

1. Tell the hospital staff that your child has just had such and such vaccine. If someone actually checks, then continue

to insist that you did have the vaccine and the forms have wrong information. Perhaps the paperwork got lost, you can say.

2. "My child went into a coma from the last vaccine," you could say. Tell them she is allergic to the vaccine. If they ask for hospital records, say it happened when you were travelling in "Spain" (pick a country you are familiar with). Say that you'd be happy to give them the hospital name, if only you could remember it.

I only offer the grey hat techniques for emergencies, in case you get stuck and don't know what to do. I have never had to use any of the grey ones. But I promise you I would not hesitate to lie, cheat, steal, break laws, or leave the country to protect my children from this crime (I haven't had to resort to any of these tactics yet). Knowing the truth and holding a clear focus and intention in a tough situation goes a long way. Usually our lack of focus or our own numbness is the enemy. Being prepared with knowledge and evidence about the laws usually will enable you to work sufficiently to stop any vaccinator. Your inner conviction when defending your child when you feel he is in danger should be something like, "If anybody gets near my child, or tries to vaccinate her, I will kill him." Yes it sounds a bit extreme, but when you are holding that level of focus and clarity I assure you nobody will question you. On the other hand, if you are unprepared, uncertain or equivocal about what will happen to your child, then you'll have a much harder time retaining any authority in the situation. After Sparkle's birth in the hospital, we didn't let anyone touch her. We told the pediatric doctor to leave the room when he came to do a check-up. He was insulted. Too bad for him and his ego, because this is our child and only we will decide if she has a "check-up" or not. We didn't want our little baby poked or prodded or touched by a stranger for no reason. Other parents may be happy to have doctors examine their baby, so it's up to you. Make sure you file the correct paperwork and documentation regarding baby check-ups, shots, vitamins, drops or whatever the law states you are supposed to subject your baby to. Unless you are in the mood to fight the entire system, sign the waiver form. We filled out several waivers at the hospital. We left without checking out.

The procedure for leaving the hospital is simple. You say, "We are leaving now. Good-bye," and walk out the same way you walked in. Remember, they cannot detain your body. Only police officers can detain you if they suspect you are going to commit a crime or if you are guilty of a criminal act. Protecting your children is not a crime. If you want to be polite ask if there are any waiver forms to fill out before you leave.

For Yeshe's birth, there was no hospital and no midwife. Nevertheless we had to fill out a "new baby screening" waiver. Michelle was very upset when we got a call from the State of California after we filed for a birth certificate. The state invaded our personal privacy just to see whether we had a new baby screening. What business does the state of California have to do that? The waiver form warned us that by not submitting our child to the screening we were waiving our right to blame the government for our baby's potential health problems.

Note: When you do certain things like refuse medical treatments that are a waste of your time and money and are invasive to your infant, you may be registered in a child abuse tracking system, because some officials believe it is child abuse to **not vaccinate** your children. You should be fine unless you somehow create other infractions.

Further Resources

video.google.com – search "Vaccination - The Hidden Truth."
www.knowvaccines.com - A parent offers this vaccination information site because of the loss of his daughter to vaccine-induced cancer.
www.vaclib.org - Organization devoted to repealing mandatory vaccine laws.
www.whale.to/vaccines.html - One father's investigations into vaccinations. Very thorough information.

www.healing-arts.org/children/vaccines - Studies on vaccine complications.
www.thinktwice.com - Offers an extensive selection of uncensored information on childhood shots and other immunizations.
www.medalerts.org –The VAERS database has been put online, you can see how real the adverse events are.

Books

Vaccination: 100 Years of Orthodox Research Shows That Vaccines Represent a Medical Assault on the Immune System, by Viera Scheibner, Ph.D.
Immunization, The Reality Behind the Myth, by Walene James, 1995.
The Sanctity of Human Blood: Vaccination is Not Immunization by Tim O'Shea
Handbook of Homeopathic Alternatives to Immunizations by Susan Curtis BA, MCH
Vaccines: Are They Really Safe and Effective? by Neil Z. Miller, 2002.

Safer and More Natural Vaccine Alternatives

While as a culture we still choose vaccinations, we overlook alternatives that may safely immunize children from childhood illness.

Homeopathy can give someone an energetic vaccination by administering such a small amount of a substance that only the energy signature of the substance is imprinted. Homeopathy generally has no side effects. This is a correct vaccine if there was one. But again, one must be careful not to thwart the body's natural responses as it can make conditions worse.

Intravenous vitamin C has stopped illnesses, although it probably works by over stimulating the glands.[561]

The universal oral vaccine is 100% safe, is taken orally, and can be made in any country in the world. Over 4,000 studies support that it works.[562] It is made by injecting substances into a pregnant cow's teat cistern, and when the cow produces colostrum it contains the substances needed to heal the illness of the individual.

What if You Have Already Vaccinated Your Child?

You might be feeling grief, shock or disbelief. Forgive yourself. And at the same time, take whatever appropriate outer world action you need to resolve the situation.

The poisons of the vaccines are still likely lodged in many places in your child's body. If, within a few days of the vaccination, your child seems in good health then the short term vaccine risk, the first hurdle, has likely been passed. The second hurdle is the long term health effects of the vaccine toxins. These toxins can be eliminated from the body. Eating a diet without any white sugar or white flour is a start. Eating a high fat diet, and a diet high in raw animal products helps detoxify the body. There are many other methods to help heal and cleanse your child's body. Fresh vegetable juices including beet juice, as well as raw eggs and raw milk bond to vaccine toxins and aid in their elimination. Raw eggs, several per day, and plenty of raw butter, are especially helpful. (See footnote for more info).[563] Seaweeds and other supplements designed to chelate heavy metals can help. Any type of protocol designed to help cure autism will likely help cleanse vaccine toxins from the body. Other treatments include chelation therapy, DMSO, oxygen therapy, homeopathy, herbal medicine, clays, and mineral supplements designed for autistic children.

Vaccinations, Tools of Genocide

If there is such clear evidence that vaccinations do not work, and no evidence that they do work, then you might ask yourself why we vaccinate at all. We are taught to believe that Western medicine operates under two ruling guidelines. The first is "Do no harm," and the second states that only medicines and procedures that have been thoroughly tested and proven to work be administered.

Let us look at why we really vaccinate

You have no doubt heard of all the campaigns to vaccinate people in poor countries. Prominent political figures gather to help raise funds and donate money to vaccinate and "save" the poor people and children in "Third World" countries. These vaccination campaigns are expensive, or at least the infrastructures that administer the programs are expensive, and require hundreds of millions of dollars. Why would we spend so much money vaccinating people when these large sums could really make a difference in supporting their basic health needs of food, water, clothing and housing? Again we hear from vaccine insider Dr. Randall:

> At the highest levels of the medical cartel, vaccines are a top priority because they cause a weakening of the immune system.

In the early 1900s, Indiana physician Dr. W.B. Clarke made an alarming point regarding vaccines:

> Cancer was practically unknown until compulsory vaccination with cowpox vaccine began to be introduced. I have had to deal with two hundred cases of cancer, and I never saw a case of cancer in an unvaccinated person.[564]

The conclusion is this: the purpose of vaccinations, besides providing immediate profit, is to cause cancer, AIDS, and lowered intelligence.

Want Some Cancer? Get a Vaccine.

We don't usually associate vaccinations with cancer, but there are many citations in the medial literature showing this link, especially with Oral Polio Vaccine, DPT, and HPV [565] which indicate or even prove that vaccines have caused cancers. It was well known in the 1800s that vaccines caused lymphatic problems such as

leukemia and other cancers, and diseases of the skin.[566] It has been well documented in *The Virus and the Vaccine: The True Story of a Cancer-Causing Monkey Virus, Contaminated Polio Vaccine, and the Millions of Americans Exposed* by Debbie Bookchin and Jim Schumacher, that as many as 98 million Americans received a polio shot tainted with a "monkey virus," SV40. In reality they were not tainted with a virus, since viruses don't exist. The vaccines contained highly toxic substances, probably from sick monkeys. University of Chicago researchers have found "genetic material" from the "virus" in a number of brain cancer victims.[567] Again, they probably found genetic material of monkey cells, not viruses. But they were able to correlate the vaccine to the brain cancer. Depressing our immune system with toxins in the vaccines increases our risk of cancer.

The question you might ask yourself is whether or not the contamination of millions of doses of polio vaccine was an accident? Today vaccines are not independently tested or analyzed, even with the ongoing large scale poisoning and debilitation of thousands. Meanwhile, raw milk, which has never given anyone cancer and is one of the safest foods available is tested regularly for pathogens by government agencies.

Want AIDS? Get a Vaccine.

What does Kenyan ecologist Wangari Maathai, the first African woman to win the Nobel Peace Prize, think about HIV?

> In fact it (the HIV virus) is created by a scientist for biological warfare.[568]

And how is this warfare carried out? The answer to that was on the front page of the London Times in 1987.

> Smallpox Vaccine Triggered **AIDS** Virus

The story developed after some employees in the World Health Organization (WHO) thought their efforts to vaccinate against smallpox might be causing AIDS.[569] An independent study they contracted showed their suspicions to be true. AIDS has been linked to the smallpox vaccine, hepatitis B vaccine, and the oral polio vaccine.[570]

Consider the story of Dr. Archie Kalokerinos, who took his medical degree from Sydney University in 1951.[571] In 1978 he was awarded the A.M.M. (Australian Medal of Merit) for "outstanding scientific research." Dr. Kalokerinos was a convinced vaccinator whose opinion changed when working with Australian Aborigines. He observed Aboriginal people dropping dead after being injected with a flu vaccine. He also saw dirty reusable needles being used in the African vaccine campaigns, even when the campaign organizers themselves said that "AIDS was carried by dirty needles." The needles were not reused out of necessity, because since the 1960s there had been more plastic syringes than anybody needed.[572] He writes:

My final conclusion after forty years or more in this business is that the unofficial policy of the World Health Organization and the unofficial policy of 'Save the Children's Fund' and almost all those organizations is one of murder and genocide. They want to make it appear as if they are saving these kids, but in actual fact they don't. I am talking of those at the very top.[573] *(Emphasis added.)*

We must mourn the loss of our fellow humans who have suffered so greatly. Many people in Africa who were vaccinated were also undernourished, which means their bodies could not handle the vaccine toxins well. Organizations that claim they are going to the Third World to save children are actually murdering them. They do this knowingly, at least at the top levels. It is common knowledge, even in conventional medicine, that it is contraindicated to vaccinate a sick or malnourished person…unless you mean to kill him.

The Darkness is Within

Within the human incarnation there is evil, so we must make changes in the outer world. This can include informing people about this crime against our children, and opposing its promoters and perpetrators. We must stop vaccinating our children.

But if we only attempt to make changes in the outer world, the inner world will remain unchanged. If we eliminate vaccinations without equivalently healing and changing our individual and collective dark inner belief systems, then a new form of evil and darkness will emerge in the world.

I tried once to share with a family member information about the evils of vaccination. This person refused to hear what I was saying and offered arguments in favor of vaccination, arguments based on the most recent news reel he'd seen. It did not matter what I said because the reporter had given a different story that completely eliminated any opportunity for outside reasoning. I felt intense anger and rage build up in me as I tried to defend my position. I noticed it. "Wow," I though to myself, "Even though I am speaking to support a good cause, and even though there is a righteous kind of anger that is fuelled by powerful truth, this is not what I am feeling." I was feeling the darkness within me, as though I could hurt another person. This evil of separation turns the other person into an object. While righteous anger would have been a powerful force for good, the force I felt was a distorted power, one that sought dominion over another. This is the same energy as in a vaccine.

When we harbor this kind of darkness within us, we promote negative creations in the world on the level of energy and consciousness. When I examine the roots of the anger I feel for vaccine promoters, I am able to get to the bottom of it. Below the anger, I really feel pain and hurt. And as I feel those emotions, I find myself feeling more free, and more at peace with life. My reaction to the vaccine promoter was based on my own unresolved pain and my defense to this pain resulted in numbness. Once I am in a numb state, I can act out, objectify, and even feel violent energy in me. This separated energy, if I let it remain, will contribute energetically to the cause of evil in the world. The other side of the picture is that the good unified in me contributes to ending evil. Through examining my responses, on a physical, mental, emotional and spiritual level, I made a small contribution to the end of evil in the world. The world is but a reflection of our collective mind, and awareness and attention dissolve negative energy.

"Resist not evil." In this context the statement does not mean to allow wrong actions. Rather, the admonition is to resist constructing a wall against the evil in you; do not turn away from it. The evil of vaccinations involves the evils of hurting innocent people (largely children), of false truth, of greed, and of oppression. Vaccines were not created out of love and abidance to Nature's laws; they were created from evil and darkness. But as I showed in my personal example, it is possible for hatred and separation to rise within us even as we try to act in the service of what is good. To eliminate darkness on the planet, we must eliminate the darkness within each of us. Where else would this darkness come from, but from the depths of our own beings? We heal our darkness with love and compassion, and through admitting and acknowledging our own truth no matter how painful it is to hear. When you feel negativity, look at it, acknowledge it, search for its origin, and ask yourself why it is there. Darkness cannot survive the light of your presence.

If we use evil and darkness to fight the outer evil of vaccinations, even if we win in the outer world we will loose the war. That conflict is within you, the choice is made in every moment: do you choose good, evil, or somewhere in between?

Why the Vaccination System Continues to Exist, and How to Stop It

How have we come to allow an unscientific practice to become an accepted norm in our culture? How have the normal checks and balances been evaded? Why is there mass vaccination when there is **no** scientific evidence to support its practice?

The answer has to do with you. This system exists because you and everyone else — the majority of the 300,000,000 or so of us United States citizens — has allowed it to continue to exist. Even further, we have created it as a reflection of our negative *imprint* of the world. We believe in negativity, hatred, and disease and thus we have unconsciously created its reflection in the mirror of the outer world. Let me use the words of the Pathwork to explain how we allow evil to persist. This can apply to many evils in the world and **within us**.

What happens when you are weak, when you do not stand up to evil behavior, when you collude with it and refrain from fighting for the truth? You encourage evil, you sustain the illusion in the person who perpetrates it that it is not so bad, that it is all right, that it is smart and that many people support it. This perpetuates the further illusion that by asserting truth, standing up for decency, and exposing evil, you will be isolated, ridiculed, and rejected. In other words, you foster the delusion that in order to be accepted one needs to sell out integrity and decency.[574]

So when each of us remains numb to the doctors who vaccinate, the scientists who make up studies to promote vaccines, the media who support the propaganda and are puppets delivering false reports, the government who makes laws to vaccinate, and the companies that bribe the government to vaccinate — we encourage evil. When we do not say "no!" to the doctor who is committing this crime, it continues. When we do not sue the government and seek to make new laws, it continues. By doing nothing, we allow evil to exist. We have but a handful of elite people and groups who make policies at the top of the bureaucratic chain. The rest of us dutifully follow along regardless of the harm done. We also have to notice how an environment has been created that strongly rejects people who speak out against the wrongs of vaccinations. This makes people afraid to speak out. Yet this fear of speaking out, of being rejected, is an illusion, and we are selling out our decency when we submit to this fear. Our fears about doing what is right and speaking out against wrongs are usually from childhood, and don't represent actual dangers.

When someone in your presence maligns another, for example, your silence is not goodness, gentleness, peacefulness. Far from it. In a sense it is more destructive and insidiously negative than outright, active maligning. Maligners expose their evil and thus take the chance of being rebuked and having to face the consequences. Passive listeners cheat by trying to have it both ways: they derive as much negative gratification from the maligning as the active one, without, however, risking any negative consequences, and even priding themselves that they really did not participate in the act.[575]

Every one of us who does not make an active effort to speak out against vaccines becomes like the vaccine promoters. We can continue to derive negative pleasure from letting it happen, and without any apparent consequences. Silence is more destructive and insidiously negative because its negativity is harder to see. How destructive is this silent collusion?

Can you see that silent collusion with evil is more abrasive than active evil? [Evil acts] required the cooperation of the traitors, the colluders, the silent bystanders who were afraid for their skin and thus allowed evil to — apparently — win. But, of course, evil can never really win.[576]

I myself am still working with my fear about speaking out, but I have taken some steps nevertheless. I have made a video on **youtube.com** of me speaking out against vaccines. How does not colluding, and not being a bystander, look for you? The video I made has made a difference in some people's lives. If I can do it, so can you.

Your mission (if you choose not to be a silent colluder) is to find ways to help stop vaccination. This could range from informing friends and relatives about the harms of vaccines, to not vaccinating your own children. It could mean filing lawsuits, or it might mean starting public organizations or support groups, or joining or donating to current organizations. Even when you do not see your anti-vaccine allies, we are here. We are working together to stop this. So go for it. Strike a blow to the darkness that has strangled our children's health, intelligence and well being.

Vaccination proponents will lose one day. But how many more lives will be taken before we stop this mass poisoning? Remember, your silence in the face of this obvious evil will not make the change happen.

Healing yourself from Vaccination Peer Pressure

Many parents will face criticism, coercion, and even subtle or overt forms of violence for voicing and acting upon their objections to vaccinations. This section is to give you some tools to help you handle possible backlash.

Your family members might accuse you of child neglect. Your doctor could threaten to not treat your child. In fact, it might be hard to find a doctor who will support you in not vaccinating. If your doctor will not treat you, consider a naturopathic doctor. Don't enter into a futile struggle with your vaccine-promoting doctor. He has been programmed by his medical school, which is controlled by special interests, not least of which is the pharmaceutical industry.

The first thing that you will notice in the undertone of vaccine promotion is the drumbeat of fear: the fear that your child will contract a deadly disease and die. The vaccination pushers claim to have your child's best interests at heart. If only your child gets the tiny little shot then she will avoid the consequences of serious and deadly diseases. Vaccines do come with side effects, admit the promoters, but isn't that small risk better than contracting a frightening, deadly disease? A secondary fear is that your unvaccinated child will become a disease carrier and infect other children. Both of these suppositions are phantom fears, and both are untrue. In fact, if you do not vaccinate your child, she will be *more* immune to diseases because her body will not be burdened and compromised by the toxic vaccine ingredients. And if vaccinations confer immunity to disease, how in the world could vaccinated children contract disease from unvaccinated children? Underneath the fear mongering, negative pleasure lies hidden within vaccine promoters. It is the motivation to see your child suffer.

People usually do not tolerate the emotion of fear very well. As a result, fear in the vaccine promoter can turn into anger. The person urging you to vaccinate your child will become angry if he believes that you are setting your child up for life in a wheel chair. His fear might easily trigger fear in you. "What if he's right?" a small voice may ask. Or you may feel that you will be punished for breaking the rules. Of course, you don't need to follow the rules. A friend or family member who promotes vaccination may try to emotionally hijack you by withholding love or acceptance if you resist their advice. Conversely, you yourself might get angry at this person because his fear and disapproval threaten your sense of self and authority. After all, this is your child, and no one has the right to tell you what's best for her. If you become angry with the vaccine promoter, notice if your anger is righteous (which is good) or is derived from fear (which has its origin in pain and separation). The fear that the other person is right can turn into anger if you feel that you must defend yourself against their assertions. Sometimes you will need to assert yourself; this is strength.

First, know your rights. You are in charge of your child's health. Nobody can decide what the best health care choice is for your child except you.

Second, understand some of the evidence. Those promoting vaccines get their "facts" from television, newspapers, magazines, government agency publications, or educational institutions. If they are willing to actually converse with you and not merely insist that they are right, then consider asking them what sources they base their claims on. How many unvaccinated children do they know who have contracted such and such disease? Ask them if they can provide you with evidence to support their pro-vaccination stance, since you would like to see if such evidence exits? If they demand evidence from you, this book provides bountiful evidence. But be sure they play fair; if you show them your evidence, they should show you theirs. Other than some meaningless charts with false figures they have none, because there is none. Nothing.

At this point the discussion has either turned to your favor or the other person is not listening to you. Ask if he might be open to hearing evidence which you believe is truthful about vaccines. Might he be open to changing his mind? What if his opinion is wrong? Is he willing to face those consequences?

People who promote vaccinations are often "rule followers," and their convictions are based on fear. We'll learn about how we all become mostly rule followers in the next chapter. The rule followers have created their sense of safety in the world by following the rules. The rule is you must vaccinate. To such people, opting out of vaccination is like driving on the wrong side of the road, heading right into traffic. In the case of vaccination, however, there is no oncoming traffic, and all the danger lies in following the rules. I myself used to be a rule follower. I would watch the TV news reports and can remember how I used to believe vaccines were good. Those were the days when I wasn't thinking for myself; the news and television programs were thinking for me.

People who promote vaccines are afraid. They are afraid to know about the lies, the hypocrisy, and the violence that goes on in the world because they are numb. Everyone can perceive, through their embodied feelings, this reality about the evil of vaccinations. But only a few of us today really acknowledge it. Western medicine succeeds in healing in a small percentage of cases, but it does not prevent disease, and certainly not by vaccination programs. Vaccine promoters must come to grips with how they have poisoned their own children, and promoted and believed in a system based on disease, death and suffering. For many people, this type of change does not come about easily, because that brief moment of awareness, when the truth is accepted, is quite a shock when it first hits. In truth, one's world seems to turn upside down.

Activity: responding to vaccine peer pressure. Notice the fear in you and in the other person. Trust the reality. Trust the truth. Trust the evidence. Trust your feelings. Vaccines are poisons; there is no evidence that they work, and there is an enormous mountain of evidence that they do not work. Vaccines are used for genocide in the Third World, and in our culture they are used to promote cancer and lowered intelligence. Do not fight unconscious behavior with your own unconscious behavior, but move toward a higher ground. Come from your heart, and notice where the other person's heart is. Does the other side really care about you or only about driving home their point? Make the choice that cares for you and your child.

Vaccine Final Words

There is evil in the world.

Evil exists in the corners of our outer world, reflecting our inner numbness. The numbness that exists within us prevents us from feeling the real life force and consciousness of our children. Our inner numbness provides the opportunity for evil forces in the world to take root, because they can do so unnoticed. Your instinctual role as a parent is to nurture and support the health of your child. Your goal is to protect your child from harm. Real child abuse is allowing your child to be vaccinated

We will now examine the forces in our world that create an imbalanced power structure. We will learn how we have become numb, how we have disassociated from our inner authority and how we were encouraged to participate in unconscious negative behaviors. In understanding these forces, you will be empowered to see some of the pillars of disharmony, and the roots of evil in our outer modernized world.

12

School:
The Enslavement Of Our Children

The broken system of our society is based on social controls in which our natural behavior is suppressed and controlled in childhood. As adults we then suppress and control ourselves and pass along this heritage of oppression to our children. This system has its roots in a theoretical model called the panopticon. *Pan* means "all," and *optic* means "of sight." A panopticon is a prison where everything the inmates do is observed (all seen). We live in such a prison, and if we can understand our predicament we can then begin to free ourselves from it.

Intention: We raise our children according to modern customs. We "educate" our children in this model and they become part of the problem, the modern plague, and not a part of the solution. You will learn important elements of how we are taught to accept being controlled, and more important, how to break free!

I wish for you to understand some of the roots of the system of corrupted power in our culture today, which has arisen from our life-destroying attitudes. I want you to see how this power structure is taught in school, and how you have become accustomed, through your socialization, to believe in a false, imaginary "authority."

Except for recess and physical education, and talking to other students, I never liked school. I did not like most of my class work or class room experience. It was real drudgery, and I even went to supposedly highly reputable schools (people buy expensive houses near these special public institutions just so their children can learn the lessons of life there). I believe many readers will have different conclusions

about the actual schooling of their children. I acknowledge that for some children school may provide wonderful rewards. I am not here to be an "authority" and impose my opinion on you and tell you how to think and be. I am here to tell you how you can choose to live in harmony and abide by Nature's abundant and generous laws. I am here to remind you of your own authority. In the end, the choices you make are yours. But first, it might be a good idea to see what school really does to our children, and what it did to you.

Panopticon - A Cold, Lifeless Prison

A panopticon refers to a building, real or metaphorical. It can be a prison, hospital, library, or the like. The original design was for prisons. The building is constructed in a circle, like a Roman coliseum. The entire interior of the structure, and every prison cell, is visible from a single point in the center, a central surveillance tower. In modern terms, the central tower would be replaced by a security room filled with the screens from hidden cameras spread throughout the building. One can monitor the entire building from one room, but the cameras are hidden in corners where people can't see them.

The principle of the panopticon underlies our modern civilization, at least partially. Through growing up in a panopticon-influenced society, we have created a "matrix" and an imprint of "authorities." Somewhat like in film

"The Matrix" (minus giant robots using us as batteries) our minds are plugged into an ethereal matrix that is distorted and disease- promoting. Most of us, in some way, are plugged into certain behavioral patterns or belief systems, yet few of us can recognize our condition because everyone thinks the same way, and these beliefs have become ingrained habits and accepted "facts."

The column in the center of the panopticon represents the *authority*. The column is designed with blinds and other lighting effects so that the prisoners cannot see into it.

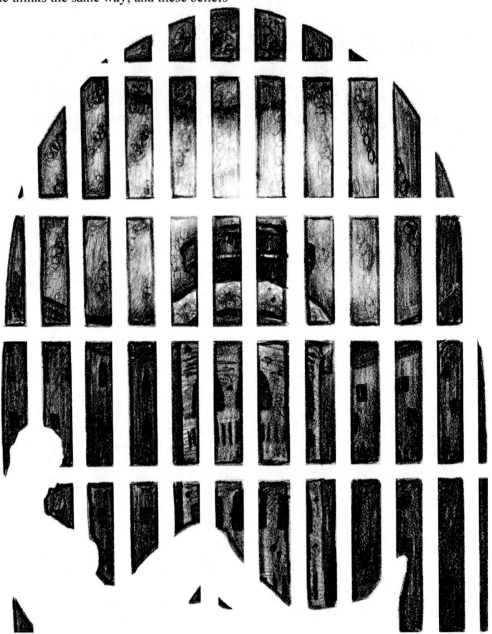

A prisoner doing penance in panopticon-designed penitentiary. In the center is the central column that represents the authority. From this looming central pillar all the prisoners can be seen.

The prisoner does not know when, or if he is being observed. In this way, there is a looming omnipresence of the authority. If the prisoner believes that he is being watched he will in fact "guard" himself and his behavior. The system is designed to save time and resources. Because the prisoner does not know when he is being watched he will always behave properly. This is just like the surveillance video cameras in the corner store. The presence of the camera tells you that you are being watched, so you behave; you think you are being monitored by authorities. Prisons built with this model didn't work out as well as theorized, as the inmates could all see each other and yell to each other. But the reality of constant observation is what is important. The guard watches the prisoners and enforces discipline, so the guard or authority defines what type of behavior is acceptable or unacceptable. The purpose of the panopticon is control of the prisoners' behavior at all times. The prisoner feels the omnipresent power of the State. What I want you to understand here is the principle, the concept, of being secretly observed by authorities at all times. The panopticon enforces the idea that you should feel the power of the State and obey the rules of authorities "out there."

Learning about the panopticon might have been one of the few useful things I learned in college. I have forgotten most of what I learned in traditional schools, including college, and I even earned mostly good grades! I have a four year college degree from the University of California Santa Cruz, which proves that I am supposedly "educated." I did enjoy yoga class, one of the most meaningful classes I took there. I did partially improve my writing in university. On the other hand, there was a specific and rigid way I was expected to write, and in that way my writing was prevented from improving. I believe my lack of memory on the subjects taught in class has to do with the fact that what I learned had no relevance to my life. In order to graduate from college you don't need to think for yourself, but rather be good at rephrasing and parroting what the professors or the texts present. In other words, you learn from the "authority," whether from a textbook or the professor, and if

you can memorize the beliefs of the authority, then you pass the class and are deemed "educated.

How much do you remember about the specific topics and lessons learned in school, especially in your early years? It would seem that you should remember a lot. After all, you probably spent at least twelve very influential years in school. Of those twelve years, what do you have left now that is meaningful and practical? Yes, yes, there were the memorable field trips and the enjoyable extracurricular projects, but I am talking about the bigger picture. What did you really learn in school? How did you spend those 12 years? In school, we learn lots of facts and theories, yet a majority of us forget these facts and theories just a few short years later. So, what is the point exactly? For example, I took an engineering math class of moderately advanced calculus and geometry in college and scored near the top of over 60 students. If you give me a simple calculus equation right now, ten years later, I wouldn't know what to do with it. I usually use a calculator to solve math problems. The only sure skills I learned in grades 1-12 are reading, writing, and basic arithmetic. An intelligent 12-year-old can learn these very skills in four to twelve months. Most adults could fit all their great and memorable learning experiences from grades K-12, the ones that were actually valuable, in three to nine months of part time classes that just focused on those special subjects. So what did you learn the rest of the time? Why were you there? What was accomplished?

Added to this not-so-funny joke called school is college. You arrive at the prestigious University and sit in the enormous lecture hall where the professor seems like an ant way down there in the front, and what does he say? He says that the history you just spent the last twelve years learning in school is all wrong. Part of being in college is learning how short sighted and mostly inaccurate the education of the previous 12 years of school were.

Have you ever wondered what the point of going to school for so long is in the first place when very little classroom knowledge is useful for adulthood? For example, I did not learn carpentry, even though it would have been useful. I didn't learn how to fix a broken toilet, or how to check for gas leaks. Other useful skills would be car repair (which you can sometimes learn a bit of in high school) computer repair, farming and gardening, raising livestock, ecological building, how to start a business, how to be healthy, how to have good relationships, how to help people, how to heal people, how to be one with the Universe, how to experience the pleasure of being alive…the list of useful things I didn't learn could go on and on. The pinnacle of my kindergarten through grade 12 education was 7th grade woodshop. I learned how to make wooden pencils on a lathe, and I still have some of them. I am trying very hard right now to remember what I learned at school. I do remember junior high school—particularly sitting at desks, bored out of my mind. I remember making up games in my head staring at the clock, fading out of reality, and suffering the endless torture of forced confinement. I didn't know why I was there; I just had to deal with it. Why do we learn almost nothing in school that serves us? The answer lies in the panopticon. We actually learn quite a bit in school, as you'll see. And as usual, prepare yourself, because it's not what you expected.

Discipline and Punishment

Along with the panopticon comes another theory. French philosopher, Michel Foucault wrote critically of the social history of discipline and control, particularly in his book *Discipline and Punishment*. The central theme of this book (and I hope I am not butchering his philosophy) is that Western society controls people's behavior by inflicting various types of violence, subtle or overt, on their physical bodies. If you break the law, a police officer can detain you in a cage (jail). If you break a serious law and are found guilty, the state is then allowed to inflict punishment upon you by forcing you to spend years of your life in a large building filled with cages (prison). The people with more might and physical power exert their control over the thoughts and actions others. If you don't behave according to the dictates of the "authority," then the authority will inflict pain on your physical

body or lock you in a cage until you yield to their imposed rules. You may be able to sense that this is really a feudalistic form of social control.

Mr. Foucault also points out the all-pervasive microstructures of power that keep the authority firmly in place. In the prison, the guard watches the prisoner, so the guards are the messengers and executors of the State's power and authority. In our culture we have messengers who enforce the dominant paradigm, who make the presence of authority become real. Without the enforcers, the authority has no power. Some examples of enforcers of the collective belief system are doctors, lawyers, judges, police officers, politicians, television, newspapers and teachers. Anyone we identify as an *authority* has the power to tell people how life is. If there are enough enforcers of belief patterns then most people come to believe what they say. The laws and beliefs in our society would have no meaning if they weren't actively enforced. People who do not believe in or support the dominant paradigm will not be allowed to take central leadership roles, so they are not in a position to influence many people's behaviors. The dominant energy form always acts to maintain its permanence and hold onto its power.

Where do the ideas of what is right and what is wrong come from? For example, who decided that Western medicine should be the dominant approach to our health care? Who decided how fast we should drive our cars? Who decided which countries we should go to war with? Who decreed that we shouldn't walk around naked in public? Ultimately, there is no central authority. Even if a totalitarian dictator were in total control of an entire country, where would his ideas of what should and shouldn't be controlled come from? Not from the source of life, but from bundles of thoughts in this dictator's head, a set of ideas which can be influenced by evil forces and likely came from his imprint in childhood. Where did this imprint come from? Well, if you continue to trace backwards in time the behaviors that are now supported in our culture have no specific origin. They arose out of nowhere, and out of nothing. The only explanation is that negative behaviors have arisen out of pain that came from a long way back, from the origin of human existence. **Therefore, enforcers of the dominant mode of thinking have little or no real source of knowledge and thus have little real power.** We mistakenly believe that those authorities are the ultimate purveyors of truth. We believe that might makes right. We believe the president has more authority than we do. This is not the truth. Most people whom we fear are totally ignorant of life. In a way, they are like robots following a set of rules. They embrace negativity. But they lack the true source of wisdom and power, so they always fail in the end. Only truth can survive; all else falls away.

Human authority can be a distortion of divine authority. Divine authority is based on your personal connection with the source of life, and its roots are truth and love. Our Constitution and our government were founded on the belief of divine authority, as stated in the Declaration of Independence.

*We hold these truths to be self-evident, that all men are created equal, that they are **endowed by their Creator with certain unalienable rights**, that among these are Life, Liberty and the pursuit of Happiness.*

The real authority is endowed to each of us by the Creator of life. Our personal authority includes liberty, which can be defined as a freedom of choice and action and a freedom from servitude, confinement or oppression. The wise declaration upon which our country was founded now stands in stark opposition to the way we live our lives and the way we arrange our society. An ideal authority figure in society would not use his position to enforce personal or cultural beliefs, but rather would be a vehicle for divine authority to shine through. This benign authority would honor the right of all people to realize their own inalienable rights.

Our society is designed around the paradigm of the panopticon. This helps explain why in the last 25 years (1980-2005), the US prison population has grown from 319,598 to over 1,446,269.[577] These numbers create vast budget problems because it costs at least $30,000 per year, and as high as $80,000 or more to house just one prisoner. The number of people with shorter terms, or awaiting trial, climbed in the same time period from 183,988 to 747,529. We now have over 2.19 million people incarcerated in correctional facilities. Half or fewer of these prisoners have been convicted of violent crimes. The United States has the highest prison population in the world, and we also have a significant bulk of the estimated 8.75 million (based on 1999-2002 statistics) prisoners world wide.[578] Our society has become more and more focused on incarcerating people and more and more focused on punishment.

The idea of a prison, a penitentiary, comes from the concept of doing penance. Perhaps a few hundred years ago, if a person stole something a priest or some similar authority would assign him penance for a few days or weeks so he could make amends and ask forgiveness for his errors. The aim of a pen(ance)tentiary is for the person who makes a mistake to be able to be rehabilitated and learn from his errors by doing penance. The original concept of a prison was to give someone time away from society to help him see and repent his errors. Today prison is foremost a punishment, with little emphasis on or opportunity for rehabilitation.

Activity: where's your authority?
Who exactly is in control of your life and your choices? Are you living by someone else's standards of what is right and wrong? Where did your ideas about right and wrong come from? Are you afraid of getting caught for breaking rules? Do you tend to blame other people for your problems in life — your spouse, your children, your boss, the government?

The result of the panopticon system is that it breeds a mono-culture. Everyone must be a conformist, and anyone who deviates even slightly finds himself a social outcast. Conformism is actually a goal that many people try to live up to—to fit seamlessly into societal expectations. In American society, men are supposed to wear a suit, drive a nice car, build a pension fund and have an attractive wife and a few children. Women are supposed to have status in society, to be productive in the world, to be professional, to find a rich man who will take care of them and to have a few kids who are well behaved. The stereotypical family wants to live in a nice house in a suburban neighborhood with two nice vehicles and the ability to afford regular entertainment and consumer indulgences. The children should earn good grades and go to prestigious colleges, then become a doctor, lawyer or businessperson so that they can carry on the very same cycle of life and wear a suit, have some kids and a dog, and live in a nice house in a suburban neighborhood.

When you break free of this system of similarity, of monoculture, people can think you are crazy, unstable, or doing something wrong. For example, we live in the mountains. Our house is a twenty minute drive from the six-million-strong land of suburbia (Silicon Valley). We have a driveway that is a mile of gravel and dirt, not a paved road. People think we are living on another planet. They don't want to come visit us. It is not because we live far away, but because we live outside of the box of how other people they know live. Even today, in other parts of the U.S., the way we live is quite unremarkable and even normal. But for most modern folk, if you don't live in familiar ways you are classified as strange, weird, or crazy. This is the power of the microstructure of authority. Each person believes the world should be a certain way, and then lives his life according to that standard while expecting all other people to live to that same standard. That mindset wouldn't be too bad if we were living in a pleasurable way and filling the world with goodness and peace. But since our lives are both highly stressful and unsustainable, something needs to change.

A Typical School

Public schools teach a set of ideas and concepts that have little or no practical application. As a result, this instruction separates your child from life. Life becomes an abstract idea, rather than something to take part in. Teachers, and even parents, do not know what is real in the world and have forgotten what is important; they are out of touch with their true and vibrant selves. And that is what they teach to children in school, how to be out of touch. But even just the

words *your true self*, or *who you really are* — that divine spark in you — can ignite something in you. And that is what is not talked about in school. The truth of who you are is contrary to the existence of the school system as we know it.

To give you an idea of what it feels like for a child to be in school, I will share a personal experience. In first grade, I remember being in class, numb to my surroundings, sitting at a small and uncomfortable desk with an uncomfortable feeling inside of me. Listening to the teacher was a great burden to me. I felt impatient; I did not want to be there. We were asked to read and fill out questions in a workbook, but the activities were impossible to me and were completely uninteresting. The answers were hidden by a covered section of the page. I felt that I had to perform the assignment, but I didn't want to. So I just lifted the cover and started to copy the answers. I didn't want to be there and do the school "work" which was really just mindless drills. It wasn't what my body, heart, mind or spirit needed. So I in fact did not do the work. The teacher saw me copying the answers and scolded me. I could not control myself any longer and started crying, "I want my mommy!" I put my head down on my desk and sobbed. What a mean and cruel world we live in, I thought. My mommy is not here and people are being mean to me. I felt alone, and sad.

Coercion. Did your child ask you to take him to school today to be left with a bunch of strangers? Did he ask you to lock him up in a room for most of the day under fluorescent lights? Did your child tell you he wanted to look at symbols on the walls and in books all day? Did your child choose these activities, or are you forcing him to go to school, daycare, or summer camp? A majority of children who have a strong bond to their mommies won't want to be away from their mommies all day. They will choose their mommies over sitting in a prison cell with other children the same age, isolated from society. If the bond has been shattered or destroyed, then the child might not mind school. Some older children may want to go to school as they start feeling independent and sure of themselves. This might happen anywhere from the age of eight to twelve; your child will let you know what he is comfortable with.

Slavery of the spirit. In 1912, Mary Montessori, the originator of the Montessori educational method, had already seen corporal punishment as a means of controlling behavior being replaced with punishment of the children's spirit. She wrote how we have replaced whipping and physical blows with systems of prizes and punishments. She describes these systems as, "the *bench* of the soul, the instrument of slavery for the spirit."[579] Our children's natural (good) impulses, their natural, full-bodied intelligence, are not just destroyed; they are crushed and annihilated in school. Children's bodies are humiliated and degraded. Children are confined in cold desks and they lose their ability to trust and honor their own impulses. These impulses represent a vast intelligence of the Universe that the Creator imbued into the fabric of your child's being. The child wants to explore the world, to play, and to have fun. That is the child's innate design and nature. Yet Nature's design for children is not honored by our modern school system, which forces children into boxes, confines them to desks for one purpose only: to be controlled. Play is frowned upon except at special predetermined times of the day when "structured" play is permitted. Loud noises and creativity are not allowed except in certain limited activities. Otherwise, children are trained to keep their mouths shut, not to speak without permission, and not to experience the pleasure of relating with other children. Children must learn to control the flow of energy in their throats. Free thinking and free will are destroyed as children are taught to behave a certain way and to cut themselves off from their roots to the Earth.

Moral degradation. Controlling children is done through imposing domination over their physical form. Montessori writes,

Today we hold the pupils in school, restricted by those instruments so degrading to body and spirit, the desk—and material prizes and punishments. Our aim in all this is to reduce them to the discipline of immo-

bility and silence,—to lead them,—where? Far too often toward no definite end.[580]

The imprint of school. The imprint of school is not education, as you may have thought it was. It is enslavement of your child's spirit. The purpose of school is to train your child to become a malleable and spiritless automaton that can be controlled and manipulated. The purpose of school is to subjugate, to teach people how to listen to the authority rather than to be an authority. Children experience forced oppression, forced submission, and learn to become victims of this act of social conquest.

While it looks as though school teaches your child important facts and information, what it is really teaching children is how to be controlled by other people. To children, teachers are authorities. More and more, state and federal laws try to restrict the freedom of teachers in the classroom. These regulations further kill off any creative spark in the well meaning teacher who might be tempted to break out of this social structure. School teaches your child to expect a miserable, silent, monotonous and confined life. School does not teach freedom, creative liveliness, and unity. **School is the place where your child's mind, body, and spirit become enslaved by false knowledge about the world**.

Obsessive and compulsive. I once tutored a sixteen-year-old girl who attended a very prestigious, private boarding school. She was constantly distracted. She complained that she could not focus because instead of sleeping at night she had to do all the schoolwork she was given and frequently stayed up after midnight completing the assignments. This was a time when a new awareness was coming to me. I eventually gave up "teaching" her because she was so burned out from "learning," and I just listened with compassion to her difficulties. Out of the one-and-a-half hour session, we probably spent fifteen minutes on the material; otherwise I just listened to her sorrows. That was the last SAT tutoring that I did.

Destroying the bond. Children are designed by Nature to believe that their parents represent the trusted authority. They are supposed to look towards their parents, and not to all adults, for what is right and wrong. Nature's design was illustrated in more detail in Chapter 9. Children merge with their parents and become one with them, and then slowly learn who they are and merge outwardly toward the world with an inward sense of self. Yet in school this natural process is thwarted and destroyed. Children have no one left to merge with but their teacher.

Public schools are provided free of tuition because they encourage mothers to work, and the school becomes a surrogate mother, yet without the nurturing qualities of a mother. While mothers are away making money, their children are taught about life, and how our society wants them to think about life.

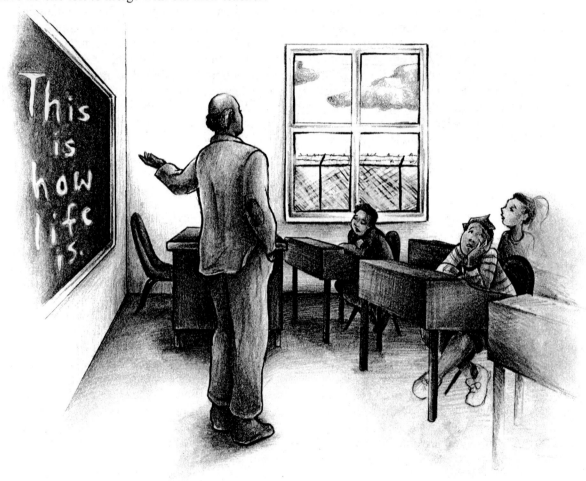

School is based upon the principle of the panopticon. The idea is that there is a central authority outside of the student, "the teacher." The teacher does not fill the student with divine truth and knowledge, which would help the student find his true nature and inner authority. The students are forced to be present and are confined to their desks, and in this way they learn that life is filled with subjugation, domination, and the denial of their natural instincts.

I think I should be fair and talk about one of the most euphoric moments of my child life was the last day of high school. No more schoolwork ever!!! (Well, at least not until college).

"Why do our children suffer?" They suffer because they are raised in this alienating way, in which the school becomes their surrogate parents. Our children's natural instincts are objectified. We have sold our children out to the State.

Our medieval schooling methods, combined with all the poisons of vaccination, fluoridated water (a powerful nervous system toxin that lowers I.Q.[581]), and all the drugs modern children are given to control their normal behavior, mentally debilitates our children. In school, your children are fed modernized foods to poison their bodies and thwart normal growth. The typical school menu of devitalized foods includes graham crackers, peanut butter and jelly, fruit juices, soft drinks, boxes of chocolate milk, chicken nuggets, animal crackers, goldfish cracker snacks, pretzels, tacos, potato chips, and if they are extraordinarily lucky, a few pieces of fruit or vegetables.

As children grow up they are taught unscientific beliefs about medicine and health. Much of what is taught in school could be classified as religion since it is required to be accepted on faith. The religion taught in school is labeled as "science" and is mostly false and fabricated. Thus, school violates the covenant of separating the church from the state. That is why many homeschoolers come from strong religious backgrounds; they can rightly see how false knowledge is perpetuated in school. School is the authority in the model of the panopticon. With the combined forces of toxic food, water, drinks, toxic buildings and forced confinement, the majority of our children become obedient to authority. School helps create a deficient child, one who will become a powerless adult. You might not believe this, but Sparkle, now four-and-a-half, asked me about the picture here. I said that this is what school is like.

She asked, "Are you joking?" And she asked who the big person was. I told her that is the teacher who tells the students how to think.

She asked me, "Does anybody tell me what to do?"

"No," I said. "Well, sometimes mommy tells you things but she tries not to."

Then Sparkle said, "People are not supposed to tell children what to do."

Again, Sparkle is not parroting what Michelle or I have told her, rather she is speaking from her own wisdom, which she has gained because we have given her space to be herself. I said, "You are right, and we are going to make sure nobody ever tells you what to do." She walked away feeling happy.

School is prison. Children and teens in elementary, middle and high schools are coerced, dominated, manipulated, confined, punished and oppressed. The students are treated like temporary prisoners. Schools are surrounded by fences, even barbed wire fences, and the children cannot escape. Ironically, another argument for the fences might be to protect children from the harm that would come in from the outer world. This fence is really symbolic of a prison and is symbolic of keeping out not dangerous influences, but life itself and infinite possibilities of fulfillment. If a child did escape and was caught by a police officer or some other "authority," he would be returned to school. Ditching class is an exciting behavior for teens because they can experience some freedom

Within the walls of the school/prison, there is a smaller type of confinement system which breaks children's connection with their bodies and the earth. These are called desks. The desks are hard, cold and extremely uncomfortable, much as you would expect a prison cell to be. Students may even need to ask permission to leave their desks to use the restroom or must hold it in. It's a true imposition on their bodies — not being allowed to respond to their own impulses for eating, drinking, urinating and defecating. Just as in the panopticon, the teacher is in a position where she can observe all of the students in class. The teachers in schools monitor children's behavior. If children misbehave, then they face the consequences of discipline: longer confinement during recess or after school, which is appropriately called **detention**. Until recently, humiliation and physical abuse were still used to enforce discipline in both public and private schools. I commonly bore witness as a child to teachers emotionally abusing students as well. Sometimes it happened to me. But as a child I did not comprehend what was happening.

Students are also taught to believe the textbooks, to place authority in what they read. These books supposedly convey the ultimate truth. I remember myself as a teenager, believing whole heartedly what was written in the textbooks I read in school. With a captive and gullible audience ready for the taking, many dark forces in our culture have gained access to school textbooks in subtle and coercive ways. The books' contents are manipulated to present certain messages about all aspects of society and how life is. This manipulation and censorship serves devious purposes, and keeps the next generation—your children—oppressed.

How Humans React towards Oppression

The system of reward and punishment — grades — does not nurture real growth in our children's spirit and intelligence. As Montessori writes, they are

> *...incentives toward unnatural or forced effort, and, therefore we certainly cannot speak of the natural development of the child in connection with them.*[582]

Humans, and I mean both children and adults, respond to falsely imposed rules in a variety of ways. The creative spark within each of us wants to be in the world, to move, to create, to play, to enjoy. But the imposed discipline practiced in schools forces the child to restrict his movement away from the world, and direct it into the mental spheres of thought. In this way the child's effort, and the natural energetic impulses in his body, will have to be channeled into different outlets of expression, and this creates an unnatural and forced will.

On the surface, the purpose of imposing authority, through rewards and punishments, is to create children who are obedient and who follow rules. And on the outer level it appears that this system works. The children sit still, form lines, recite memorized passages and so forth, and their parents pretend to be happy at their cute little subjugated children. However, on the inner landscape of our children's hearts and bodies, other responses form that are less visible but no less real.

Eventually, children subjected to enough "discipline" will do one or both of the following. They will develop characteristics of either the rule follower, never disobeying, or a rule breaker, constantly fighting the rules. Most children exist somewhere within this spectrum. A rule follower knows the right thing to do; he knows how to avoid punishment. However, on the inner landscape he is consciously battling with himself. He must create secret worlds and secret compartments in his psyche into which all the energy currents that want to break the rules can be channeled. Children really are not physiologically designed to follow imposed rules. They are designed to play and copy their parents and older children. As an adult, the rule-following child will subconsciously constantly thwart his own pleasure principle, and his own desire to be in the world, because restraining himself in this way allowed him to obey the imposing authority in childhood. Yet subverting the natural outgoing movement in children creates an inner rebel. The inner rebel must sneak to the surface, and the side effects of the oppression spill out in subtle ways. The side effects of rule following usually become more dangerous because the energy movements and currents have become suppressed and forgotten. As an adult this person will either live an extremely constrained life, or somehow their rebelliousness will come to the surface in very self-destructive ways. Rule following also does not ultimately produce the desired outcome of obedience, because of the altered energy currents. For example, a child might sit still at his desk, and hum to himself and appear to be listening, but really not be listening. Perhaps he will ignore the teacher, and draw or color if it is allowed. A child will do **anything** to fight the imposition of authority against his own natural desires, so long as he can do it and not get caught. Oppressing children through outer discipline teaches them to learn subtle and sophisticated methods of rebellion that we ignorant adults either do not have the energy to do anything about, or we pretend to not see. Outer discipline will never create absolute self discipline. Only inner discipline, chosen by the child, will create true discipline. A true support system would encourage children to pursue their own inwardly-driven goals and desires, and over time they will develop self discipline.

At the opposite end of the spectrum we find the rule breaker. Remember, this is a spectrum, and children generally break or follow rules based on their mood and situation. The rule breaking children control their life force as well, but they are unable to hide their self control well. They are too much in contact with the pleasure of physical life, and of being in the world. The rule breaking child will feel good when he does bad things. He will be happy to get thrown out of class and face another meeting with the principal. Until I became a "good boy" in fifth and sixth grade, I would purposely get thrown out of class. After sixth grade I became excessively shy and I could not continue to be a rule breaker. This shyness was probably due to inadequate nutrition making me feel weak and not confident. An effort might be made to crush the rule breaking child by all means necessary: physical violence, isolation, and other threats that are severe to the child. While the rule breaking child keeps his life energy, it becomes untamed, reckless, perverse and destructive because he was not allowed the natural growth and maturation process to learn to channel his energy in healthy ways. His outward movement towards life, towards love, towards the Creator, is channeled into fighting the authority. There is a place in our society where we honor the rebel. We admire the rebel because we all have the reckless rule-breaking rebel within us, and we would love to set our inner rebel free. But rebels are caught in a bind: because this rebel has not been honored and nurtured, he will desire to be rebellious in ways which are destructive, because that is what the underlying method of his schooling years taught him to do. Releasing the rebellious energy might lead to destructive and inappropriate acts, but holding onto it means controlling the stream of life. Here, the rebel needs to be carefully let out, so that his free energy can be reincorporated into the adult psyche without causing too much destruction.

Activity: let the rebel free. There is an inner rebellious part of you, and it would be extremely rare if you didn't have one. This is the hurt, punished, coerced and manipulated part of you. Not letting it out leaves the feeling of obstructed life force. Letting it out might lead to destructive behaviors. This is a bind. What can you do? Imagine the rebel in you. Give the rebel what it always needed: freedom to be. The rebellious child really was the child who wanted to play, to be innocent, to be free. Remember the David Whyte poem at the end of Chapter 1, Sweet Darkness? "You must learn one thing: the world was made to be free in." Invite your inner rebel forward, and give her what she didn't get as a child — space, compassion and caring. With nourishment, you will heal the impulse to be destructive. You can allow the rebel to start to come out again, in her true self.

Enforcing The Rules

If a teacher has a "no talking" rule, one child in a classroom eventually might enforce the "no talking" rule with another child, so as to protect the other child from the stress and humiliation of punishment. In this way, children start enforcing the rules of the authority figure. The children mimic the authority as an escape or a survival mechanism.

In school we are socialized. The teachers know how the world is, or believe they do. So they teach the children that it is good to be obedient, to be rigid, and teach how to keep safe by not acting out too much. In the school environment, the child takes this snapshot of life as an accurate representation. After twelve years, children internalize their schooling environment. Just as the infant imprints the world she grows up in, children imprint the schooling and socialization that they have learned.

A few underlying assumptions that many of us have learned in school are:

- Natural human behavior needs to be controlled and monitored.
- Truth lies in the authority figures and/or books.
- If you rebel, act out, or attempt to release your creative energy you will be punished through physical abuse, ma-

nipulation, humiliation, betrayal and/or abandonment.

- You must ask permission to be who you are, even ask permission to respond to your body functions.
- Breaking the dominant paradigm (the cultural oppression), breaking the mold of what is acceptable, is taboo and other peers will stop you from doing it.
- Rebellion is acceptable and tolerated when it is not observed. That is, you are allowed to break rules if nobody catches you.

What is the dominant paradigm? What is the way our culture thinks, feels and believes? Where did it come from? And why do we continue to uphold its values?

As adults, we continue to subtly control and discipline others. This conformity is upheld in part by laws. I want to be clear though: I do not support criminal behavior, violating other people, or violating the planet. But our legal system insidiously teaches people how to be out of balance with life by subverting their own inner authority, an authority based on goodness. A false authority is installed, which ultimately encourages wrong attitudes and actions. It is this imbalance of never looking inward to the self while conforming to the dictates of an outer authority that strangles the human soul, and as a result, evil actions occur in the world.

Michelle says: "Criminal behavior, people violating other people's boundaries, the destruction and violence, disrespect of each other on the planet are results of controlling and trying to 'teach' children. They are the result of not taking the time to heal ourselves and our wounds from our displaced upbringing.

One way we perpetuate evil and numbness is in and through school. In school we have numbed our children out of life, and out of their natural development. Not everything children learn in school is wrong or bad. However, the overall scheme is fatally flawed; it is a reflection of a culture of madness."

As adults we unconsciously act like the authorities we had in school and at home as children. We have internalized this false authority, this false belief system. In our small ways, we enforce these expectations towards others, much like the child in class who acts as the authority figure by shushing another student to prevent punishment. Ultimately, by enforcing the rules, we encourage people to avoid looking inward, to avoid feeling their own pain, because we can't feel ours. As a result, we have created an outwardly driven society that has lost its real vitality and meaning. Life is fearful in such a place, because many of us are driven by fear, the fear of being who we really are.

The greater the degree of discipline enforced, the greater the conformity in the society, as well as the greater the rebellion that is created. The less discipline, the less conformity; and conversely, the more freedom and free thinking. The less discipline, the more joy and happiness people will experience. You might actually fear the idea of less discipline because you fear the subtle punishment you have been receiving your whole life for being your Self. So you fear being yourself. Of course, there is the extreme of not enough discipline, in which there are no boundaries in society; this is not healthy either. Here, I am referring to a lack of inward discipline, in which you align your internal energy channel towards the light, and accept your human realities and limitations.

When people assume positions of power and their behavior becomes overbearing, this is an example of not enough discipline in controlling their thoughts and attitudes. Children controlled by outer authorities seem to be disciplined and behave, but they don't learn any internal discipline. When they find themselves in positions of power they easily become the subjugators and seek to control others for their own personal gain. A healthy use of power was not taught or modeled in schools, so now the subjugator is able to mistreat others just as he was mistreated, continuing the vicious cycle. Healthy authority comes from imbuing children with a sense of goodness and rightness about themselves and the world. Children who have role models of healthy authority will become enforcers of goodness and rightness, because that is what they believe in.

The Origin of the Panopticonal System: Loss of our Mothers

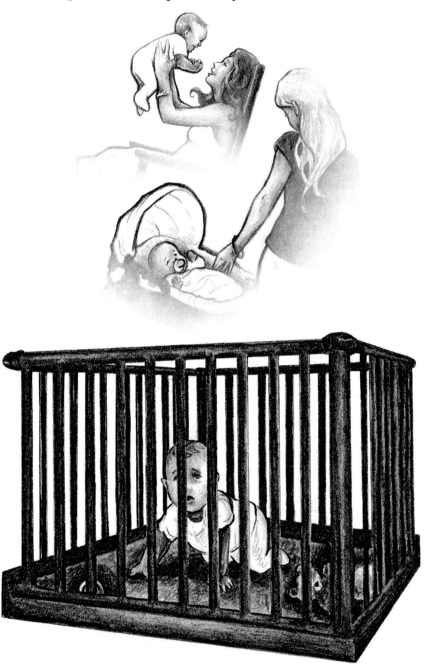

This picture shows various levels of physical separation that children face in our culture. First, there is unity with the mother. Second, there is the moderate form of separation a child experiences by being physically disconnected from an aloof mother. Finally, the child is confined alone in a child's prison: a playpen. Physical separation is a necessary condition when creating the illusion of an outer authority. Confinement of our spirits and souls starts at an early age through confinement of our bodies.

Other than reading, writing and arithmetic (which can be taught to an intelligent child in a few months' time), I cannot see what is useful in schools. Yes, children need to socialize, play with each other, learn about life, and explore their creative outlets. Yet a majority of the real nurturing and creative activities are thwarted in our normal schooling methods and replaced with completely dreary nonsense. In today's culture, at least here in California, a school, even an elementary school, filled with students earning high test scores is praised, while a school filled with joyful children is of little importance or concern to the majority. The forced, subjugated way children are allowed to relate to each other eventually seems natural. As we get older, we come to half-heartedly accept these circumstances and to participate in our subjugation willingly. As adults, in many situations, we tend to find work in which we experience the same or similar type of subjugation we felt in childhood. This is our imprint; this is how we believe life is, so we subconsciously recreate it. The goal of many employees who are subjugated is to eventually become the boss, so then they can become the oppressors and subjugate others and possess the illusion of control.

The child stuck in his playpen-cage will soon become frustrated. To a child, his mother is the kind Mother to place his trust in. Without the bond with her, he will constantly look for this bond elsewhere. These systems of authority will replace his mother, because he never completely moved into the stage of autonomy in a healthy way, such that he could become inwardly driven.

Remember the concept of the second womb? When children are isolated from their mothers they are never allowed to complete their developmental processes. They usually go through life with thwarted developmental stages. Attendance at school separates children from their parents. Placing children in school facilitates mothers going to work. Having mothers work inhibits communities. If mothers were not working they could easily form their own "schools" with other mothers—thus creating community. In school, the child still longs for a loving and nurturing space where she feels loved and accepted, even if she does have this at home. School, in a majority of cases, is a reflection of distorted mother energy. Rather than nurturing, schools attack and destroy our children's innocence. Rather than loving, schools punish and inhibit children. Rather than teaching community, bonding, conflict resolution, and communication, school teaches useless facts. Many years of school may have only a few meaningful moments of knowledge and growth. **The purpose of school is to isolate the child from the mother, and it enforces the prison-like idea of society: life is about being separate, alone, and even punished.**

Because traditional schools represent the opposite of what mothers stand for, and because their purpose also allows children to be separated from their families and communities, I conclude that the purpose of school is to enforce a separated way of existence.

Unfortunately, when you leave your children at schools, they are subjected to a variety of vile forces. This includes the government and private corporations who sell your children drugs called soft drinks, and poison called candy bars, right on your public school property. Is our school system really still for the people? Or is it for the corporations? Ironically, vaccinations, one of the most despicable forms of evil against our children, are required to place your children into schools. (There are exemptions.)

This puts parents into a dishonest bind, which really must be unconstitutional as it is a clear attempt to violate our personal freedom and choices. It is required by law that children over a certain age (six years in California) must attend school. Schools then require vaccinations for attendance, even though you can file waiver forms. This system coerces parents into vaccinating their children.

School Attendance is Not Voluntary. It is the Law

Are you still not convinced that the purpose of school is to manipulate and control your child? Just look at the laws. It is the law that your child must attend school. If your child is not in school, the government has the ability to force your child to attend. The laws vary from state to state. The California Education Code states:

All children between the ages of 6 and 18 must attend a public full-time day school unless otherwise exempted.[583]

Our laws clearly spell out our false and misguided authority. Legislators who passed these laws have assumed that parents won't know what's best for their own children, and so the State invades our personal privacy and tells us what to do. Once their children are attending public schools, parents lose their right to control or otherwise have an input in what their children are taught. In a case that was denied review by the Supreme Court, a court of appeals made its position about school very clear: once your child has been submitted to the public schools for his "education" you lose the ability to control the course of instruction.[584] This sounds like a terrible dictatorship and not a free country. That a court can decide that parents cannot guide their child's education is a real violation of our parental rights. Yet this is the law of the land today.

For now, there is a legal solution to this system of imposed social order — home schooling, or starting your own charter "school." There are also many alternative schools that are much better than public schools. Of course, these schools usually cost quite a bit of money, which disqualifies most lower income parents (unless scholarships are available). So, if you don't have a lot of money your child will be subjugated in public school for lack of a better alternative. But there are some alternative public schools and some schools that even want parents to participate in their child's education. To find more information about the laws regarding schooling for your state, I suggest the Home School Legal Defense Association, www.hslda.org. This also is an excellent example of a group of individuals taking responsibility for what they feel is important in the world, and working together for a positive intention. The core group of attorneys is composed of fathers of children who are homeschooled. On their website they write, "Defending homeschoolers is not just a job for us. It is our very way of life and our heartfelt conviction."[585]

This is a good example of what I discussed in Chapter 9 about men and fathers working together. Here, the men who are lawyers are using their legal knowledge to protect their children. They are protecting the bond between the mothers and their children, as well as protecting their children's minds from invasion from outside forces. Just a few men working together to protect the health and well being of their children create a powerful force, along with a feeling of safety in the world. In this case safety refers to the right to home school. Imagine what a larger group of well-intentioned men could do to create peace and safety on this planet?

In Germany it is illegal to home school. Their laws claim that the state has a compelling interest to *educate* children in the manner that it wants them to be educated. What are these children taught in Germany? How did schools come to supplant the transmission of knowledge as it originally occurred, from parent to child? This is a scary system that appears to be an attempt to control the way people think through indoctrination. I only mention this example to shed light on one of the real intentions of public school.

We are lost in a maze. We exist in a state of darkness. We cannot find our way out. To whom shall we turn?

You must see and feel your oneness with the divine laws of Nature, and your own inner authority. Authority comes from presence, from knowing truth in your being, and through accepting and abiding in who you really are. Knowing yourself makes it possible to separate false, distorted knowledge from true, right knowledge and right action. What does it mean to know yourself? Listen from the inside, honor your feelings, trust your gut, and take responsibility for your life.

Our Life Based on Outer Authority

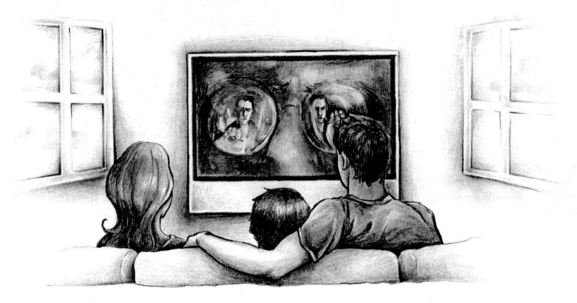

After a lifetime of self confinement, from play pen, to classroom, to life, we learn to enjoy, embrace, and even pay lots of money to have a fancy confinement system (house). We make our confinement comfortable, with nice large couches and lots of food. We stare at the outer authority who tells us how life is, or who entertains us away from our own life, from our own feelings in our bodies. (The image on the television screen is based on the scene from The Matrix where the hero chose to take the "red pill" of truth and knowledge of the world, rather than the "blue pill" of numbness and ignorance.)

The third dimension of power and three levels of social control. This is a political concept which explains how people can become controlled.

1. The first level of power and control is when people have a free choice, but are persuaded by the power of outer world forces, elect a leader, or make a choice that is not in their best interest.
2. The second level of power is when the dominant party sets the agenda. The party members are in control of the rules of the game. They set up rules to benefit the dominant class and decide what is talked about and what is not talked about. They decide, for example, what your children are indoctrinated with in public schools.

3. The third level of power is when the subjugated class chooses to subjugate itself based on the manipulation from elites and social classes. They vote for their own oppression.

The family pictured watching the movie are victims of the third dimension of power. They now subjugate themselves, after a lifetime of being told what to do. They waste their lives watching television, and playing video games. They are unconsciously choosing to live in the panopticon system because they were raised in it and have become accustomed to it. Rather than living our own life, we live through fictional movie characters. We live vicariously through the adventures of the hero on the screen, rather than taking the fearless leap to being the hero in our own lives.

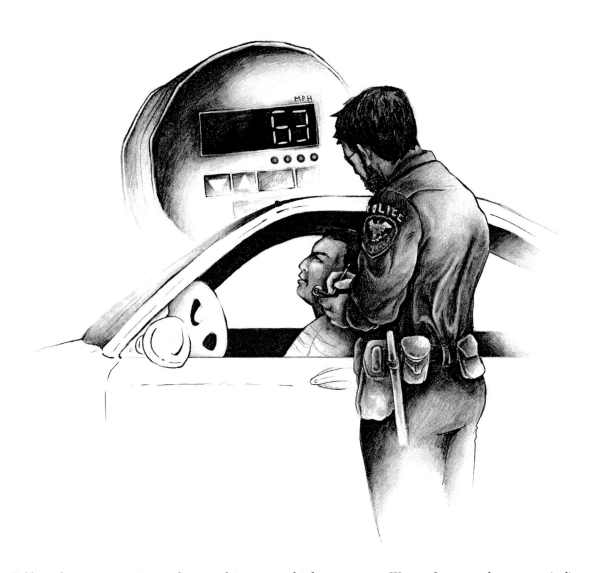

Self-confinement continues when we drive in our highway system. We confine ourselves to our individual vehicles. The ominous highway patrol looms about, on the lookout for law breakers to apprehend and punish. Just as in the panopticon prison, you never know if the police officer is spying on you with his radar gun. Deeply negative feelings underlie how we police ourselves. The police officer enforces discipline on the violator, and remains hidden behind his uniform and reflector glasses. He is a tool of coercion, he enforces the State's illusion of authority over its citizens.

Living with the knowledge of the Panopticon

Most of us do not live in actual prisons, but we do have our prison cells. But because these cells are voluntarily chosen and are not forced upon us, their confinements are more subtle. Our prisons are our living rooms, our cars, our classrooms, and our offices. Our authority figures are not unseen prison guards watching from a cen-

tral tower. They are the images that we see on the television and in the newspaper. We are also imprisoned by the internalized images and beliefs we have about life. These imagines convince us that life is a certain way, and many times the images of the media create feelings of fear and excitation, and thus we feed our own fears. Our images constrain us into fixed beliefs that men behave in certain ways and that women behave in certain ways and that the world is a certain way. Our internal world, our emotional landscape, in conjunction with these images, informs the ways we move about in life. Both outer and inner images encourage us to control how we think, feel and act in the world. Changing the images requires that we first compassionately accept them as they are.

We actually choose to remain in our "prisons." We choose to be isolated from life, isolated from fellow humans, and isolated from the inner knowing that we are one with all that is. We were taught that this is the way to live as children. We cage ourselves in our living rooms and stare at the television, the news broadcaster—the nice looking, well-groomed authority—who tells us about life. Or we receive both subtle and overt cues and product placements in commercials and television drama shows. We volunteer ourselves to be controlled. We volunteer our children to be subjugated. We choose and support ignorant and life-destructive ways because it is what the authority says is right. We allow our minds to be literally poisoned (with pharmaceuticals or food additives) and manipulated by those authoritative institutions in our culture. Today, it is both expected and tolerated for the leader of our "free" country, the president, to lie habitually and consistently as part of a scheme of manipulating the public.

Just as in the panopticon prison, the threat of observation is considered an acceptable way to control our behavior. Speed limits are a good example. Our cars are like miniature prison cells: we strap ourselves into the seat, we can even lock the doors, and we are supposed to follow rules. Generally, nobody is enforcing these rules, so you have a choice of whether to follow them or not. For example, perhaps 95% of the time you can drive over the speed limit, yield rather than stop at stop signs, make illegal U-turns and no one is right there to stop you. Only occasionally is there a highway patrol officer, who is generally hiding, just like the guards in the central column of the panopticon. So you limit your behavior because of the possible threat of being caught. In other words, many people do not speed not because they believe speeding is wrong or dangerous, but because of

their fear that they will be observed, caught, and then punished with a fine. This system of phantom observation creates a kind of paranoia. In a more evolved culture, in which people participate in the rules of society and rule making, they would voluntarily police themselves because driving too fast is unsafe. The rules would also be different and reflect the inherent nature and goodness of the citizens. Yet, we do not trust or respect people's inner authority. Sometimes we do this rightly, and it is appropriate. But our only response to rule breakers of any kind is to control them through punishment.

Most rules are only indirectly agreed to. You did not make the rules yourself or vote for them directly; rather, you are obliged to follow them because you happen to live in this country. Our system of financial and physical punishment is flawed. The fear of imprisonment does not prevent enough people from committing crimes, as is evident in the rising prison population. People still break laws despite the consequences.

Furthermore, our methods of discipline, the death penalty for example, are forms of violence in themselves. We act in criminal ways to criminals, dehumanizing them, and thus on a holographic level, we are committing cultural acts of violence. To be clear, I am not advocating that violent people not face severe consequences for their actions. I am saying that our entire system promotes violent behavior and that we need to eradicate the undertones of violence in our justice system if we want to create more safety in our society. Other than this threat of physical punishment and confinement, our culture does little to prevent criminal behavior. There is no focus on the cause of why people commit crimes, and thus the world is less safe for our children. In the interest of making the world safe for our children, we need to address crime at the causal level, and excessive threats of punishment will not significantly deter crime.

Real Authority

Outer world authority seems very real, especially when it unjustly affects our lives, or seems to. The real authority is not government employees or someone with billions of dollars, though. Real authority lies with the Creator. Real authority therefore comes from within us, because real authority comes about through honesty, truth and love all endowed by the Creator. We become powerful by spreading truth, and by living in truth. The truth is who you are. This truth is whatever is real and alive for you in this moment.

Unplug yourself from your television. Unplug yourself from the media and plug into the truth within your own core. Through this, you will begin to reclaim your authority and your right for health and healing. Slowly but surely, the system of corporatism will collapse as people begin to reclaim their inner power. They will insist on a government, and also energetically create a government, that supports people, rather than a government that is engaged in supporting the criminal behaviors of war, economic imperialism, and medical genocide (for which vaccines are but one example).

Divine and Loving Authority

We can easily become trapped in the vicious cycle of looking for authority, for guidance and direction outside of ourselves, and miss our loving presence emanating from within. It is okay to look outside of yourself for answers to problems, but ultimately, the decisions about your life, or even where to look for help, come from you. When our developmental stages are incomplete, when we did not get the love we so needed as children, then many of us become trapped in a pattern of seeking this lost love and nurturance in the world, where it does not really exist. Or we give up seeking this entirely, and end up feeling cynical about life.

In your search for your real inner authority, the womb of compassion in your heart, the infinite wisdom of bliss that can only emanate from your being, you can use a temporary, harmless, or loving authority. There are teachers who exert a positive and loving authority, and even a life-sustaining discipline. But these authorities are rare in our culture, even though they are desperately needed now. The panopticon model itself is not necessarily negative. You can also place

your authority in a guru, a wise teacher or a symbol. An altar, for example, can be a positive symbol of outer authority. Place on your altar a reminder of a divine authority figure who is in contact with his true nature within himself. Through devotion to their authority, you will eventually learn to see the real authority within yourself. In this way, one can become a master and creator of the universe. And when we are masters or creators operating from our higher internal values and standards, then we can take action that creates peace throughout the world.

The real authority is the Creator. The real authority is the energy, the force, the intelligence, and the consciousness that created the manifest reality and that created the possibility for our being on Earth. Most religions subscribe to some kind of higher power, and this is what I am referring to. This authority and this power is not only in you, but it is no different from who you really are. Most of us do not believe this truth, because we do not feel it in our flesh and bones. So I encourage you to not just blindly believe in what I am saying, but to search within for the experience of your personal truth no matter what it is. Your truth is not a narrow idea, but a vast experience.

Rigid social structures are not built on the foundations of goodness and peace, and therefore are meant to crumble. Misaligned structures in our society, which seem so impenetrable and vast, must crumble because they careen out of balance. Although this disillusionment can be painful or even disastrous, in the wake of these ashes, a new force will rise.

The Ultimate School

An alternative style of learning can be seen in Nature. Animals do not have their children attend school while the parent is away hunting. Animals generally teach their children through example. Indigenous people throughout the world do not have schools as we do, yet their children learn to survive and become capable adults. The children learn by playing, by mimicking the behaviors of the adult. For example, playing with a bow and arrow teaches a child to be a hunter as an adult. Playing with cooking utensils teaches children to cook. As adults, they know the patterns for survival that they learned by mimicking their parents. As adults, their work — hunting, cooking, or whatever the task may be — is fun and pleasurable because it was allowed to happen naturally; it was not forced when they were children. Many indigenous groups do not believe that they can tell other people what to do. If there is a work party, for example, building a hut for a family, then people are allowed to participate for as little or as much as they like; there is no obligation or expectation of what another person should do, and each person operates out of free will. The native society operates in general out of free will for the individual. You might look inside yourself if you feel fearful imagining a society in which people behave freely. I can only assure you that the reality of such a society would not match your fears. When our natural tendencies to be sociable, generous, giving and life preserving are not interfered with, people naturally want to help out their fellow humans.

In many indigenous groups, children are rarely or never told what to do or not to do. They are allowed to play and experience life as they wish. As adults, they then have positive associations with doing work. They are never forced to sit at desks and be uncomfortable day after day, although there are in many groups short periods of stress that accompany a rite of passage at a particular age of maturation. Typical indigenous life is involved with cultivating and activating communication with Nature and embodying the life force.

The ideal school then is a mirror of these conditions. In a more ideal school, children would not be separated from their parents, or from older children or society and locked in buildings (even this mere act of separation could lead a child to believe that he is wrong, flawed or bad). In this hypothetical unified society, children would have a spacious freedom to play. Being included in society the children would see the role modeling of success in their parents, and as they grew, they would naturally copy their parents' patterns as well as have opportunities to participate without being forced. Children, for good and for bad, mimic and copy their parents' behaviors. A more ideal school does NOT need to spend much or any time teaching children factual knowledge and academic skills since these can easily be learned in a non-oppressive, non-judgmental and supportive space when the child wants to and feels ready. A real school would be based upon the principles of truth, love and compassion.

Many parents might fear that if they do not force or encourage their children to read or write at a very early age, then their child will be unintelligent and be unable to learn. But in each stage of growth the child is capable of being the best that he is. An infant cannot be a three-year-old, and a three-year-old cannot be a six-year-old. [586]

If children are forced to read and learn symbols too early, when their minds are not sufficiently developed, these forces can break reality into fragments so their minds then will perceive life in an unbalanced manner. Forced education also can drive away and thwart their natural interest in what Sparkle calls, "play, play, play, play." For my Sparkle, we will not have to teach her how to read, because her natural inclination, after we read her some books, is to want to read more books. While she cannot read the words, she feels positive and motivated to learn how to do it. Without any effort on our part she started asking us the meaning of each of the letters. As of now, she has been able to memorize the words of most of the books we read to her, so she knows what each page says. In fact, the pressure is more on us as parents; because she likes reading so much, we need to read her several books every day for her to feel satisfied. This is with absolutely no prodding, imploring, or forcing on our part. We simply just read her books. Our teaching is through example, through care, and through our compassionate and present actions in which we seek to understand how she really feels, and what she really wants and desires.

Life is our classroom. The ultimate school would not have a classroom, and we would teach children about the laws of life. We would teach them about personal responsibility, the law of brotherhood, how to communicate with each other, how to express feelings, and mostly, the school would be focused on creating an optimal learning environment. This means its foundation would be, "play, play, play, play." Children need to be given opportunities to learn about things that are important, like childbirth, and how to make peace, and how to care for the environment.

At the very least, a child should not go to school before the age of 6. The law does not require a child to be in school before this age (please confirm the law in your own state). Children should definitely socialize and have contacts with other children, but to force them to learn "facts" about our culture and to separate them from their parents, and confine them in prison-like edifices is painful. Here's what Joseph Pearce writes in the *Magical Child:*

> *Learning to take our cues from the child and make a corresponding response means learning to heed and respond to the primary process within ourselves as well...Hospitals for delivery, bottles for feeding, cribs for sleeping, playpens and strollers for isolation, day-care centers for not caring, nursery schools for not nurturing, pre-schools – all create abandonment and weaken the bond.... To nurture the magical child is a full-time responsibility.*[587]

The term *primary process* refers to life, the source, the creator, our inner primary experience of life.

For more "learning" about how school is toxic, I suggest the many books written by former school teacher, John Taylor Gatto. His most recent book is *Weapons of Mass Instruction.* Other titles include: *The Underground History of American Education,* and *Dumbing Us Down: The Hidden Curriculum of Compulsory Schooling.*

The Oppressor and the Oppressed

In many ways, there are outward oppressive forces in our country. There are state and federal governments that make and promote laws related to schooling, food, and vaccinations. People like or dislike certain aspects of the govern-

ment, or they just withdraw and pretend not to care about what the government or authority does. And we have the corporate media, which transmit certain messages to us, and we have the pharmaceutical industry that controls our standard health care system, and there are many larger corporations which manufacture food. There are also a variety of known and hidden special interest groups setting their own agendas.

The people who get to call the shots and make decisions in those organizations are not conscious. They have a distorted sense of what is best and right. They are not really present to how their decisions affect other people. They feel a twisted pleasure as they exert their power and control. When people in these organizations make decisions that affect the rest of us negatively, it is important to understand that they are not making decisions that come from presence; they are not acting out of love, and a desire for a greater harmony. They act out of hatred, ignorance, greed and other negative energy forms.

We experience what appears to be a dualistic state of consciousness: on one hand we have the oppressors, who seem to have all the power and, and on the other hand, we have the oppressed, who seem powerless to make changes in life. Many of us feel that we are victims of the policies and behaviors of these large institutions. We feel powerless to make changes; what can one person do, you might think? The oppressors and the regular citizens are opposite ends of a core and central distortion: the distortion of freedom, free will, and divine will.

Activity: breaking free of oppression How do the oppressed become free? By realizing that their feeling and experience of life as being oppressed, thwarted and trapped creates the opposite energy current, the oppressor. Without the oppressed, the oppressor has no one to oppress. So our rigid social structures exist because we believe in the reality of being oppressed. They only appear to oppress us, and we believe in that reality because we oppress ourselves in hidden ways. The shackles that you think come from the world, in most cases, are really self imposed. When you realize this, then you can release them.

Breaking Free of the Prison of Society

The prisoners and the guards in the panopticon model are symbols of the oppressed and the oppressor. They are outer reflections of common threads of dysfunctions that many of us face throughout our personal — emotional, mental and spiritual — worlds.

Our institutions, our prisons, our schools, our buildings, our food and our automobiles, the many facets of our modernized way of living, have evolved over time out of a fear of our more animal and instinctual urges.

> *You see, my friends, the life that is inherent in nature is also in you... Only the feeling life, the natural life, can indeed bring you the fulfillment without which life is a sorry affair indeed.*
>
> *Now why has humanity lost touch with the source of its own life, the source of its feelings, the source of its instincts, the source of its own nature, deep inside the self?*
>
> *Only because you are so terrified of your destructiveness and do not know how to handle it. So civilization has for millennia denied the instinctual life in order to preserve itself from its dangers. But by doing so humanity has cut off its connection with the essence of life itself. It had not realized that there are other ways to eliminate the distorted, perverted, natural forces, ways that need not deny life itself. The instinctual life has always been wrongly equated with destructiveness. Only as humanity matures is it capable of learning that the instinctual life does not need to be denied in order to avoid evil. Indeed, it should not be denied, for doing so defeats life every bit as much as the feared evil itself. Only within the deep core of the instincts can God be found because only there can true aliveness be found.*[588]

Much of the way we live can be seen as a reflection of our caged instincts, and our dissociation from Nature and the stream of life. Our modernized lifestyle is a clear reflection of how we have chastised ourselves. As the Pathwork excerpt above stresses, we have cut off our instinctual forces because, in their unpurified form, they can cause destruction and pain. But we are given part of the key to unwinding this riddle: the Creator, the source of Life and of pleasure, lies within the core of those instincts. We begin to release our instinctual drives when we see them, honor them, recognize them, and tease out the negative streams that surround them through our compassionate self-observation.

The process of purifying instinctual drives is much too broad a topic for this book. But you can begin to live by a different set of rules. Life and the experience of a painful existence exist because life is a school.[589]

Modern Food, Crime and Prisons

Today imprisoning people has become a profitable industry. You might see how we treat our prisoners like the caged animals in a zoo. In a holographic metaphor, a prisoner is someone who has acted out of a distorted instinctual drive and caused harm in society. Prisoners are the outer reflection of our instinctual drives. Instincts are driven into dark corners of our psyche, and prisoners are driven into the depths of confinement in prisons. Our entire society is built on a model of the panopticon to reflect the imprisonment of our souls. To create a society that is safer for our children we want to have less crime, not more prisons and more punishment. More prisons and more punishment mean that crime has not been addressed at its source.

With the arrival of the white man and his plague of modernization to native peoples came not only death and disease, but also crime. Dr. Price writes:

> *After one has lived among the primitive racial stocks in different parts of the world and studied them in their isolation, few im-*

pressions can be more vivid than that of the absence of prisons and asylums. [590]

I am not speaking here of a utopia or a fantasy vision of ignoring violence, I am talking about a society in which crime does not exist, so that there is no need for prisons. Speaking of the Loetschental Valley, Dr. Price explains that there is something in

> *...life-giving vitamins and minerals of the food that builds not only great physical structures within which their souls reside,* **but builds minds and hearts capable of a higher type of manhood.** *(Emphasis added.)*

What Dr. Price is speaking of is a deep and abiding truth. If we live in harmony with Nature we will create children who will not grow up to be criminals. There will be more bonding in this society, and less numbness. Without numbness, and with healthy, well functioning individuals, crime will be almost non-existent. Dr. Price continues.

> *Criminal tendencies in isolated primitives are so slight that no prisons are required. I have referred to the Loetschental Valley in Switzerland, which, until recently, has been physically isolated from the process of modernization. For the two thousand inhabitants in that valley, there is no prison. In Uganda, Africa, the Ruanda tribes estimated to number* **two and a half million,** *had no prisons.* [591] *(Emphasis added.)*

What has so radically changed between these societies and ours?

- The bond between mother and child is broken.
- Children learn from schools rather than from communities and family.
- Children are poisoned with pharmaceuticals and vaccines.
- Children and pregnant mothers eat foods not fit for life.

We must not overlook these critical factors. We can never build enough prisons, or destroy enough of our perceived or real enemies, to create a feeling of safety. We cannot make the laws strict enough or penalties severe enough to protect ourselves and our children from the violent and ignorant behaviors of others. So we must change what we are doing, and how we are living.

Disease is a result of our discordance with Nature's laws. Disease is not a germ and it is not a virus. It is our unhealthy way of living— the plague of modernization. In this plague, we in ignorance create a fertile terrain for disease through poisoning ourselves and our environment. Deficiencies in our soils produce deficient crops and animals and lead to further deterioration of our internal terrain. Could it be that those who are most susceptible to our diseased way of living are the most likely to fall into the trap of criminal behavior? Has Nature designed us in a flawed way, made us capable of destroying ourselves and turning earth into a hellish world? Or, has Nature designed us with a potential for perfection, and given us a formula for creating peace on earth?

Nature has never been flawed, and we are not doomed to a certain predetermined fate. But rather, we modern folk have strayed too far from our divine heritage, and so we create suffering.

When Dr. Price visited the Ohio State Penitentiary, he found that many criminals showed signs of prenatal nutritional deficiencies. He did not see one individual in prison with properly formed facial development. [592] There must be a connection between proper physical growth and the tendency to see the world from a mature place, and thus participate in society in ways that benefit others rather than harm them.

Dr. Price's grand conclusion to his book:

> *There is a nutritional basis for modern physical, mental and moral degeneration.* [593]

There is a nutritional basis for criminal tendencies. That is not to say that people are not responsible for wrongdoing. But people are much less dangerous and less prone to dangerous behavior if their bodies and minds are sound and content with good nourishing foods. This is our calling, to stop our insane food and dietary habits, to contribute to the creation of a more sane and safe society for our children-to-be. Crime and other negative behaviors are aggravated by improper nutrition. If you have ever been hungry, you know that starvation of nutrients in the body can create violent and irrational moods.

Could inner pollution, a body congested from a lifetime of vaccines, pharmaceuticals, and processed foods lead to polluted behaviors? Dr. Bernard Jensen thinks so:

> *We can only begin to guess the number of people incarcerated in psychiatric facilities, prisons, and other institutions because of socially unacceptable behavior associated with mental dysfunction ultimately due to filthy, toxic and malfunctioning bowels.*[594]

And what do we feed our prisoners in this country? Absolutely the cheapest food imaginable. I once saw a documentary on prisons in which a guard said the food for their guard dogs costs more than the food they feed the prisoners. Prison is, both on the psychological and physical level, a breeding ground for dysfunction. I learned in my college criminal behavior course that some criminals spend their lives in and out of prison, each time committing more and more violent crimes. Some prisoners who are unstable will become worse through their prison stay, their deficiencies exacerbated by association with other unstable prisoners and the inhuman prison system itself. As Western medicine causes disease, prison could very well breed and help to create violent people. In other words, prison can create far worse and more violent

criminals than would exist if there were no prisons. (Again, I do not support a lack of consequences for violence, but rather wish to highlight that our society is so dysfunctional that the very institution meant to stop crime causes crime.)

Emotional, Mental, and Spiritual Degradation in Our Modernized Society

Perhaps most people do not become criminals, but this depends on your definition of a criminal. Many of us break laws occasionally or even regularly. This includes speeding, going through red lights or stop signs, being dishonest, petty crimes of theft, illegal copying of software and music, use of illegal drugs, lying on resumes and applications. What's more, many of us have harassed other people (usually our spouses), hit, pushed, or otherwise physically confronted other people, perhaps in our younger years, and possibly engaged in inappropriate conduct at one time or another. All I am saying here is that most of us tend to break rules, and it is very hard not to do so because a majority of us don't even know even a fraction of the laws in our state. We only know a few basic rules. That's why the government invented signs. Everywhere you don't know the rules, signs are posted explaining the rules. Most of us don't know or understand in any detail the laws of our culture. We don't know much of what is legal, or illegal. For example: What are food labeling laws? Can you collect rain water? Does the government have legal precedent to spray chemicals on people?

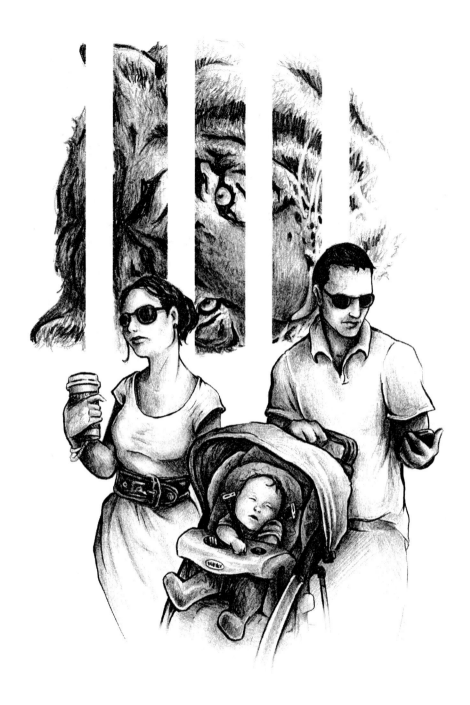

Day at the Zoo: *This scene is typical of our modernized lifestyle. The man and woman are actually seeing a reflection of what they are doing to themselves. They see the tiger, and are entertained by it. The caged tiger in this picture represents our animal instincts. The child, caged in his stroller, is learning about life's realities. The parents are distracted, looking for the next stimulating activity to mask their dissatisfaction with life. As exciting as the zoo is, the parents are afraid of the tiger breaking free of his cage. The root of the fear is in them; it's the fear of unleashing their own animal desires and instincts.*

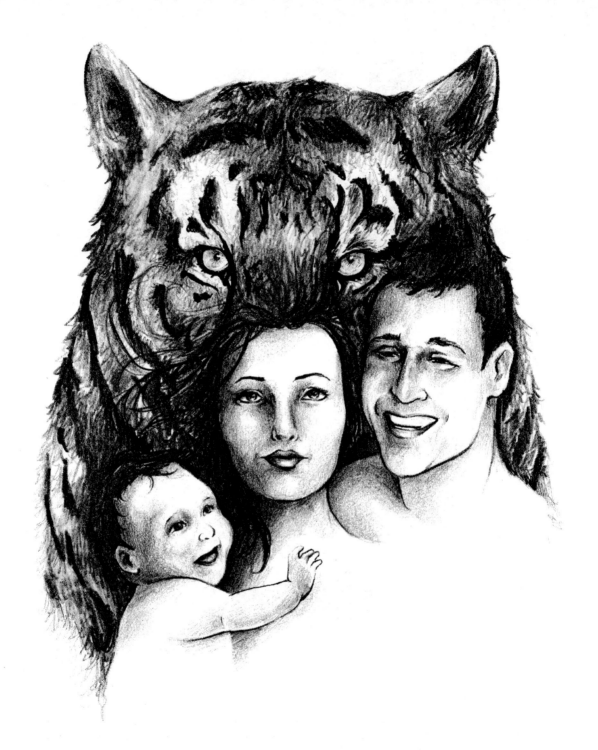

When we can free our caged selves and our instincts, life will flow freely again. This is not evil or violence, but a higher order of reality. Here, the image is a symbol of transformation. The separated family, separated from life, unhappy and lacking meaning, has the potential to find meaning in every moment. They will still face conflicts and challenges, but they have the potential to feel whole and to live together in harmony. How much joy this will bring their child is immeasurable.

Each individual must take responsibility for any perpetuation of violence he creates. But as a society, we cannot ignore and must take responsibility for how we treat each other. We tend to treat each other like garbage, operating out of our own self interests while only pretending to be compassionate, caring, or understanding. Under the façade of our fake caring and fake smile, our own anger, darkness, and repressed feelings lie. And under that, our real soft pain, our hurt and wounded child waits. And under that, the gold at the bottom of the "Well of Grief" (see poem on page 250) the source from which we drink, the secret waters of life can be found. Without the gold at the bottom of our own internal wells, we cannot become channels for goodness and light to enter into this world of partial darkness.

Like caged animals, we suffer. We can make changes and we can make life far better. It starts when we begin to take care of ourselves and take care of our children by really being there for them. The higher standard of parenting described in this book is not just an idea. It is your higher potential, your grace, your love, striving to burst to the surface and into the world.

Final Thoughts

By bringing awareness, love, humility and acceptance to your negativity and inner darkness, while not indulging it, you can help release your caged "animal" instincts, and become capable of attaining a higher type of humanity.

The world that we see, the smoke stacks, melting icebergs, the unfair laws and policies, is not a result of a cruel accident. These things are outer reflections of our inner landscape. You must look into yourself and find how you pollute your own soul with negative feelings, emotions and desires. Honor them with compassion in order to heal them, but do not avoid them. You must find the iced walls of resistance that prevent you from returning to a state of love. You must find how you were treated unfairly by life, by your parents, siblings and so forth, and feel the pain that has welled up in you as a re-sult, so that you do not unconsciously continue to cause harm to others.

The panopticon, the idea of the separate outer authority, the rigid social structure of domination and subjugation, exists as a reflection of our own fragmented internal authority. Real authority comes from truth, love, compassion and divine inspiration. In a broad sense, we do not see this type of authority in the world, because it has not been activated within all of us. It lies as a seed with the potential to burst to the surface. It simply needs water and sunlight.

You are the authority for your child. And while it is usually a lengthy process to embrace your own higher authority, it is also a part of the learning process of life. In other words, the challenges of life will help you learn how to be a better authority. Life will show you your weaknesses and your strengths. Our children need us to be present for them, to show them our love and compassion, and to take the higher path towards grace.

13

Feeding Our Children

The parents of healthy children know what to feed their children.

Intention: Learn what to feed your children to make them strong and healthy. Learn what not to feed your children.

How we feed our children is a direct reflection of what we think about life. When our subconscious and underlying belief about the world is, "Life is suffering," then that belief manifests itself as an unhealthy lifestyle. Thus, we don't feed our children foods that will make them strong. Feeding our children is very much about how we care for and honor our children.

Diet for Children 5 months to 6 Years

The best information that I have discovered for feeding babies and children is to feed them healthy fat. In India the special food for babies is ghee, which is essentially 100 percent fat. For other groups, bone marrow is a preferred food for babies, and again is largely composed of fat. Others have told me that an excellent food for babies is avocado. Again, fat.

Here are many of the most essential foods to offer your children in their early years:

Yellow grassfed raw butter

Raw grassfed milk

Grassfed liver

Raw or cooked grassfed bone marrow

Eggs that are raw or soft-cooked, especially the yolks (hardboiled is okay)

Mineral-rich bone stocks (beef, chicken, fish, and so on).

Cooked or raw caviar or wild caught fish eggs

Raw, marinated or cooked wild fish

Raw, seared or cooked, beef or lamb

Fermented vegetables

Other organ meats

Oysters, clams and other shellfish that include the organs

Freshly juiced vegetables.

The keys to health for children are the same that we have already learned for healthy adults. Activator X is available in yellow butter, in fish eggs, and very likely in certain organs of animals from the spring, summer and fall seasons, and in the organs of crab and lobster. Your child's diet needs to regularly include foods high in Activator X. Other fat-soluble vitamins are found in liver, bone marrow, and other organs. They provide vital nutrients for a growing body that are not present in the typical diet. The optimal trio for infant health is: **liver, bone marrow, and yellow butter.**

Foods such as cereals, grains and breads are very challenging for little ones to digest. It is best to hold off on grains until at least the age of one. Some sources suggest waiting until age two. **Grains must be soaked, fermented, and debranned prior to eating**. Your baby's earliest foods should be animal foods such as fats or proteins. [595] There may be some indigenous cultures that feed specially fermented grains to children under the age of two. I have no recipes to share with you on how to do this, so I suggest you avoid grains entirely until your children are between one to two years old.

Michelle and I are still learning how to feed a baby in a healthy way. At almost exactly five months, Yeshe became ravenous for solid food. She would try to grab everything that we would eat and start whining. Yeshe now eats an incredible amount of food. While some parents feed their babies foods that we should generally not eat in large amounts, such as bananas and other fruit, healthy parents feed their babies with fat and protein. Yeshe's diet at just over five months includes a high quality yogurt (full fat), raw butter, ghee, raw liver, soft boiled egg yolks, raw fish (previously frozen), raw beef (previously frozen), oysters, raw cow's milk, occasional fruit smoothies that include raw milk and cream, avocado, vegetable juice, and probiotics. Rarely does she eat plain fruit, although she is extremely excited by it. She has some fruit in smoothies every two to three days, and only because it is summer right now and these fruits are in season.

A parent commented to me that formula or breastmilk has plenty of protein for babies. Clearly, from experience, this is not the case. However, some babies might eat less when they are little, or their appetites may grow more slowly if their mother has a richer breastmilk. After feeding Yeshe lots and lots of food she is mostly calm, peaceful, and easy to care for. When she is hungry, or doesn't get enough to eat, she complains and whines.

After Yeshe has eaten, we know we have done the right thing because she makes very loud cooing noises and seems very happy and content. Yeshe sleeps well at night, is growing and maturing very fast, and everyone comments on what a beautiful baby she is (not necessarily because of her genes, but because of her rosy cheeks and well-formed, even proportions). Although Yeshe was somewhat congested for a little while after birth, the congestion soon cleared. She's never been sick, and eating all of those raw foods has been of no danger to her, contrary to the popular but flawed belief that raw milk, or other raw foods, are dangerous for babies (of course, it is your own responsibility to ensure that you eat high quality raw foods).

Also, your baby's bowel movements carry clues as to the success of the foods you are feeding her. The bowel should not be clumpy or appear to contain undigested matter. It should be smooth, come out without too much difficulty and have a frozen yogurt type of texture. If the stool is irregular in any way, your child may need either more easily digestible foods or the addition of high-quality probiotics, or perhaps both.

All foods that you offer your child should be natural, and free of pesticides, hormones and antibiotics. All animal products should preferably come from animals allowed to roam and eat their natural diet. Nothing should be manufactured in factories. Make your own baby food at home.

The Twelve Covenants of Children's Health

I call these covenants because these guidelines need to be ardently followed to support the solid health of your children.

1. Do not vaccinate your baby!
2. Do not give your child fluoridated water.
3. Do not give your child prescription drugs, antibiotics or medications unless an emergency requires it.
4. Do not give your child white flour or processed flour products.
5. Do not give your child white sugar, or processed sugar products.
6. Do not give your child pasteurized or excessive amounts of fruit juices.
7. Do not give your child unfermented soy foods, such as soy formula, soy proteins, soy milk or tofu.
8. Do not give your child commercial infant formula.
9. Do not give your child margarine or rancid vegetable oils like soy, canola, corn, and so forth.
10. Do not give your child pasteurized commercial dairy products.
11. Do not give your child low fat products.

12. Do not give your child food with additives.
13. Do not apply chemically laden soaps, shampoos, sun blocks or other body products to your children's bodies.

Pasteurized milk and commercial infant formulas, which are commonly available in our society, are especially dangerous to your child's health. Dr. Bieler explains in his book, *Food is Your Best Medicine,* that heating makes milk indigestible and as a result it putrefies in the child's body, creating toxemia and eventually illness. The heating process used in making baby formula has the same result. Modern baby formulas are loaded with processed ingredients like sugar. Many times the first ingredient on the label is corn syrup. Remember, infants are designed to drink raw breastmilk. Any type of modified milk will be reacted to as an allergen because of your baby's undeveloped digestive system. Giving your baby commercial foods will give rise to sniffles, frequent colds, tonsillitis and croup.[596]

Grains fed to children should be fermented and not contain the bran or the germ. Grain bran and germ is usually toxic to children. Brown rice soaked with a starter, quinoa, and buckwheat may be exceptions for that rule, but be aware that they may contain potent anti-nutrients. Watch out for store bought whole grain products, including ones that are sprouted or soured. Learn more about grains is at:
www.healingourchildren.net/wholegrains

Always avoid: Commercial dairy products (especially ultra-pasteurized), modern soy foods, margarines and shortening, excess fruit juices (infrequent consumption of freshly made fruit juice is acceptable), reduced-fat or low-fat foods, extruded grains and all processed foods. Avoid commercial rice milk, soy milk and almond milk, even organic varieties. Don't feed your babies granola bars, breakfast cereal, or other processed grains.

Nutrition for Children

These nutrition guidelines for children are a work in progress, which means that I offer some tips that have some minor contradictions. Some of these suggestions may not work for you or your baby. But children have a natural wisdom regarding food. If they do not like the food or it is not right for them, they spit it out. The exception to this natural wisdom is sweets. Children will indulge in sweets beyond what is healthy for them. Based on the temperament of your baby, and many other factors, some of these food suggestions will work for you. Your intuition will tell you which guidelines need to be modified. Never ever force your child to eat anything unless it is an emergency. A particular example of a commonly rejected food is vegetables. Sometimes children do not like them, and this is because their body cannot yet utilize them well. You can offer your child vegetables, but do not force him to eat vegetables if he rejects them at first. Wait several weeks or months and calmly try again.

You can trust your own instincts about when to start to give your baby food; and watch his cues. When your infant begins to bring his hand to his mouth while you eat, that eager gesture could mean he is ready. Babies begin eating solid food generally at around 5-6 months of age, and regular breastfeeding continues with the introduction of solid foods. Almost everything we feed Yeshe she loves and she opens her mouth and reaches out to indicate that she wants more.

Breastmilk alternative

While I ardently support breastfeeding your child for many years, there will be a few cases when breastmilk may need to be supplemented.

There are two natural formulas, a dairy-based formula and a bone stock-based formula. The dairy-based formula uses certified raw milk. These recipes can be accessed online at www.westonaprice.org/children/formula-faqs.html The ideal breastmilk replacements use whole and unprocessed milk from grassfed cows or goats. Animal foods, such as these formulas, are suitable replacements for breastmilk and can be used regularly. Bear in mind that these formulas do not replace the emotional nurturance of breastfeeding. They are, however, better than other store-bought formulas or fruit. Never buy packaged infant formula no matter how natural they claim to be. If you are totally strapped for time, see if you can have a friend make homemade foods or natural formulas for your growing baby, or hire someone to do it.

First foods

The majority of your child's first foods should be animal fats. Your child's first foods can be egg yolks, liver (raw or cooked), raw butter or ghee, bone marrow (raw or cooked) and yogurt.

Fruits are okay to eat, provided they are cooked and are used as a vehicle for cream or butter. High pectin fruits like peaches, apricots, apples, pears, cherries, and berries should be cooked for babies.[597] Do not feed your child excess fruit.

The typical parent feeds her child fruit, potatoes and grains as first foods. In general this is a bad idea. While it is fine to give your young baby some fruit and potatoes, these are not the most nourishing foods and their use should be limited to supplemental status.

Fermented sweet potato and taro are good for babies, as they are easy to digest and help support the baby's beneficial bacteria.[598] The fermentation process consumes many or most of the simple sugars in these starchy foods and increases their nutrient content, making the foods more healthful for baby. Cooked vegetables normally should be prepared and served with lots of butter. And lots of butter…means a lot.

In at least some indigenous cultures, the parents chew the child's food before they give the food to the child. In our modern culture, we are told that this practice is unhygienic and even dangerous. There is fear that parents can pass *Strep mutans* bacteria to their children. In light of our new awareness about bacteria as Nature's helpers, we know that giving your child chewed food won't confer disease. Clearly, from an anatomical point of view, food chewed by parents will be more digested than food blended in a blender. Beneficial bacteria are transmitted from mother to child. Giving your child food from your mouth will not give your child cavities, as only a nutritional deficiency or body chemistry imbalance will.[599]

Special Native Foods for Babies

I am not aware at what age these foods were fed to babies in native groups. Nor do I know the amount of foods that were used. But I cannot emphasize enough the importance of using some or all of these special foods listed here, as well as organ meats and other special foods listed in Chapter 6. These are vitally important foods.

Bone marrow. "When I asked what the bone was for he said for the marrow to use for food for the baby."[600] (Canadian Indians)

Wall of stomach (tripe) milk. "The Indian explained how the moose eats buds of trees which were strong foods. The strength goes from the buds into the wall of the stomach and he explained that the Indians clean the stomach and pound the wall up fine to make milk for the baby."[601] (Canadian Indians)

Fish juice. "The waters draining towards the arctic do not have the running salmon of the Pacific coast rivers but do have pike and white fish. The Indians spear some of these through the ice in the winter. They are difficult to catch in the summer with their meager equipment, for white fish cannot be caught with a hook and line. *They make a nutritious milk for babies* by grinding and squeezing the juice of the fish muscles." (Canadian Indians)

Liver. In some parts of Africa mothers give their infants liver as their first food; they chew it up for the infant. [602]

Fish eggs. "On the logs below the hanging fish are the fish eggs being dried for food for the **babies**, young children, and mothers when raising families."[603]

4 months+

An egg yolk that has been soft or hard boiled. [604] Also yogurt or ghee (clarified butter).

6 months +

Feed your child lots of fat.

Recommended foods:

Raw or cooked grated organic liver.

Whole-milk yoghurt or kefir.

Room temperature whole raw milk.

Ghee (clarified butter).

Soup from bone broths.

Yellow butter, preferably raw.

Do not give your child a low-fat diet. Low-fat diets have been linked with failure to thrive in children.[605] Do not give your child processed salt or excessive salt. Coconut cream (the cream from juicing mature coconut meat) or a small amount of coconut oil may be of benefit due to the presence of lauric acid, a fat that is present in breastmilk.[606]

8 months +

To the list for six-month-olds you can add some mild cheeses, cream, custard, and blended vegetable soups.[607] Babies can also eat smoothies made with raw milk, raw eggs and a little bit of fruit. Alternatively, pâtés made with fish or liver are also nourishing.

If you are not feeding your baby liver, very small doses of high-vitamin cod liver oil is probably a good idea. Think dropper sized. Somewhere from 1/32 to 1/8th of a teaspoon per day; consult with your health care practitioner for the exact dosage.

9 months+

As I have mentioned several times in this book, raw milk, from certified high quality grass-based farms, is health-giving and life promoting. Raw milk is far safer to consume than pasteurized milk. A smoothie prepared for your baby can include ¼ cup raw milk, 1-2 ounces of cream, and one raw egg yolk.

Raw or cooked liver, fish, or organic meats or chicken that are appropriately mashed or puréed may also be good foods.

Activator X: Children should continue to eat foods containing Activator X.

Foods to Avoid:

Cooked egg whites: It is probably not a good idea to give your young child cooked egg whites as some may have difficulty with the protein in egg whites.[608]

Avoid until **6 months of age:** Certain foods such as spinach, celery, lettuce, radishes, beets, turnips and collard greens, may contain excessive nitrates, which can be converted into nitrites (an undesirable substance) in the stomach. Leafy green vegetables are best avoided until 1 year. When cooking vegetables that may contain these substances, do not use the water they were cooked in to purée.

Avoid until 9 months: Citrus and tomato, which are common allergens.

Avoid until 1 year: Because infants do not produce strong enough stomach acid to deactivate potential spores, the prevailing belief is that infants should refrain from eating honey.[609] (This may not be the case for a good quality, unheated raw honey.)

A further resource is "Nourishing a Growing Baby" found under children's health at: www.westonaprice.org

Diet for One Year +

Grass fed animal foods: fish, meat and poultry, ocean-caught fish, and shellfish. Until the child is older he may not chew his food thoroughly, so keep this in mind in your preparation methods. Raw grass-fed cream, butter and bone marrow support healthy growth and are nourishing fats. Make sure to give your children lots of foods with organ meats and plenty of raw milk. These special foods don't exclude grains that have been freshly ground and soaked for 24 hours, vegetables, vegetable juices and fruit.

Remember the three special food categories, and feed your child two of these three at least in some amount every day; and twice daily is preferred. If you cannot offer these foods every day, try to provide them very often.

1. Raw dairy from grassfed animals (milk, cream, butter, cheese).
2. Organs of pasture fed land animals.

3. Organs and head meat of wild-caught sea animals and shellfish.

Food Preparation

Raw or rare-cooked sashimi style fish and meat are the easiest for children to digest.[610] If this concerns you, cook the food to the degree with which you feel comfortable. Also, freezing or marinating meats or fish in an acidic medium can disable supposed pathogens.

Special Foods for Children in The Formative Years

I do not have clear data indicating at what ages these different types of foods were fed to children in native groups, or how much was given. I'm sure the parameters were somewhat variable. Many indigenous cultures only used some of these special foods, as the other special foods were not obtainable in their immediate area. Many of these foods can be beneficial for a breastfeeding mother to eat as well. Feed your child as much of these foods as he would like; pay attention to any kind of odd reactions, and adjust dosages accordingly.

Bone marrow. "I found the Indians putting great emphasis upon the eating of the organs of the animals, including the wall of parts of the digestive tract. Much of the muscle meat of the animals was fed to the dogs. These Indians obtain their fat-soluble vitamins and also most of their minerals from the organs of the animals.

An important part of the nutrition of the children consisted in various preparations of bone marrow, both as a substitute for milk and as a special dietary ration.[611] (Canadian Indians)

Fish eggs. "I presented data indicating that the Peruvians, who were descendants of the old Chimu culture on the coast of Peru, used fish eggs liberally during the developmental period of girls in order that they might perfect their physical preparation for the later responsibility of motherhood."[612]

Fish and fish eggs. "Fish eggs were dried in season. They were used liberally as food for the growing children and were recognized as important for growth and reproduction."

"The fish are hung on racks in the wind for drying. Fish eggs are also spread out to dry… These foods constitute a very important part of the nutrition of the small children after they are weaned."[613] (Eskimo)

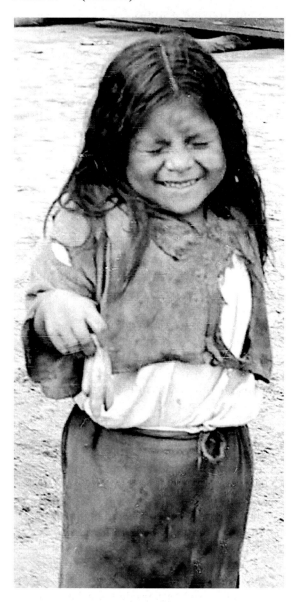

© Price-Pottenger Nutrition Foundation, www.ppnf.org

(Picture Caption) During the period of great growth, the girls are taught to eat fish eggs liberally in order to complete the building of excellent bodies for highly efficient reproduction. The little girl shown has been down to the beach where the women were cleaning the fish. She is holding her ration of fish eggs in her hand. She is on her way back to her cabin to have them cooked for her breakfast.[614]

Plant ashes.

*"In Africa I found many tribes gathering certain plants from swamps and marshes and streams, particularly the **water hyacinth**. These plants were dried and burned for their ashes which were put into the foods of mothers and growing children."*[615]

The ashes were probably high in minerals and calcium. Spirulina or blue-green algae may be a suitable replacement.

Raw milk, raw cheese, raw cream, raw butter, raw yogurt, and raw kefir. During the growing period, approximately ages 8-16, it is a good idea for children to get at least one gram of calcium per day. This is a general figure, and it varies greatly based on the age and size of the individual. Four cups of raw grass-fed milk with 1-4 ounces of a high quality raw cheese, as a good measure for safety, will provide the required amounts of calcium.

Shellfish such as sea urchins, clams, scallops, mussels, oysters, and sea cucumber.

It was a very common experience for us to see the children following the tide out and picking up the sea forms, including

scale fish and spiny forms, eating these raw after scraping the spines off with a piece of coral, which provided a handy grater.[616]

Examples of scale fish are cod, salmon, sea bass, mullet, shad, grouper, red snapper.

The children in the South Sea Islands were taught to follow the tide out and obtain every day oysters, clams, bêche-de-mer, etc., and such other sea forms as were available."[617] *(South Sea Islands, Bêche-de-mer is a sea slug.)*

Defibrinated blood.

When available, each growing child receives a day's ration of blood, as does each pregnant or lactating woman. Formerly, the warriors used this food exclusively. These three sources, milk, blood and meat, provide them with liberal supplies of body-building minerals and the special vitamins, both fat-soluble and water soluble.[618] *(Masai, Africa)*

When infants and older children are fed well they will develop thicker skulls. By inference, we know that thicker skulls likely represent a body built with thicker and more well-formed bones. In childhood, children many times fall and bump their heads. They throw their bodies in all sorts of ways and will hit their bones fairly hard at times. Having more well-formed bones and a thicker skull will make them more impervious to trauma. When they fall, it will hurt and sting less. As a result of eating a healthy diet, children will feel safer in the world because their bodies will be less delicate and fragile.

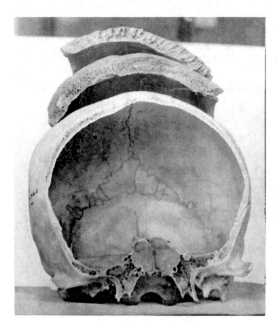

Example of greater thickness of pre-Columbian Indian skulls in Florida. The modern skull is below, and has half or less of the thickness of the more ancient skull fragments above. This is not from a genetic difference, but a factor of nutrition.[619]

School Lunch

The typical school lunch today is deplorable. Lunch is usually convenience food made in a hurry. It is essentially empty food: it might look and taste good for a moment, but provides little nutrition. Is what we feed our children a reflection of the superficial relationship we have with them? Does our modern diet reflect both how we think and feel about our children, and ourselves? Have we also become accustomed to sacrificing our higher values in life for the quick and short-lived pleasure of the convenience food?

The typical lunch menu for our children leads to improper physical development, which includes an elongation or lengthening of the child's body, a much higher chance of developing disease and illness, poor mental concentration, poor physical strength, poor vision, and lowered overall vitality and intelligence. This occurs because the foods we normally feed our children are almost totally devoid of nutrients. In Chapter 5 I discussed how our modern diet is deficient in many essential nutrients. So how can we expect our children to grow strong and healthy on this deficient fare? With our modern diet, we literally are poisoning our children, and they are starving for nutrients. This leads to sugar cravings and bingeing and snacking on sugary foods: the body's attempt to obtain nutrients. Let's look a bit into what you can do.

You will have to adapt your school lunch to what your child likes, and what you feel is healthy. That is, of course, if you send your child to school.

Deplorable Typical Lunch Items	High Vitamin Replacements
Peanut Butter and Jelly Sandwich Provides no nutrients, the phytates in the peanut butter make the nuts indigestible; if the peanut butter is not organic it is chock-full of pesticides, and the jam causes a sugar rush which pulls minerals from the body to neutralize. The child gets about 0.0% of absorbable nutrients from the bread. If you are lucky, maybe your children can absorb 0-10% of nutrients in typical whole wheat bread	**Butter and Cheese "Sandwich"** Give your child large amounts of yellow butter, with a large piece of raw cheese, on a sourdough piece of bread made with freshly ground grain. Or the same combination with no grains. **Organ Sandwich** One or two slices of homemade sourdough bread from freshly ground grain, spread with a pâté made from liver or other organs, or spread bone marrow, butter, or other animal fat all over the bread.

Deplorable Typical Lunch Items	High Vitamin Replacements
Cheese and Crackers, or Peanut Butter and Crackers Pretty much the same as above: the crackers are processed at high temperatures and contain phytates; they will gum up the interior of your child's body. Processed wheat will pull nutrients out of the body.	You can make a typical cheese or meat sandwich, just make sure they are made from home made cuts of meat, and then load the sandwich with animal fat, butter (avocado can be good too). **Raw, rare cooked, marinated, or dehydrated beef or fish** Pemmican is made with dehydrated beef ground up and mixed with beef fat. Add honey and some cranberries and it's very tasty! Salmon and other types of fish can be smoked, dehydrated and/or fermented. They can be eaten with butter or cream cheese. Lox is one example. **Beef, lamb, chicken or fish stews and chowders are excellent meals.**
String Cheese Your typical string cheese is loaded with processed vegetable oil and has been pasteurized. The overly heated cheese turns into a poison, particularly because the cow has eaten foods laden with chemicals and pesticides which wind up in the milk. Your child's body is gummed up and shocked by the broken protein strands. The cheese may have MSG and other toxic chemicals added. Commercial milk contains synthetic hormones and antibiotic residues.	Raw, grassfed goat, or cow cheese (there are many varieties). Grass fed raw butter Grass fed Bone Marrow, raw or cooked Organic avocado Soaked and low temperature dried organic nuts.
Fruit Juice/ Fruit Punch Loaded with sugar and pasteurized, this will send your child's blood sugar level over the top. Likely filled with chemicals, preservatives, and MSG which pull calcium and phosphorus from bones, and over- stimulate the glandular system, making children hyperactive. The hyperactivity from the fruit juice is a toxic response to this poison.	**Raw grass fed milk and/or raw grass fed cream.** My daughter loves the "baby milks" which are the bottles of cream we have. She just drinks the cream straight out of the bottle. This will create a happy and calm child. Vegetable juice that is freshly juiced and doesn't include too much excessively sweet vegetables.
Potato chips, or corn chips Fried in the lowest quality, rancid oils, the chemicals generated by the denatured potato, corn, or whatever else the chips are	**Lacto fermented vegetables**, like poi, sauerkraut, or fermented potatoes. **Homemade french fries**, with duck fat, lard,

made out of are a sure way to clog your young child's arteries, and irritate the inner mucous lining of their digestive track. Flavored with MSG and other poisons, these toxic foods will alter your child's brain chemistry and lull your child into a chemically induced trance.	or coconut oil. **A baked potato**, loaded with raw grassfed butter, and/or sour cream.
Pudding Made with denatured pasteurized milk, sugar and a slew of chemicals to disguise the rancid taste, the pudding will do nothing but cause intestinal discomfort. Many foods also have synthetic vitamins added, and some of those synthetic vitamins that are supposed to be healthy, are very toxic. MSG is likely added to create an addictive impulse.	**Suet pudding**, that is pudding made from animal fat. **Rice pudding**, homemade pudding made with cream and rice. **Whipped cream** with a little unheated raw honey and carob powder. Made from raw unpasteurized grassfed cream. **Custard**, homemade with egg yolks, cream, and milk.
Cookies Processed flour and all kinds of unwholesome processed, powdered, denatured, sugared, and toxic ingredients make up the typical cookie. MSG and other chemicals are usually added.	**Crispy nut cookies**, make cookies with arrow root powder, and soaked and dried peanuts or almonds.

Fruit, such as apples or oranges, or vegetable sticks, like celery and carrots
These foods fit in both categories. They can be health building if used wisely, and at the same time, they may not provide enough absorbable nutrients to make your child healthy. Basically, do not count on carrots or apples to be a healthy staple in an otherwise unhealthy diet.

A typical parent will feel less guilty about all the unnatural foods that they are giving to their children if they give them something wholesome and unprocessed, like a nice piece of fruit or some vegetable sticks. If these choices are not organic, you are giving your child the RDA of pesticides that have never been tested for safety on children. Raw fruits and vegetables have nutrients that can be difficult to absorb. The absorption depends on the individual's digestive capabilities, the food eaten, and the method of preparation of the food. Oranges and other very sweet fruits can quickly create too much blood sugar fluctuation, causing body chemistry imbalances.

Wise parents give their children fruit as a side dish, not as their main healthy food. The fruit is best prepared or eaten with animal fats, such as luscious strawberries with cream and apples with cheese. Serve mashed potatoes with plenty of butter. You do not always have to eat fruit with animal fats, but it should be a norm to do this.

Fruits and vegetables create balance in a diet, and provide needed nutrients. Never force your child to eat them, though, or count on them to provide the full nourishment your child needs.

Fermented vegetables are good to use as condiments and increase your child's digestive strength.

Take the time to feed your child foods dense in nutrients. Parents, who have healthy children, have healthy children because they know what to feed them.

14

Amazing Grace

Amazing grace! How sweet the sound
That saved a wretch like me!
I once was lost, but now am found;
Was blind, but now I see.

This book was not created by accident, or by an act of coincidence. The unnamable truth whispering through the centuries made it possible for this book to come to be. It did not even seem possible to write this book when I started. The necessary time, money, and resources that it required, and the conditions under which I wrote it, can only mean that this book arose out of grace. And it has entered your hands, and likely touched your life, also by an act of grace. Grace is not something outside of us that is given to us once in a while. Grace is the space within you, your timeless essence, being invited to come here into a new world. A world filled with hope, faith and healing. This world is in our midst, and it is one of the infinite possibilities of life that we can choose. We just need to reach for it, to long for it, to pray for it, to desire it. Grace is not outside of us. Look into the depths of your soul and find that unconditional "yes" to life.

Intention: To feel, acknowledge, and experience grace moving through you. To see the simple and elegant solution for ending a majority of diseases, and how we create truly vibrant children. Because your child matters!

Yes, there is amazing grace on this planet. We may not see it too often, but it exists here, for all of us. I feel inspired by the last line in the familiar hymn above: "Was blind, but now I see." This has several meanings. It applies to me, for I was blind to the many ways that I was creating ill health in my life. But now I see. I see that I can change this. This is grace. And I believe that my inner light will find truth and clarity through those spheres of darkness where I am still blind, so those blind parts in me will one day see.

"Was blind, but now I see," also applies to you; it applies to our country, and to our planet. "Was blind" to the many causes of suffering, but now you **see** the causes, and **see** how to make changes. The light of truth is shining compassionately upon you. This is grace.

Once you were lost like I was, huddled in a maze of darkness. Disease was the inescapable enemy. And now a helping hand is reaching out towards you, saying, "Grasp onto me. This is where you can rest yourself."

"Was blind" because we once could tell ourselves that we did not know why our children, and our mothers and fathers suffered. We see that suffering comes from our wrong way of living, that the pain of miscarriages, birth defects, mental deficiencies, physical imbalances, chronic diseases, and early childhood death is created by us and can be healed. "Was blind" because we did not know why some children are weak while others are strong. It seemed that all attempted solutions only caused more suffering. "But now I see" means that you now can see, although perhaps have a difficult time wholeheartedly believing, that you are not powerless in the face of these causes, and that in fact in a majority of cases, our way of living is the cause of the condition.

Our culture was blind, and our ignorance has kept us living in a diseased manner. We have blindly created systems of destruction in our country: government organizations, laws, institutions, policies, and mega-corporations have all created suffering on a vast scale. Our ancestors, brothers and sisters, did not realize what they where doing via their poor choices, choices that dishonored their children and life on this planet. They did not understand how they where polluting and destroying the Earth, and harming sentient beings. "Was blind" refers to our own suffering. We were not aware of it, but now we begin to acknowledge it. We constantly blamed the outer world for our problems rather than looking at our own inner attitudes and numbness to life. And finally, "was blind" gives us compassion. **If you saw a blind man stumbling on the street, not knowing which way to go**, you would want to help him, you would forgive him for his mistakes because he could not see. In the same way, the people who harm our planet are indeed extremely blind. They cannot see the pleasure of doing good. We must forgive the people who were and are blind, who have caused and contributed to our health massacre. They must still be held accountable, but we must realize that such acts come from blindness, weakness, pettiness, and from a diseased state of consciousness. Only our own blindness would not hold these people accountable. But now you see, accountability begins with your own choices and actions, and grows from there. By itself, "Was blind" is complete, because it means that you have acknowledged, and continue to acknowledge, where you can make mistakes. Redemption lies in merely seeing the blindness. Seeing is the intelligence, is the grace.

Your task now is to use this book and other resources to help you **see** the blindness in yourself, and to help you see it in others so that you can make a positive change in your life and in your children's lives. Sharing information with others supports change in the world, and the people you reach no longer need to be wretches; they too can be "found."

Amazing grace is the grace available to us now. It has provided us with the knowledge that we can now prevent a majority of the diseases related to pregnancy and early childhood. And when it is too late to prevent them, there can be natural treatments for many conditions. "Now I

see" gives us hope for the future. We now have the vision, and the wisdom, and we can create the world we long to live in. This is the world we longed for as children. The world where we were seen, honored, loved and cared for as we needed to be. A peaceful world of communion with our brothers and sisters.

The Time for Healing Is NOW

It is our own blindness that keeps us stuck in the story that says, "one day this disease will be cured." That one day is today. We do not need more time, more science, or more money to awaken to our deeper loving selves, to awaken to living in a higher degree of harmony with Nature. The cure for our illnesses is not more technology; it is more awareness, more love, and more compassion. The cause of disease is the way we live. To cure diseases we need to change how we see the world, which means we need to change how we feel about ourselves. We need to unplug our minds from the false authorities that distract us through the newspapers and television. We need to plug into the divine authority—the enlivening presence that constantly electrifies the Universe into existence. In applying Nature's technology, by aligning with and realizing some of the fundamental laws of creation, you can find some degree of peace. I hope that you can find total surrender to peace, satisfaction and health.

Throughout this book, I have been focused on a central underlying theme: robust health is a result of living in harmony with Nature, which corresponds to being in harmony with the divine laws of the Universe. To the degree that you abandon these laws, you will experience suffering, and your children will suffer as well. Our misalignment with Nature, reflected in our unhealthy way of living, is magnified in its effects on our children, because they are more sensitive and their bodies are less developed than our own.

When one child suffers, the world suffers. When one child cries, the world needs to hear it. Evil enterprises take advantage of our ignorance, and even murder our children with vaccinations and other birth-related medical procedures — all in the name of profit. All of us suffer as a result. When someone is sick, it means we are all sick in some way.

The problems of health will continue to worsen if we, as a society, do not change our habits immediately. And this change begins with you. It is very much an all or nothing situation. If you are not eating correctly, as outlined in this book, you will suffer, sooner or later. Dr. Weston Price documented how many diseases arise as a result of improper nutrition. On a diet composed largely of sugars and white flour, even children contract degenerative diseases like arthritis and tuberculosis. Even in 1936 Dr. Price observed:

> *Modern civilizations are progressively breaking down* in many districts through the increase in both the incidence and the severity of several degenerative diseases, among them dental caries.[620] (Emphasis added.)

Scottish surgeon Sir Arbuthnot Lane, in studying both modernized and indigenous groups of people, concluded:

> *Long surgical experience has proved to me conclusively that there is something radically and fundamentally wrong with the civilized mode of life, and I believe that unless the present dietetic and health customs of the [Western] Nations are reorganized, social decay and race deterioration are inevitable.[621]*

As the result of our ignorant ways, child birth has become difficult for the majority of women. Tens of thousands of children die before the age of one. Children suffer from supposedly unexplainable illnesses. I identified one of the key misperceptions causing this situation: the belief that "life is suffering." We are so entrenched in this belief that it causes widespread blindness to how we can heal and prevent our suffering.

It has been quite a journey. I can imagine reading a book like this is much like riding a roller coaster, with many highs and many lows. As I near completion of this book, I realize the utter simplicity of what I am advocating. On one hand, there is the depth of suffering that results from our wrong lifestyle habits — the deaths of our children, painful separation, painful medical procedures, and deep grief and loss as parents. And on the other hand, it is so simple to replace low-quality, deficient foods with their raw or specially cooked alternatives, to spend more time and more effort with our children, eat more satisfying full-fat animal foods, avoid mass-produced foods, avoid medications and vaccinations, and be open to alternative health approaches. It really is not terribly complicated. Why not give it a try? Imagine what can be gained! And what is there that can now be easily let go?

We can create a new story. We leave the depths of despair and climb to a higher level. This story may not be as satisfying for our superficial selves, and it might cause little concern or excitement from our friends and neighbors; but there is a deep and underlying truth here. We are free.

Your child was not meant to live a life filled with suffering. And it does not have to be filled with suffering anymore. Your child's life can be filled with health, happiness and joy. And it is completely your choice.

Promote the Prevention of Childhood and Pregnancy Conditions

What follows is a general overview of how the principles you have learned here relate to certain health conditions. Because you now know what makes us sick, you can go a long way towards creating health and limiting disease. You may not eliminate disease entirely, but significantly reducing the frequency of disease and its impacts is a realistic goal for a majority of readers.

In the long term, even in one generation, illness will all but vanish.

Remember the child we saw in Chapter 3? The boy's mother was told by a doctor that he would not recover. He had been in hospitals, had fever and arthritis, and was suffering from severe tooth decay. Despite being bedfast and crying constantly he was healed through nutrition by Dr. Price:

Before and After

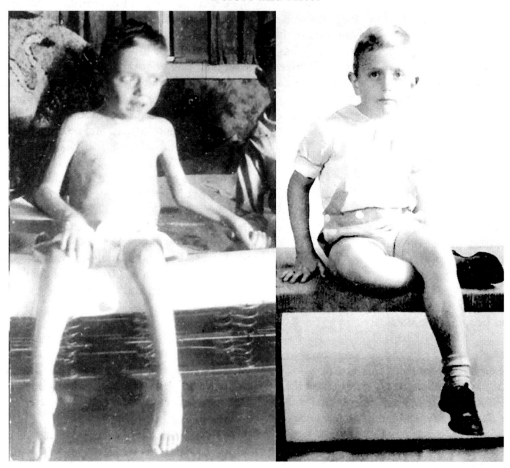

© Price-Pottenger Nutrition Foundation, www.ppnf.org
***Left**: Before, **Right**: After*

I made in this boy's dietary program was the removal of the white flour products and in their stead the use of freshly cracked or ground wheat and oats used with whole milk to which was added a small amount of specially high vitamin butter produced by cows pasturing on green wheat. Small doses of a high-vitamin, natural cod liver oil were also added.... With the improvement in his nutrition which was the only change made in his care, his acute pain rapidly subsided, his appetite greatly improved, he slept soundly and gained rapidly in weight..." At the right, the same boy is pictured, one year later, after following the dietary program. "This occurred six years ago. As I write this a letter has been received from the boy's mother. She reports that he is taller and heavier than the average, has a good appetite and sleeps well.

It is important to emphasize the changes that were made in our modern dietary program to make this boy's nutrition adequate for recovery. Sugars and sweets and white flour products were eliminated as far as possible. Freshly ground cereals were used for breads and gruels. Bone marrow was included in stews. Liver and a liberal supply of whole milk, green vegetables and fruits were provided. In addition, he was provided with a butter that was very high in vitamins having been produced by cows fed on a rapidly growing green grass. The best source for this is a pasturage of wheat and rye grass. All green grass in a state of rapid growth is good, although wheat and rye grass are the best found.[622]

Here is another story from the edge of death.

A minister in an industrial section of our city, during the period of severe depression, telephoned me stating that he had just been called to baptize a dying child. The child was not dead although almost constantly in convulsions. He thought the condition was probably nutritional and asked if he could bring the boy to the office immediately. The boy was badly emaciated, had rampant tooth decay, one leg in a cast, a very bad bronchial cough and was in and out of convulsions in rapid succession. His convulsions had been getting worse progressively during the past eight months. His leg had been fractured two or three months previously while walking across the room when he fell in one of his convulsions. No healing had occurred. His diet consisted of white bread and skimmed milk. For mending the fracture the boy needed minerals, calcium, phosphorus and magnesium. His convulsions were due to a low calcium content of the blood. All of these were in the skimmed milk for the butter-fat removed in the cream contains no calcium nor phos-

phorus, except traces. The program provided was a change from the white flour bread to wheat gruel made from freshly ground wheat and the substitution of whole milk for skimmed milk, with the addition of about a teaspoonful of a very high vitamin butter with each feeding. He was given this meal that evening when he returned to his home. He slept all night without a convulsion. He was fed the same food five times the next day and did not have a convulsion. He proceeded rapidly to regain his health without recurrence of his convulsions. In a month the fracture was united. Six weeks after this nutritional program was started the preacher called at the home to see how the boy was getting along... He was restored to health by the simple process of having Nature's natural foods restored to him.[623]

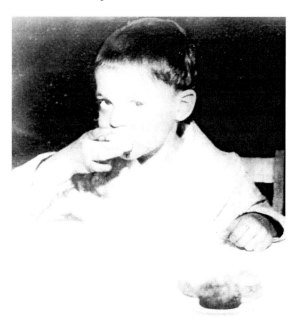

Here we see this boy after he was splendidly recovered and was living on a properly balanced diet.[624]

Disease is Not an Accident

There is something about living in harmony with Nature, with the divine, that inspires us to live a life without disease. Disease is caused by three things, and nothing else.

1. Toxins
2. Deficiencies
3. Emotions, and feeling separate from the Creator/Life

The only reason why we cannot find the cure for disease in the mainstream thought is because the mainstream is itself the disease. We create the diseases, and as long as we uphold our diseased lifestyle disease will continue. While this does not mean parents are at fault, or are to blame if they have a sick child, it does mean that we are now responsible for our children's health. It is rarely a cruel fate, or the hand of a higher power causing illness. There is no black plague; there is only a modernized plague. It is much easier to prevent disease than to cure it once it has taken hold.

Promote the Prevention of Birth Defects

We have studied three key causes of birth defects: lack of essential nutrients, particularly fat-soluble vitamins, lack of trace minerals, and too many toxins in the body from food, the environment, drugs, vaccines and toxic emotions. By addressing these areas seriously, prior to the time of conception, in both the mother and the father, the chance of a child having a birth defect will significantly decrease. Rather than using modern technology to check for birth defects or birth problems, we can use ancient technology to prevent them.

Preconception health is essential to help prevent birth defects because significant congenital malformations can result from imbalances within the germ cells—the sperm and the egg—prior to the time of conception. That means that some birth defects begin when the particular sperm and egg are forming, during the 3 month time period before conception. Improving the health of the future mother and father prior to conception, both by removing toxic influences and by increasing nutrient dense foods,

will decrease the chance of birth defects in their offspring.

I have outlined a program of preconception health, which includes various cleansing and rejuvenating methods that need to be employed by both the mother and father-to-be.

The Foresight program (www.foresight-preconception.org.uk) is very successful in creating healthy babies. Many of their guidelines have been discussed in this book, in a general sense. Their program also includes testing of blood and hair to determine levels of toxins in the blood. With their program, only two children out of 534 births had birth defects. On their website, they post a 0.47% rate of birth defects.[625] Compare this to the national average for birth defects in England, which is 6-7%. The Foresight rate is especially exceptional since many couples who are in the program are already high-risk families.

To summarize the cause of birth defects: deficiencies or toxic substances present in the mother or father, particularly prior to conception and during pregnancy, are the primary cause of birth defects.

Promote the Prevention of SIDS

There are two key explanations for Sudden Infant Death Syndrome or SIDS, and I believe both of them are true.

First, SIDS is a toxic reaction to vaccinations. The body goes into shock and the child dies. Vaccinations have a cumulative poisoning effect and most likely the multiple vaccines interact with each other, forming more dangerous and potent toxins. The answer to why SIDS affects some vaccinated children and not all has to do with other factors that could be affecting the child's health, such as hidden defects in the internal organs, or toxic accumulations gathering from the mother's body during the time in the womb. Nutrient deficiencies and a lack of comfort and holding can all together create an environment where a child could die.

The second cause of SIDS was discovered in New Zealand and has been ignored in the US.

Fire retardants added to children's mattresses have caused a significant number of cot deaths. Dr. Jim Sprott identified this problem.

I believe SIDS is caused by gaseous poisoning and the poison comes from the mattress where the baby sleeps. The gas is formed by the action of an otherwise harmless fungus on certain chemicals within the mattress. [626]

The gasses form when this fungus combines with the fire retardant chemicals put in many infant mattresses. The gasses identified are phosphine, arsine, and stibine, and are extremely toxic. [627]

In New Zealand and in England, this information has been widely circulated. The SIDS rate is now just 10% of what it was a few years ago in England. There have been no new SIDS deaths, out of over 100,000 babies born in New Zealand who have slept on specially prepared mattresses.

Dr. Sprott has designed mattress covers called Babesafe covers. These can be purchased on various sites on the internet. Mattresses in general can be very toxic. Try to use mattresses that are either older and have had time to outgas, or ones made without chemicals, which unfortunately are more expensive. We use a three inch thick blend of organic cotton and wool futon on the floor. For extra padding we could buy a natural latex rubber underpadding. Of course, breastfeeding and avoiding infant formula will help increase your baby's immunity to toxic exposures in the world.

The question arises: why in the United States are we not told what causes SIDS? We are told that doctors do not know what the cause is. To pursue this question, Dr. Jim Sprott wrote a book called *The Cot Death Coverup?*

To summarize, SIDS death is not out of our control. It is caused by toxic exposures to gasses from mattresses and chemicals from vaccines.

Promote the Prevention of Mental Disabilities & Learning Disabilities

Improper nutrition and the toxic additives in food can lead to learning disabilities. The infant's brain is formed from the seed nutrients of his or her parents. For the brain to fully form and develop properly, a child must have proper nutrition as described in this book.

I gave one example how a deficiency in vitamin E can disable the pituitary gland. Without the proper functioning of the pituitary your children's brains cannot develop properly. If their bones do not fully form, and the cavity of their skull is too narrow or malformed, this can lead to mental dysfunctions. This is clearly evident, as the whole face and body of a mentally disabled child is almost always significantly out of harmonic proportion. You can see their disability in their entire body and being. As I have stressed before, these conditions are not a result of faulty genetics; they are a result of *intercepted* heredity.

These conditions would be extremely rare on a dietary program that creates proper bone growth and development. With proper bone growth, there would be no mental disabilities due to physical malformations of parts of the brain. In an interesting example in *Nutrition and Physical Degeneration*, Dr. Price widened the dental arch of a mentally disabled child by correcting some of the imbalances in the cranial bones through surgery. The child immediately matured several years and became much more functional (however, this also added some difficult behavioral problems).

I have seen that some learning disabilities are caused by severe physical or emotional violence. Terrifying life circumstances, such as a violent parent, a significant medical procedure done during at an early age, or an emotionally disturbed parent or sibling, can lead to different types of learning disabilities. This is because the child becomes so numb, or is in such a state of shock, that he defends himself against pain in a very constricted way, so that his body (and mind) will not function fully.

Typical learning disabilities are created by our culture. They come not from a disabled or deficient child, but because the child's environment is not made for his stage of growth and development. Consider attention deficient disorder. These days I don't know even many health adults who don't have this disorder. They cannot concentrate more than 20-30 minutes on one topic. Television viewing also causes attention disorders because the television is constantly trying to entertain and stimulate the mind and emotions. When a child is loaded with sugars or other drugs, he exhibits behavior that is labeled a learning disability. Most learning disabilities are a consequence of the modern plague, resulting from a culture that is almost completely lost and disconnected from all that has real value and meaning in life. Less severe learning disabilities, like most diseases, are a result of modernization—our wrong way of living—which affects children's lives primarily through a poor bond to the mother and father and poor food selection. By choosing foods wisely, and by giving children emotional nurturance and placing them in an environment appropriate for their level of development, learning disabilities can be healed, reversed, and prevented.

The end of learning disabilities comes with the beginning of preconception health practices. To summarize, learning disabilities come from a deficiency of nutrients for glandular growth. The deficiency begins before conception and continues through pregnancy, and is amplified after birth by repeated exposure to toxins in chemically laced water, antibiotics, vaccines, food additives or other environmental poisons like pesticides.

Promote the Prevention of Autism

If you don't want your child to have autism then don't allow him to be vaccinated. Autism, like other diseases, is not caused by poor genetics, but by a heredity that is *intercepted*. An autistic child (or one with a similar disease) is one whose potential for normal growth has been thwarted.

The primary way his growth is thwarted is through exposure to heavy metals, the main source of which is vaccines given to the child. Vaccines given to the mother even remotely near the time of conception could also influence the prevalence of autism.[628] Secondary sources can be dental work (metal root canals, fillings or crowns), industrial pollution (living near toxic waste that you are not aware of), large high-tension power lines, fluoridated or chemically treated water, western drugs, pesticides, and food additives.

The result of autism is dysfunction related to the brain and nervous system. Along with other mental disabilities, the soul or spirit of the child cannot become fully present on Earth because the spirit communicates and participates on Earth through the body (which includes the brain). If the brain of the child is damaged it is not that his soul or spirit is not present, but only the vehicle for his soul or spirit is not properly functioning.

The article, *Deadly Immunity* by Robert F. Kennedy Jr. helps show the connection between autism and vaccinations. It can be read at **www.robertfkennedyjr.com/articles/2005_june_16.html**

Kennedy points to a dramatic rise in autism corresponding to a commensurate rise in the number of required childhood vaccines. Dr. Andrew Wakefield, also an opponent of vaccination, found components of the MMR vaccine in the guts of autistic children. Governments and scientists vehemently deny Dr. Wakefield's discovery but I will tell you, he is absolutely correct; don't listen to any other false information that tells you that "we don't know the cause of autism." The cause is known, and knowable.

Autistic children basically suffer from heavy metal poisoning. There are many programs to help with heavy metal detoxification. These include raw foods, raw eggs, raw vegetable juices as well as special supplements and chelating substances designed for autistic children. It can be tough to get those heavy metals out of the body. When the heavy metals are removed from the gut and the body can regain its balance, many of the symptoms of autism decrease or go away completely. I have met a mother who cured her child of autism using a program similar to Max Gerson's cancer-curing protocol.

Another documented autism cure uses a specific carbohydrate diet: *Gut and Psychology Syndrome* by Dr. Natasha Campbell-McBride essentially traces the illnesses to a diseased gut which, of course, is triggered by vaccines. A raw foods diet that includes animal foods is described in *Recipe for Living without Disease* by Aajonus Vonderplanitz. Mr. Vonderplanitz cured his own autism.

It should be of no surprise to you now that vaccinations are accountable for many childhood diseases. This is because **vaccines cause disease**. Children's bodily defensive functions are not fully developed. This includes having only partially developed protection against toxins entering the blood-brain barrier, which helps protect the brain from absorbing toxins in the bloodstream. The brain and the spinal column have their own circulation system and their own type of fluid, called cerebrospinal fluid. Our brain actually has several somewhat small cavities, located near the center of our head between our ears, in which this fluid circulates. This inner circulatory system is highly sensitive, and it does not have a central purifying organ as our bloodstream does. It is reasonable to assume that when a child's body is not strong enough to protect itself from the poison in vaccines or other highly toxic substances like western drugs, the blood-brain barrier would be compromised. The toxins from the vaccine or drugs would then enter into the brain and the spinal column via the cerebrospinal fluid. Because these toxins would be lodged so deeply in the body, they would be difficult to remove. Also, high-pitched screaming, and other unusual emotional behavior caused by vaccinations, is a sign that the brain is being affected in some way.

A confidential study by the Centers of Disease Control (or the Centers for Disease Causation, as I like to call them) showed that exposure to mercury in vaccines significantly increases the likelihood of the child developing autism, stuttering and ADD.[629] The pharmaceutical companies can easily see this from animal and human tests they've done — so they purposely put the poisons in the vaccines. Even our government's own EPA has certain standards for safe levels of heavy metal exposures, and vaccines far exceed them, making them both illegal and highly toxic (that is if environmental laws have any meaning). The primary causes of autism will be vaccines, preconception and pregnancy exposure to heavy metals and antibiotics, heavy metal pollution in the air and water, and chemicals from the electronics industry.[630]

Supposedly, no one born within the Amish community has developed autism. The explanation posed for this is that they do not vaccinate their children.[631]

I have also seen references that linked autism to both pasteurized milk and white sugar. One boy had a recovery from autism after being placed on a grain-free diet with lots of raw goat milk, raw butter, raw cream and kefir. He was also given chlorella, a single-celled alga.[632]

www.autismwebsite.com - Autism is Treatable
www.healing-arts.org/children/ - Alternative Therapy for Children with Brain Injury
autism.org – center for study of autism

In *Impossible Cure: The Promise of Homeopathy* author Amy L. Lansky describes how she healed her son's autism with homeopathy. I have also heard, during a lecture on homeopathy, of a case where homeopathy was used to cure mental retardation.

The success of the cure depends on how much you understand the current condition that causes autism.

If your child has a learning disability, I want to say this: Have faith. I walked down the dark road of hopelessness, fighting through the veils of darkness, not knowing how to make the impossible (healing teeth) possible. But I found a solution. So too, I wish for you to find a solution to any health crises your child might face. Other mothers have done it, and I feel an assured sense that it is possible.

Promote the Prevention of Colic

Colic is a generic term to describe a baby who is fussy, and the fussiness seems to be related to meal times and digestion. Many times it can be indigestion or gas. An additional indication would be frequent clumpy, watery, and what appears to be partially undigested bowel movements rather than the healthier smooth, creamy and less frequent bowel movements. If you are breastfeeding your child, the odds that he will be fussy are lower. I discovered recently, and I am very sure of this, that my daughter's fussiness was caused by a lack of nutrients and fat. I saw a video documentary about the Masai people, whose diet consists mostly of animal foods. They drink significant amounts of raw cow's milk, eat beef, goat and mutton, the animal organs and drink steer blood. Their babies are plump and mellow; these calm little people are not fussy at all. The Masai diet is very high in fat. In the documentary, the babies sat, hardly moving, they were so filled with contentment and rolls of baby fat.

I finally realized that although this contentment does come from parenting methods, more important, it has to do with the fat and nutrient content of the mother's breast milk. Colic is primarily caused by infant formulas and the other toxic foods that are fed to children. Along with a lack of nutrients and fat, colic can also be caused by a bacterial imbalance in the mother's milk or baby's gut.

To our surprise, when Yeshe was a few days old, she started having more and more difficulty falling asleep in the afternoon. First we had to sing to her. Then we had to take her on walks. Eventually, she was very uncomfortable every day and would sometimes cry for longer than a few minutes. She also began not sleeping well at night, although initially she slept well. We tried a variety of solutions: herbs, homeopathy, breastfeeding longer on one side, diet adjustments. We finally found the cause, and the cure.

Infant probiotics. We used the brand Natren; other brands may also be good, so take the time to investigate your options. They must specifically say they are for infants on the label. Apparently, even after following a good health program for many years, Michelle's bacterial balances in her body were still off. So Yeshe's gut never got seeded with the healthy ecosystem necessary to easily digest breastmilk. As a re-

sult, breastmilk would cause her indigestion, and she wouldn't be able to sleep, or nurse. She became very fidgety and flailed her arms and looked uncomfortable. Within less than one day of using the probiotic, Yeshe improved significantly. In a little more than a week, she returned to being a solid sleeper. No more fussiness, and a lot more smiles. What more can a parent ask for? She usually falls asleep very easily, sleeps through the night, and never has the late evening colic. We have continued to give her probiotics for several months. At this point she got better, and we discontinued probiotic use, and now are trying some probiotics for older children in small amounts.

"Calming Cry of Colic" at **www.westonaprice.org** contains more guidance on calming colic naturally. Colic is caused when the foods eaten become toxic to the baby, as they are unable to digest it properly. Enhancing the quality of the baby food, or giving a baby probiotic, will help solve the problem. When their bodies are out of balance, breastmilk is more difficult for some babies to digest.

Promote the Prevention of Tooth Decay

Tooth decay is caused by a deficiency of nutrients needed to build healthy teeth. Sugar, which is a highly processed food, encourages calcium to be pulled from the bones, and therefore does not cause tooth decay by its direct contact with teeth.[633] Rather, sugar causes an increased amount of nutrient deficiency which the body then tries to correct through pulling nutrient reserves out of the teeth. We saw examples of this borrowing process in Chapter 3, where nutrients were being pulled from the bones of children, as well as from a monkey, in order to save the more vital organs.

Tooth decay begins as a deficiency in the mother and father before the child is conceived. *The child's first teeth are formed in the womb of the mother.* Tooth decay really begins as a deficiency many generations back, with each successive generation becoming weaker and weaker through an improper diet.[634]

By practicing preconception health, the mother's body will be full of the nutrients needed for the child to build strong teeth and bones. This child's organs will be robust and be able to assimilate nutrients well. This preventive measure, with the addition of breast feeding, should make your child immune to tooth decay, provided you are following most of the dietary guidelines outlined here. Remember, the key is fat-soluble vitamins.

As a review, breastfeeding is the key means to deliver nutrients to your child. Breastmilk also has beneficial bacteria and decreases the levels of harmful bacteria. Do not listen to anybody who tells you breastfeeding is wrong or bad, or that it causes tooth decay. Dr. Brian Palmer has extensively studied this question and shows strong evidence to support the fact that tooth decay is not caused by breastfeeding, **www.brianpalmerdds.com**

Even if your child's teeth do decay, you can still fortify their nutrition enough to where the dentin—the middle tooth layer—will cover itself over and protect the pulp chamber of the tooth. In this way, we can avoid unnecessary medical procedures which could be scary and traumatizing to young children. Even after the enamel disappears, the well-nourished body heals the tooth with a black scab. This healing process may not occur unless your diet and your child's diet are superb. Otherwise, an infection could result, which is the body's attempt to expel toxins that it could not remove through usual channels. But if a child is well nourished, I imagine letting the tooth just decay is a better alternative to a root canal. Even with a root canal, the gums and tooth area still have to heal. Why do we think nature, with the right building blocks, cannot do it herself?

Tooth decay is not only unnecessary, but an indication of our divergence from Nature's fundamental laws of life and health.[635]

In a group of children whose mothers had the special nutritional reinforcement during gestation and lactation and who had been provided with the same dietary adjuncts during the winter and spring months of infancy and early childhood, not a single carious cavity has developed. A number of these children are now in public schools. Their physical development is distinctly above that of the average children of their age, as is also their efficiency in school work.[636]

My first book, *Cure Tooth Decay,* is devoted to this subject. Many of the guidelines in *Cure Tooth Decay* arose out of this book. As a side note, some children's bodies can be poisoned from any kind of steel or metal dental work; if your child is sick, this may be the cause.

Promote the Prevention of Post-Partum Depression

Post-partum depression is a mild to severe depression that mothers sometimes experience after birth. Post-partum depression is caused either by a birth trauma, such as an unexpected emergency medical procedure, from a deficiency of nutrients, or from a reaction to western drugs taken during the birth.

First, depression can be caused by imbalanced feelings. If the birth was somehow traumatic for the mother (which is determined by how the mother feels, not by the outer world circumstances) and the shame or pain is stuck in her, then she might have depressed energy. Because of the traumatic experience, a mother is now in the fight, flight, or freeze response, and her body is in shock. In this case, her feelings need to be unfrozen, and a skilled trauma therapist can do this. Feeling disassociated from life, lost or alone is a sign that you are experiencing a trauma. See Appendix A for suggestions for emotional healing therapists who could be good at releasing such trauma.

The key cause of post-partum depression, I believe, is the large amounts of hormones that are released both immediately prior to and during the birth, which can result in a deficient condition. Usually, vitamin stores in the body, along with other powerful hormones, are tapped for energy needed to push the baby out. A feeling of euphoria comes after the release of tension of birth, and joy, love and bonding with your newborn follows. This requires the glands, especially the pituitary gland in the brain, to release hormones. The release of these love hormones does not always happen; in fact the converse, an entire lack of hormonal release, may occur with resulting depression. A diet high in processed sugar will increase the tendency for depression.

Orthomolecular medicine, which uses vitamins and minerals to help heal mental disorders, suggests that depression is caused by a deficiency of vitamin C. Many sources suggest omega-3 oils from fish also help prevent depression.[637] These oils are best utilized from simply eating fish, rather than taking them in capsule form.

After the birth, the body has much repair and reorganizing to do. Without vital nutrients, a woman's body cannot come back into shape well. If you have ever been starving, you know that this can lead to irrational moods, anger, and then finally depression, as the body runs out of blood sugar and begins to shut itself down. The cure, in this case, is following the preconception health guidelines in Chapter 7, and the diet for pregnancy and lactation in Chapter 6.

Depleted glands cannot secrete the hormones necessary for life. They cannot secrete the hormones of being full of pleasure and joy — the after birth glow — so the mother will experience depression. Of course, this depression may in some cases be mostly or purely psychological. But even if this is the case, the mother likely indulges in the wrong types of food to medicate herself from the psychological condition, which of course adds to the problem.

One secret for restoring glandular health is zucchini and string beans. This was given as a recipe (Bieler's broth) in Chapter 7. You can also juice zucchini and string beans (though zucchini makes better juice) with other vegetables, and this will also help restore glandular health.

Promote the Prevention of Miscarriage and Other Illnesses of Pregnancy

Infections, abruption of the placenta, anemia, toxemia of pregnancy and miscarriage are all pregnancy conditions connected to diet.

Miscarriages do not happen by chance, but are the body's response to a set of conditions, many of which are knowable. The presence of toxins, along with vitamin deficiencies, disable the body's ability to produce a healthy template to grow a child, and a miscarriage is a result. Dr. Bieler said, "[M]iscarriages, are so frequently brought about by assaulting the system with toxic foods."[638]

By eating whole and unrefined food prior to pregnancy, by building up your nutrient stores, and by cleansing the body well before pregnancy, you will create a healthy ecosystem and thus significantly reduce the likelihood of birth complications. The Foresight preconception average for miscarriage is 1 in 32 pregnancies, while the national average in England is 1 in 5 pregnancies.[639]

Promote the Prevention of Premature Birth

Malnutrition and substance abuse are some of the known causes of premature birth. Premature birth, like other conditions, is primarily caused by the physical environment of the mother's body, which was contributed to by the father.

While we call a birth before nine months premature, the birth was prompted because the biological intelligence of the mother's body decided it was time to happen. That means that there were likely too many toxins, toxic emotions, or not enough nutrients to continue the pregnancy in a healthy way. Exercising prior to and during pregnancy to improve the well being of the mother, in addition to the preconception cleansing and nutrient building described in Chapter 7, along with the diet for pregnancy in Chapter 6, should reduce the incidence of premature births. The Foresight program average for premature births is 1 in 41 pregnancies, compared to England's national average of 1 in 13 pregnancies.[640] Again, this shows that with the right changes in the parents' environmental habits, a reduction in premature births is inevitable.

Promote the Prevention of Scoliosis

In order to grow during the early years of childhood, from the ages of 2-6, the body needs a tremendous supply of highly potent fat-soluble vitamins and minerals. If these nutrients are not given throughout this period of growth, and they were not eaten by the mother while the child was in the womb, then it is very likely that by the time this child hits his teenage years, with the attendant developing hormones and growth spurts, his body will lack the nutrients it needs to grow. In addition, modern foods, especially foods that have sugar added, will contribute to deficiencies. As a result, some children with this deficiency will develop a curved spine. In Chapter 3 we saw how bones weaken and become soft and flimsy when nutrients were pulled from them to support vital organs. The x-ray of the monkey showed this process clearly with its soft and bent bone structure. Just like the unfortunate monkey, a child or adolescent with scoliosis is suffering from soft and weak bones caused by a nutrient deficiency, which may be aggravated by a malabsorption problem. It is possible that a curvature of the spine can also be aggravated by emotional problems. If the child has a healthy diet, the curvature caused by emotional patterns will be less severe and even unnoticeable. Just as plants cannot grow up straight and tall in deficient soil, so too children cannot grow without a full supply of body-building nutrients. My friend's daughter has scoliosis. She feeds her daughter a nutrient-poor diet, with too much processed sweets and fruit juice. As a result, her daughter's spine became misshapen during the rapid growth of her teenage years. Surely a deficiency of calcium and phosphorus has an important role in creating scoliosis. Scoliosis is not a genetic defect, but a condition of *intercepted*

heredity, where this child's full genetic potential of a straight spine is not realized. As with other diseases, we see the primary cause here is a deficiency condition.

Promote the Creation of a Child who is Super-intelligent

A significant portion of our intelligence is biological. In other words, Nature's map for our brain and level of intelligence was for a very high and evolved type of intelligence. However, when this plan is *intercepted*, many of us do not become as smart as we could be. The brain acts as an automatic mechanism, like a microchip, firing through its complex pathways, automatically sorting and filtering data streaming in from the environment. Its clarity and efficiency depend, not on its genetic make up, but on the inheritance of power gained by eating the right types of nutrient-rich whole foods. While the efficiency of the brain function is biological, how this intelligence is applied has to do with the circumstances and spirit of your child. Your child will be super smart when she is given enough nutrient-rich foods to provide her brain with a vibrant energy supply, her nerves will function well, and all the parts of her brain will be fully developed at each stage of maturation.

For example, when Michelle first added a very high quality, nutrient-rich cheese to her diet, Sparkle, through drinking her now more nutrient rich breastmilk, became noticeably more intelligent in just one or two days following this dietary change. That is because good food, particularly high fat food and high mineral food, feeds the brain.

Weston Price was able to improve both the intelligence and the behavioral mood of school children using a diet based on the indigenous principles he learned.

I asked the officials connected with the Board of Education having charge of the dental phase to select for me about twenty-four children suffering severely from dental caries and who where backward in their school work... The treatment given consisted in providing them with additional fat-soluble vitamins obtained from very high vitamin butter, mixed with equal parts of a high vitamin cod-liver oil, together with the addition to their dietary of sufficient milk to make a total of a quart a day...A number of the teachers reported voluntarily to the school nurse that there was a marked improvement in the learning ability of the boys and girls. The caries shown in the x-ray pictures have apparently ceased.[641] (Emphasis added.)

The converse is also true when it comes to intelligence. The more nutrient-void foods you give your child, the more vaccinations, the more fluoride poisons and other heavy metals, the less your child's brain will function properly. In addition, his glands will not function properly, and his brain and nervous system will not have a constant and even supply of energy. Our modern medical paradigm of drugs, vaccines, low fat and deficient diet, along with the absence of brain-building foods like fish and raw milk, is a recipe for sub-intelligent children.

It is ironic that in schools, where parents send their children to become "smart," the school programs feed the children terrible food, which will make their minds dull. Many schools inadvertently allow corporations to addict children to junk food by offering low quality food in their cafeterias. Children in many schools also have free access to soda machines, candy bars and other vending machine horrors. Schools themselves are often toxic, too. School buildings many times have toxic materials insulating ventilation ducts or are made with toxic building materials. The indoor lighting systems often use fluorescent lights, which cause neurological problems and upset body chemistry after prolonged exposure. Children need sunlight to be healthy, not synthetically made light. We also force children to thwart their own biological design by making them sit inside, confined to desks, which was discussed thoroughly in Chapter 12. Conclusion: one of the purposes of

school is to make children sick and unintelligent.

Children who are emotionally well cared for will have a natural curiosity about life. When they are not abandoned, and are nurtured fully with breastmilk and holding, then their internal body circuitry will work well, and they will always seek ways to expand their ability to influence the world; this is learning. Parents who physically hold their children and express compassion for them will help their children develop a strong emotional intelligence.

Promote the Creation of a Child who is Strong, Attractive, and who has Straight Teeth

In Chapters 2, 3 and 4 I provided examples of how a distorted facial form results from improper bone growth, due to our modernized diet. The modernized diet creates unattractive facial features such as a narrow face.

With proper nutrition, your child will develop a wide dental arch, which means a wide and fully formed face. People with wider faces in general are seen as more beautiful. With ideal foods, your child's teeth will come in completely straight with plenty of room, including the wisdom teeth.

With healthy bone growth from healthy nutrition comes a feeling of confidence, self assuredness, and a willingness to explore and experience life. A well-formed face will be proportional and conform to the golden ratio, and therefore your child will look significantly more attractive. His features will be well developed in a way that many cultures consider beautiful.

Like the children of the Loetschental Valley frolicking barefoot at dusk in glacial waters, a child fed a wholesome diet will feel strong, and full of life. Sparkle has a very high tolerance for cold, and enjoys playing in very cold water that I cannot tolerate at all. At night her body stays warm with a fraction of the blankets that Michelle or I use.

Promote the Creation of a Child who is Highly Immune to Disease

By following a preconception program before your child's birth, and later avoiding vaccinations and a deficient diet by building up her body with your healthy breastmilk, your child will be highly resilient to disease. We understand now that most diseases only become severe when the internal chemistry of the child's body is unhealthy. I proposed that disease is caused when our bodies try to get rid of decaying matter and other toxins. If there is no decaying matter, and no toxins, and the body is strong from rich, unprocessed food, then there will be little if any disease.

With the proper nutrients, given in alignment with Nature through lifestyle and emotional habits, your child will rarely become ill, because immunity to illness comes from good nutrition and avoidance of toxins. This was further demonstrated in a recreated chart from Dr. Price in the vaccine chapter, in which immunity to diseases was high in relation to the vitamin content of grassfed butter. Dr. Price explains:

*A teaspoonful [of ½ butter oil, and ½ high vitamin cod liver oil] a day divided between two or three meals is usually adequate to prevent dental caries and maintain a high immunity; **it will also maintain freedom from colds and a high level of health in general.** This reinforcement of the fat-soluble vitamins to a menu that is low in starches and sugars, together with the use of bread and cereal grains freshly ground to retain the full content of the embryo or germ, and with milk for growing children and for many adults, and the liberal use of sea foods and organs of animals, produced the result described.[642] (Emphasis added. Note: Dosage suggested may not be suitable for very young children; also note that the cod liver oil and butter oil are taken more than once per day.)*

Diseases rarely come from the world around us. That is, we are not attacked by a contagious organism that we have little control over. Diseases that do come from the environment are usually or always from poisoning, not from a virus or bacteria. The poison is from toxic and putrefying substances that our bodies cannot handle well. Diseases largely are a result of modernization, and thus, if you do not participate in the practices of modernization, disease will be rare. For example, Sparkle once had a fever that was around 100-101 degrees; it was very mild, and that was the worst she has been ever been sick. Living close to a tourist attraction for several years, she was exposed to germs from all over, and again was rarely sick, even without preconception planning. Sparkle touched germ-ridden places, rode on rides and walked barefoot where I would never even walk barefoot, and she never got sick from "germ" exposure. Yeshe, now five months old, has never been sick. I recently read of a very natural mom who tried to give her children chicken pox from other sick children. No matter how hard she tried to expose her very healthy children to sick children, they never "contracted" the chicken pox.

Promote the Creation of a Child who has vision equal to or greater than 20/20

Most of the poor eyesight of today can be prevented by eating foods that give the body what it needs during the growing years.[643]

Delighted were archaeologists to discover a prehistoric cave wall painting of the Pleiades star group, 'Seven Sisters' But surprised were they that the ancient artist painted ten stars, four of which we need telescopes to see. Natural guess: stars were brighter then. Astronomers said 'No.' ... the artist had seen all ten stars with his naked eye. Correct assumption: cave men had better eyesight than modern men.[644]

Problems with eyes are not hereditary in the traditional sense, but like the other conditions mentioned in this book, are a result of *intercepted* heredity in which Nature's map of perfect eyesight cannot be completed due to inhibiting life conditions (such as toxins and a deficient diet).

It is highly likely that young children who need glasses are suffering from a vitamin deficiency and a glandular deficiency (particularly a deficiency of the kidneys and the adrenal glands). A natural form of vitamin A, which is necessary for the health of the eye, can be obtained from animal fats. Proper development of facial bones and features will mean that the eye sockets form correctly, and as a result, the eyes themselves will be the correct shape for optimal vision.[645] I believe that if the program I have outlined is followed carefully from the time of preconception, most children will rarely if ever have poor vision. Children sometimes develop eyesight problems because they have "seen" violence or some form of severe cruelty which makes them want to not see. But generally, it is possible not only for poor vision to be prevented, but in some cases to have vision better than 20/20, as illustrated by the example of the caveman. While in our modern culture the phenomenon of vision that is better than 20/20 is rare, when people begin to return to a more natural diet, we will regain our acute eye sight once again. As a side note, an acquaintance who is an eyesight expert would want you all to know that eye glasses for children do not help and are likely detrimental. There are several books written by eye doctors and experts advising against glasses for children. If your child has poor vision, I suggest looking into the facts before giving him glasses.

Promote the Creation of a Child who is Calm, Peaceful, and Compassionate

The more we give to Sparkle, the better she feels about herself. This is the amoeba principle in action. When you give children real, present, and nurturing love and attention, they feel that they are powerful and important to the world. You become a channel for Nature's divine light. Hold your children, and do not abandon them; breastfeed them, and feed them well and nurture them. When you do this, Nature's program for an agreeable child takes root. In other words, your children will want to help you, want to behave, and want to participate in life. When we don't give to them fully we thwart their potential to grow, and as a result they end up not behaving well. Children learn by example, so how you are is how they will be.

When I say calm, I mean that your child will be inwardly calm. At a young age, they will be peaceful and pleasant. Now, when you do all these things for your child, you might also find that your child will at times be on turbo charge. They will have so much strength, energy, and vitality that they will be going wild all the time, running around, and playing and embracing life to the fullest. An energized child full of life is natural and means you are doing a good job. It is not hyperactivity, but a more balanced sense of movement and excitement in life. And this also means, in general, less napping. Since the age of two, Sparkle has not napped. Yeshe is already significantly reducing her napping at just 5 months of age.

A bonus observed in the Foresight program, which includes preconception health, is that the children are bright, calm and happy.[646]

You will experience a flowering of enjoyment in following Nature's laws, as a higher degree of moral character will develop in your child. And in avoiding the toxic foods, their bodies won't be filled with gunk. Many times, a person's spirit must travel through the physical medium (the body) to express itself in life. So if the body is full of high vibration from life-giving foods and nutrients, so will their spirits be.

Integrating the Principles of Promoting Disease Prevention for Our Children

Disease in your children is a result of your divergence from life. I have never yet met someone who, after having written to me concerning a problem with their child, could not eventually identify the cause of the illness. In other words, illness and disease are not mysteries when you understand their true causes. The causes includes toxins which the body is exposed to through foods (even sometimes foods we think are healthy), drink, drugs, household cleaners, pesticides, vitamins and supplements and so forth. The cause is deficiencies from a modern diet that makes even children's bodies susceptible to decay due to nutrient-devoid foods. And the cause is our toxic emotions, in which we rush around, lose track of the present moment, and create chaos and suffering in our lives. The result is our tiny precious infants are neglected, and they feel pain and suffering. Sometimes disease happens to our children and it at least appears to be out of our control. However, in knowing the true causes of disease we can remove our fear of illness in our children, since we do not have to wonder why they are sick or if we can stop it.

Let's begin with the principles taught by some wise health practitioners.

First, disease is not caused by viruses, and it is not caused by bacteria. Viruses have never been found to exist outside of simple life forms. What we attribute to being caused by a virus is really caused by a toxin, such as a heavy metal or a chemical, for example. Disease in most cases does not just strike a helpless victim like a lightning bolt; it has knowable causes which can be indentified with careful scrutiny.

The great herbalist, Dr. Christopher:

One who has childhood disease could be without them, and have no fear of sickness if he had, in the beginning, a good strong body. Disease germs are scavengers and can live only on weak 'wasting-away' cells, mucus, and toxic conditions. Never

can germs exist in a healthy and clean cell structure.[647]

Dr. J.H. Tilden, author of *Toxemia Explained*:

So-called disease is nature's effort at eliminating the toxin from the blood. All so-called diseases are crises of Toxemia.[648]

Hippocrates the Father of Western Medicine:

Disease was the result of some mismanagement of the environment.[649]

Rudolf Virchow, 17th century physician:

The health of the body cells depended on their chemical make-up, and this chemical make-up in turn, depended on the kind of food eaten by the individual.[650]

Maverick physician Henry Bieler:

*I came to the conclusion that **germs do not initiate a diseased state of the body,** but appear later after the person becomes ill.[651] (Emphasis added).*

***The true cure comes from within**. Nature effects it; the physician is only a collaborator with nature, guiding his patient through the sometimes mystifying steps necessary to the handling of his specific problem.[652] (Emphasis added).*

Nobel Prize-winning Dr. Albert V. Szent-Gyorgyi:

Should then, man be the only imperfect creature kept alive in the face of all his imperfections only by means created by his own mind? If not, where do all these ailments come from?[653]

In other words, if the cell is perfect, and nature represents a form of order and perfection, then it must not be Nature (i.e., germs, viruses, etc.) that is to blame, but something of our own, human doing.

I described the thing that causes nearly every disease in pregnancy and in our children as *the plague*, which is the way we now live on Earth. It represents a difficult, separated and painful existence. In feeling this pain, we then make it real, and create it semi-consciously and subconsciously in this world. Western medicine labels the symptoms of this pain as a disease, and helps us avoid knowing its real cause, which is the way we live, and who we have become.

The Body Has Lines of Defense:

The body uses the liver, kidneys and skin to protect itself from disease. The liver cleans the blood. If the liver is healthy it is **impossible** for disease to develop.[654]

Usually a breakdown (disease) occurs after prolonged and heavy use of processed sugars and flours. After a longer breakdown, the adrenal glands might try to eliminate toxins through the lungs, which could result in bronchitis or pneumonia. The thyroid controls the skin; if the skin is trying to release toxins, then skin diseases arise.[655]

When you correct problems with a health-giving diet, the body can get sick as part of the cleansing process. So rather than a new illness being created, old junk stuck in the body is pushed out, which temporarily looks like the cold, flu or even food poisoning, but it's not really those things. Sparkle used to have some type of minor allergies, and have some nasal congestion. After a few detoxifying sicknesses brought about through consuming raw eggs, her congestion went away, and her allergies disappeared! But on her very sick / detoxifying days (just two or three days in total), she did vomit several times and felt weak and tired.

From Sickness to Health

Illness is also an opportunity. Whenever Sparkle was sick, I thought about and experienced many feelings towards her. I considered deeply how I spend my time with her, and our relationship. Illness seems to pull my awareness towards certain personal issues that I need to look at. Even though I felt concerned and even worried as a parent when my daughter was sick, I also embraced the fact that her illness helped me be a better father for her. I became more present and available to her, because illness stripped away my ego, my negative self identity, and brought me closer to the core of my being, where there is truth and love. You too can use illness as an opportunity to awaken to a deeper reality, to change unhealthy lifestyle patterns, and to find out how you have been misaligned with creating peace and harmony for yourself and your children. For many parents, severe illness in their children becomes a gateway for their awakening. Even what seems to be a terrifying moment, when faced as it is, can somehow bring us an experience of a deeper faith, and a more whole reality.

When there is an illness that I am concerned about, I use the following three books as references. Usually, after reading them all for the particular illness, worries go away. While these books do cost money and take time and effort to read, this kind of reading is important. I find that many parents don't even take the effort to read one good natural health book. Keep in mind not all of these books agree completely on treatment programs, so use your best judgment and the nutritional wisdom provided here to help you select the best remedies from each.

Food is Your Best Medicine, Chapter 9 by *Henry Bieler* (for naturally treating Measles, Tonsillitis, Polio, Rheumatism, Chicken Pox)

Herbal Home Health Care by Dr. John Christopher (for naturally treating many other conditions using herbs)

We Want To Live by Aajonus Vonderplanitz, (the second half of the book discusses living healthfully and addresses many treatments for a variety of illnesses)

No parent should have to face the helplessness of having a sick child alone. But I have talked to many parents who do struggle with their child's illness alone because most health practitioners, even alternative ones, are totally inept. At best, you bring your child to the doctor and they do nothing. At worst, the doctor prescribes medications or treatments and then gives your child new diseases and health problems because most western medications are highly toxic. Some parents are fortunate, and they find an excellent health care provider who seems to know everything and have treatments that work. These types of health care practitioners are in the vast minority. But many of them can be found through the Price-Pottenger Nutrition Foundation practitioner list, www.ppnf.org and the International Foundation for Nutrition and Health, www.ifnh.org. They will soon have a practitioner list on their website, otherwise call or e-mail them. Also see appendix A for alternative treatment modalities.

In the Coming Generation Learn How We Can Eliminate Birth Complications & Childhood Disease

Are we the sole arbiters of our fate? Yes.

Are we doomed to a life of suffering? No.

We will likely face pain in our life. This is inevitable, and is just part of being human. Suffering is how we respond to a painful condition. While pain will happen, suffering may or may not happen, as it is our response to the pain. We can choose to embrace our suffering as a gateway towards a higher truth inside of us. We can embrace the ideas behind, "not my will, but Thy will," or we can ignore the pain, and continue to struggle along in our mediocre lives.

Nature designed humans as its highest achievement. We are Nature's greatest masterpiece on this planet. We are the caretakers of this Earth. With our intelligence and our hearts, we can dream a new Earth. Using Nature's technology, as described in this book, we can in the coming generation eliminate both birth complications and some or all of childhood diseases.

Yes, there could be some rare exceptions to this. But the vast majority of cases are preventable. When mothers practice preconception health care and their bodies are in a high degree of health, then their children will be vitally healthy. When these children grow up and become mothers and fathers, they will be able to give birth free of complications, like the indigenous peoples described by Dr. Price. Their children will be free of disease, or disease will be extremely rare or only caused by emotional conditions, rather than physical conditions.

We do not need more vaccinations that do not and cannot work. We do not need more modern marvels of technology. We ONLY need to come back into ourselves and back home to the longing within us, to be whole again. If you align with harmony with Nature, through right ways in living, you can free yourself from certain forms of suffering. When you begin to look within for answers rather than looking towards our wrong and limited conclusions about life, you can change. If many of us work together, physically or etherically, then we will create a foundation for a new Earth. An Earth filled with peace. An Earth free of disease and mostly free of physical suffering. This is not an event in the future, but it is something that is creating itself through us, as we dare to dream, now.

The Poor, Sick, and the Needy

In the Western world and in many other parts of the world, the suffering that is ongoing right now is tremendously painful. Many mothers across the globe cannot take care of their children, cannot give breastmilk to their children, not because of the so-called disease of AIDS, but because they are suffering from malnourishment. In the West, the poor and the underclass citizens suffer malnourishment of an improper diet. Government food subsidies almost exclusively provide the lowest quality food available, and most or all of the food is on the "Avoid" list of modernization (described in Chapter 6). In other words, government provides food that will make people sick. A poor single mother on the welfare system can get full health insurance for all her problems, which probably comes at a high cost to the state government. And yet nobody teaches her how to avoid health problems with proper foods, which in the long term would be a more cost effective approach since it would prevent the almost inevitable mass of health problems in her and her children.

Many of us entertain the misconception that if we take care of ourselves, somebody else in the world will suffer more because we selfishly took what they were supposed to receive. This concept is based on a belief of lack and deprivation. It says, "If I have my fullness, I must be taking it away from someone else." While there may be examples of this in the world today, where the ruling class takes away from the "peasant" population, this is not the ultimate reality. This is a human-created reality based on our false belief systems and misuse of our natural resources.

There is a way we can live in abundance in our country and honor the underlying truths upon which our constitutional government was formed: "We the people of the United States… promote the general welfare, and secure the blessings of liberty to ourselves and our posterity…" It begins with you. When you take care of yourself and your family, you resonate to the planet a feeling of joy, peace, hope, and fullness. When you give to yourself fully, and to your children fully, you honor the needs of their bodies. These needs are not just yours or your children's in a global sense; you were born with them, and so they were bestowed to you by a greater power.

The first step towards change is almost always an inward or personal step. On the outer world, there is much we can do to ensure proper nutrition. We can return to enforcing the Pure Food and Drug Law of 1906, so that poor people are not stuck with eating inferior food that is improperly processed, filled with chemicals, and lacking nutrients. We can stop wasting some of our most precious nutrient rich food resources. Thousands if not millions of pounds of foods are thrown away today, specifically the prized organ meats of land and sea animals. Even worse, many of the best organs from grassfed animals are **literally** fed to dogs and made into dog food. Other revered foods, like the tripe that our ancestors paid tribute to, are illegal to purchase unless they have been bathed in highly toxic chemicals. If not made into dog food, our best foods are regularly dumped into the sea or into landfills. The organs can be eaten, the meat around the head salvaged, and the bones made into a nutrient-rich, life-supporting broth. This includes also the fish eggs, that in many types of fish are just thrown away. This includes the bones and the marrow of grassfed animals, which are underused and can also be made into nutrient-rich broths. This includes green tripe and other organ meats, whose sale to the public our laws virtually forbid. These millions of pounds of foods are rich in vital substances that could heal people and promote the **general welfare**.

Our own constitution declares that the intention of our government is to promote the general welfare. Rather than do this, our government promotes disease and death. It is time for a revolution. And we don't need to overthrow the government; we only need to topple the regime within us. We only need to topple the inner illusion of authority that allows for and creates the false outer authority. We only need to stop standing by as our health, rights, and livelihood are taken away. We only need to say "no" more often. The violence, abuse, stealing from the poor, the destruction of the land perpetrated by government and corporations…we only need to say we don't want it any more, and start living in a new way. We have to disconnect ourselves from the panopticon, the matrix that is telling us how to be, and we need to focus our hearts and minds to a higher more divine authority.

Why not take these "food wastes" and feed them to homeless people instead of to dogs? Why not give the poor and underclass the rich foods that will give them health and life instead of dumping them in the ocean?

When we start living wisely we can see how easy and simple it is, if it is our collective wish, to help people live fulfilling and nourished lives. There is freedom and abundance for all when we are willing to look through the clouds of darkness and see the rainbow of hope that is so tangible, yet so hard to grasp when we don't want it.

And they Ate the Fruit from the Tree of Knowledge of Good and Evil

Your child was not born to live a life filled with suffering. And yet a key cultural image and belief in our modern culture is that we have eaten from the tree of knowledge of good and evil. This means that we believe that we are doomed to a dualistic existence (in suffering, in sin) personified by the existence of good and evil. In this distorted perspective, our bodies are considered sinful, and there is an undercurrent of a belief that says that who we are, our feelings, our flesh, our sexuality, our blood and bones, are wrong and bad, simply because we are human. Thus our children, in their blood, flesh and bones, and with their needs and cries for love and nurturance, are also deemed bad or sinful. We then "punish" them with our modern way and delude ourselves into thinking that this punishment, which is our separated way of living, is good, or right. We now continue to make the choice: do we act from our "good" part, or do we act from our "evil" part. If we really have the knowledge of good and of evil, then we can use the knowledge of good to put ourselves back onto the right path. The suffering in this dualistic world is not a divine order but a misperception of the divine world we live in and thus a self-inflicted wound. Consider these inspiring words about divine grace from the Pathwork:

> *"Every substance of life, on all levels -- from the finest vibrations and radiations to the crudest matter -- is permeated with it. The very world you live in, the universe, all of creation, the way divine law is constructed, all are an expression of divine grace. You live and move and have your being in a universe that consists of such tenderness, such love, such personal care of the living God, of the eternal presence in all that is, that it simply defies description. You are surrounded by a universe in which there is simply nothing ever to fear -- no matter what the momentary appearances may be."*[656]

The Creator of this universe and this world did not intend for you to suffer or to experience pain. The kind Father, and the kind Mother, wish for you to be reborn into a new reality. A reality filled with life, joy and health. Yet we have to take that small step towards wanting, feeling, and realizing a new reality in each moment, and every day.

We are living in the Garden of Eden, **it is right here.** We don't need to wait to experience this peace, or joy, or tranquility, as it exists as an inner potential. Already, it is occasionally glimpsed in some peak moments of life when we feel that all is well. And at the same time, I can understand why you would not feel peace, joy or tranquility. We live now at the end of a long chain of events that has led to internal imbalances. So we are on Earth to learn how to realign our bodies, minds and spirits with a higher power, as it once was, and it takes time, and it takes intentionality, and it takes work and effort. The outcome of the hard work makes the effort and focus worthwhile. Each and every positive step you make towards self-understanding, every time you take the assertive right action to listen to your inner voice, to face hidden and dark feelings, and to choose to act wisely as a parent, you bring the reality of Eden through you and out into the world.

Where Do We Go From Here?

I hope I have explained myself clearly in this book, and you have gotten one of many important messages: **you are the one responsible for your health, and your child's health**. You are also responsible for promoting change in the world. This change may only happen in your personal life, but many of you will feel compelled, as I did, to spread this knowledge you gain. You have to make the choice for yourself; do you want to be a bystander to life, to sit back and watch bad things happen and claim you had nothing to do with it because you didn't initiate the action? Why live that way? Why not risk fearlessly living in a new way? Take a simple step towards change. One way to do this is to share this book with other people. I encourage sharing this book because its purpose is to help open people to a different reality, one that is here before us, but that we are blind to. Sharing this book with others can make a lasting impression in their lives. Even if you don't share this book, share what you have learned by reading it. Talk with your friends, relatives, neighbors. When you communicate with others in an honest way you engage the law of brotherhood. The evil shackles on this planet lose their grip, and the inevitable collapse of disease and suffering is hastened by your attentive actions. Strike a spear into the numbness and stagnation to reach the parts that do care. Part of you does care. Part of you does want to change. This is so, and this is the truth. You have everything to gain and very little to lose by making outward and inner changes.

Having this knowledge makes it difficult, for me at least, to sit still and watch parents set up their children for a life of disease and suffering. I can't sit by and watch them feed their children the wrong foods, not hold and nurture them, or inadvertently poison them through vaccination. So I have dedicated an important part of my waking life to bringing this out into the world. I hope that you will find speaking out against these behaviors to be contagious. You can spread the word. You can make changes. Start with your personal sphere of influence, which you can use to make a difference. Start at the local level with laws, ordinances, school regulations. For example, should schools be allowed to feed children foods with additives known and proven to cause learning problems and disease? Do not just sit there. Do something meaningful with your time here! Make a difference!

Remember, when trying to influence other people, or trying to share knowledge, come from your heart. Love is the answer and the way. Instill the seed of grace in them. At the same time, the most important change you can make is within yourself. You cannot make others change, but you can help them to initiate their own change. Your inner attitudes and feelings need to be honestly examined and brought into the light. The primary experience of life is

within us, and we have the ultimate power to exert change in our lives. You can radiate the change you want to see in the world. For example, while my family members don't live in a way that I completely agree with, I don't feel much need to change them. I point out the truth where I can. I rather try to view their choices with compassion. After a few years, they eventually began to copy what I do in one way or another. That doesn't mean that is your way, but I suggest not getting caught up in trying to change or fix others. When you feel good in yourself, you probably won't have your emotional livelihood and focus on changing other people. If other people change, or you can help them, that is good, but you can only help them when they want to receive your help.

The Golden Children

The Golden Children refers to both a real and metaphorical event. Gold is considered one of our most precious metals. Like the sun, our children are our gold. They are what is most precious to us.

When you align yourself with Nature's laws, you are channeling and calling forth a wisdom, energy, and power much greater than yourself. In the midst of a natural force, a magical child will be born whose true colors will shine forth. A child whose spirit is forged in a strong body because her parents ate and gave her the right foods, and whose heart is open and willing because she has been cared for and nurtured as this force of Nature intended. The very existence and presence of this child will represent a betterment for humanity. What could be more precious, more real, and more meaningful than creating a space for such a child?

My Vision

I want to live in a world where people care about each other, a world where we acknowledge that a part of our brother's and sister's pain (everyone's pain), is also our own. I want to live in a world that is full of compassion and love. I want to float back and relax in an ocean of bliss. I want to live in a world where we promote peace and celebrate our diversity. I want to live in a world without crime, war, or violence. I want to live in a world where we are one with the Creator, and where each of us can experience joy, freedom, and communion. And I realize that this world does not require me to change everything, or to change anything at all. I only have to let go into my Self.

In the Name of Love, Creating World Peace

You are that man or woman who has come in the name of love. While you may not be leading a public revolution, you will be leading a quiet revolution which to most people will be unrecognizable.

It only takes one person to stand in the name of love, only one person to stand for what is right in the world, to make a difference. This book is dedicated to you. When you take a stand for what is right for your child, you have brought the planet closer to peace. While you may not see many outer reflections of your efforts, there is one small person who will benefit from your positive actions, whose wide open and innocent eyes are looking towards you to affirm their goodness — your child. And while adults are usually stuck in their ways and in their beliefs about the world, your magical child is not. She does not know how the world is. She does not know what to expect from life. She is an infinitely blank template upon which your actions carve a portrait. Choose the actions of the divine, and paint the masterpiece of your child's life with love. Show her a world that is filled with more than suffering and a few fleeting pleasures; show her that her birthright is to vitality and to health and to life, so she can experience herself as love, and the world as the manifestation of love.

We are all waiting for a savior, a hero, for someone to help us. You are that person. You are the savior the world is waiting for, at least for your child. Be the hero that he or she has been waiting for. Make the remaining days of your life the days when your light shines into the world, so that your child will have an imprint of the divine. Give your children an imprint that says they are important, cared for, cherished and loved, as every child deserves to be.

A prayer. I ask for help from the highest plane and the Ineffable Kingdom. Kind Mother and Kind Father, show us where we have strayed from the path. Come live within us, enter into our hearts, and never leave us. Help bring our planet back to a state of grace, for the sake of OUR children. Help us see the divine always, and experience a tangible feeling of being loved and cared for, here and now, and for all of our days. Victory to the goodness within.

We are all sons and daughters of the Creator, and we are all therefore brothers and sisters on this path. Together we are interlinked, and we share this planet and are one with Her. We can create the peace we seek through our own inward changes, and thus fulfill our destiny.

The divine in me has written this book in reverence to the divine in you.

Mitakuye Oyasin - We Are All Family

Ramiel

About The Author

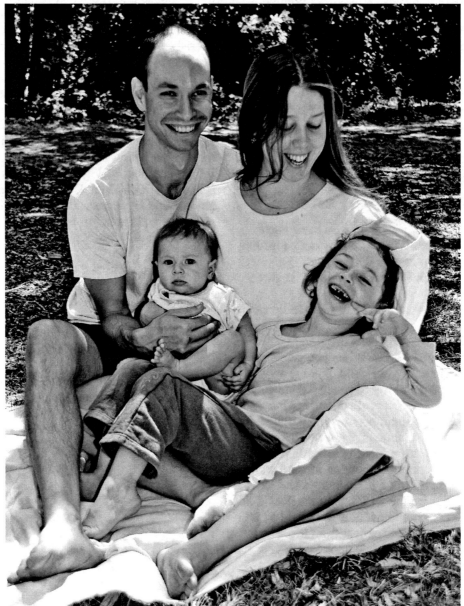

From left: Ramiel, Yeshe, Michelle, Sparkle (9/2008)

Ramiel Nagel is an internationally published author whose tooth decay research has been featured in *Nexus Magazine* and the *Townsend Letter for Doctors and Patients*. Nagel has a BA from the University of California and has a decade of training in emotional and spiritual health care. An advocate of balanced, healthy lifestyles, Nagel is also a yoga practitioner. He lives in California with his spouse and two daughters. *Healing Our Children* arose from Nagel's consistent prayer to the Universe, "Help me be of service to humanity, I know I have something good to offer the world." Nagel's next project is a movie script that will give people a tangible experience of grace for the purpose of healing.

Appendix A - Health Practitioners

Not every person listed here will give you the best health advice. Many nutritionally minded experts, might have different recommendations than the ones I have in my book. Other health care providers, do not use nutrition and are not well versed in it. Perhaps in the future, we can find a way to improve these inconsistencies. Meanwhile, you must trust your wisdom on what advice to follow, and what advice requires a second opinion.

Naturopathic Doctors – "Naturopathic medicine is a distinct system of primary health care that addresses the root causes of illness, and promotes health and healing using natural therapies. Naturopathic doctors are highly educated primary care providers who integrate standard medical diagnostics with a broad range of natural therapies."[1] There are many Naturopaths who are experts in cleansing the body, high quality supplementation and dietary changes. Make sure the naturopath has attended an intensive four or five year program.

www.ccnm.edu - Canadian College of Naturopathic Medicine

www.naturopathic.org- American Association of Naturopathic Physicians

Anthroposophically Extended Medicine – "Anthroposophical Medicine is a holistic, human-centered approach to medicine. Its basis is in modern medical science. Its concepts are broadened through a study of the laws of the living organism, of the soul and the spirit based on Anthroposophical Spiritual Science as founded by Rudolf Steiner (1861-1925)."[2] Anthroposophical Physicians are all Licensed Medical Doctors, some of them may be able to provide extraordinary good healing for your illness.

www.paam.net/outline.htm - The Physicians' Association for Anthroposophic Medicine

Homeopathic Physician – "It is a scientific therapeutic method which embodies a philosophy of understanding people and illness in an holistic context with the goal of promoting optimal health and healing… A homeopathic physician is a medical or an osteopathic professional who has added homeopathic medicine to his/her armamentarium through organized education and/or self-study."[3] Homeopathy is an excellent type of treatment to work on the energetic body, and to work on conditions that are supposedly incurable and untreatable.

www.homeopathyusa.org- The American Institute of Homeopathy

Chinese Medicine – "Acupuncture: Oriental medicine is an effective, low cost medical treatment that works in harmony with the body's natural healing ability."[4] Chinese medicine is a powerful approach to healing which is highly successful, especially when combined with correct dietary measures.

www.aaom.org- American Association of Oriental Medicine

www.nccaom.org - National Certification Commission for Acupuncture and Oriental Medicine

Acupressure - A type of Oriental healing art based on ancient Japanese and Chinese medicine. A practitioner puts pressure on specific points on the body with his or her fingers in order to relieve pain and discomfort, prevent tension-related ailments, and promote good health.

www.aobta.org - American Organization for Bodywork Therapies of Asia

www.acupressure.com - Acupressure Institute of America

Network Chiropractor – "Network Spinal Analysis™ is an evidenced based approach to wellness and body awareness. Gentle precise touch to the spine cues the brain to cre-

---

[1] http://www.ccnm.edu/about.html
[2] http://www.paam.net/outline.htm

[3] http://www.homeopathyusa.org/faq/
[4] http://qi-journal.com/tcm.asp

ate new wellness promoting strategies. Two unique healing waves develop with this work. They are associated with spontaneous release of spinal and life tensions, and the use of existing tension as fuel for spinal re-organization and enhanced wellness."[5]

www.associationfornetworkcare.com - Association for Network Care

Osteopathic Physician– "Developed 130 years ago by physician A.T. Still osteopathic medicine is one of the fastest growing healthcare professions in the U.S. and brings a unique philosophy to traditional medicine. With a strong emphasis on the inter-relationship of the body's nerves, muscles, bones and organs, doctors of osteopathic medicine, or D.O.s, apply the philosophy of treating the whole person to the prevention, diagnosis and treatment of illness, disease and injury."[6]

www.osteopathic.org - American Osteopathic Organization

www.jamesjealous.com – Osteopaths who have completed a course "Biodynamics of Osteopathy." Some on this list may be able to help with birth traumas.

www.cranialacademy.com – Cranial osteopathy information and referrals.

OrthoMolecular Medicine– Orthomolecular medicine describes the practice of preventing and treating disease by providing the body with optimal amounts of substances which are natural to the body. Orthomolecular medicine is especially useful for treating mental problems and psychiatric disorders.

www.orthomed.org - Orthomolecular Medicine web site.

Standard Process– "For 75 years, Standard Process has provided health care professionals with high-quality, nutritional whole food supplements. Our extensive collection of products supports the healthy functioning of the endocrine, cardiovascular, digestive, hepatic, respiratory, skeletal, renal, and other physiological systems."[7] Standard process was founded by the nutrition pioneer, Royal Lee, who believed that whole and unrefined foods where keys to health. Standard process makes supplements that are to a very high degree whole and unrefined and aligned with nature's principles. Their supplements are very strong and effective. If you are having problems finding a natural health care provider. Look for someone who uses standard process products.

www.standardprocess.com - Standard Process web site.

Cranial Sacral Therapy– "CST is a gentle, hands-on method of evaluating and enhancing the functioning of a physiological body system called the craniosacral system - comprised of the membranes and cerebrospinal fluid that surround and protect the brain and spinal cord.

Using a soft touch generally no greater than 5 grams, or about the weight of a nickel, practitioners release restrictions in the craniosacral system to improve the functioning of the central nervous system."[8]

This type of therapy is excellent for helping relieve any types of birth traumas or other physical traumas that may have occurred in early childhood.

www.upledger.com - Cranial Sacral Therapy was created by Osteopathic Physician John Upledger

Biological and Holistic Dentist– If you need some type of dental work, particularily dealing with the removal of mercury fillings, you must go to a dentist who takes extra and special precautions to remove the mercury. If you do need dental treatments, holistic or biological dentists can offer alternative and complimentary treatments to dental surgery. If you must see a dentist, consider what your lo-

---

[5] *www.associationfornetworkcare.com/whatisnsa.shtml*
[6] *www.osteopathic.org/index.cfm?PageID=ost_main*

[7] http://www.standardprocess.com/overview.asp
[8] http://www.iahe.com/html/therapies/cst.jsp

cal biological or holistic dentist has to offer in terms of treatments. Many of these dentists follow strict protocols for removing mercury fillings, and also have alternative's to dealing with the potentially dangerous root canals.

www.holisticdental.org - Holistic Dental Association

www.talkinternational.com/directories/dentists-usa.html - Mercury Free and Biological Denists list

Natural Hygiene Physician- Natural Hygiene doctors use only fasting, food and optimal lifestyle to restore patients to health. No drugs/medicines are used since these typically only suppress symptoms and give an illusion of health, while making matters worse. (Most of these doctors support vegetarian or vegan diets, those diets might help temporarily to aide recovery from disease. Vegetarian and vegan diets deplete the body and are I am against their use any time remotely near pregnancy.)

www.naturalhygienesociety.org/doctors.html

Nutritionists- Some nutritionists preach the wrong kind of food, not based on the traditional diets of our ancestors. Meanwhile, other nutritionists, might be your doorway or gateway to creating a healthy and balanced diet and body chemistry based on whole unrefined foods and supplements. Look for nutritionists who are familiar with the work of Weston Price, or Francis Pottenger.

www.ifnh.org – International Foundation of Nutrition and Health

www.ppnf.org – Price-Pottenger Nutrition Foundation

Colon Therapist- There are some colon cleansing therapists that specialize in doing high colon enemas, exactly the same as Dr. Jensen uses. I am unaware of the details of different types of colon therapists. Only that if you find one who does a gentle type of cleansing combined with massaging the abdomen to free the mucoid plaque, that this might be a good therapist to go to, if you are in your pre-pregnancy phase of health building, or after you are done lactating.

Ayurvedic Medicine- Ayurveda deals with the measures of healthy living, along with therapeutic measures that relate to physical, mental, social and spiritual harmony. Ayurveda is an intricate system of healing that originated in India thousands of years ago.

Health Insurance- Health insurance is a fraud designed to support allopathic medicine. Even though many natural treatments are more successful, and less expensive than the allopathic treatments, your health insurance will not cover these treatments. This is not a reason to avoid alternative treatments, which are many times a fraction of the cost of allopathic treatments. For example, a full 1 hour session of acupuncture might cost $50, with herbal medications costing $6. Meanwhile an allopathic physician might charge $200 for ten minutes ($1200 per hour), and $100 or more for medication's which usually have dangerous side effects. In the case of the midwives, even though I have presented scientific studies that show that midwives are remarkably safer with better birth outcomes, many of them are not covered by insurance. This does not make sense, because you would think, insurance companies would take efforts to lower their costs. They must know that overall, because of less side effects, midwives will cost less than conventional doctors for births. The only explanation for not supporting less expensive treatments, is that health insurance exists to a large extent, to promote a business with disease, profiting off of illness. Consider your health insurance needs seriously. Yes there are some cases were drugs save lives, and surgery benefits people. In the vast majority of cases, drugs take hundreds of thousands of lives and surgery is a needless assault on our bodies. There are alternative scheme's, such as a self made health insurance which can be done through different companies, where you pay money to a fund, where you can control who you see, or getting a health insurance with a very high deductible, or that applies only for emergency care.

Healing the Body and Emotions

It is important to be open to feeling ones feelings and allowing the flow of life energy through the body. Being a parent and having a child often brings up feelings in the body. These feelings must be felt and examined in a healthy matter. Here is a list of some specialists who may be able to help facilitate emotional healing.

There are also practices and healing modalities which can support healing our emotional body, such as: Yoga, Tai Chi, Chi Gong, and Bio energetics or Core Energetics

Core Energetics- CORE ENERGETICS® (CE) is the dynamic force in the evolution of our core - CORE ENERGETICS® (CE) The Core represents the individualized universal life energy and with that, our essential being. CORE ENERGETICS supports the unfolding of our essential being on all levels of existence.
www.coreenergetics.org
www.coreinstitute.com
www.core-energetics-south.com
www.annbradney.com

Bioenergetics- Bioenergetics is a way of understanding personality in terms of the body and its energetic processes. Bioenergetic Analysis is a form of therapy that combines work with the body and the mind to help people resolve their emotional problems and realize more of their potential for pleasure and joy in living. Source: www.bioenergetic-therapy.com

Pathwork– "The Pathwork is a body of practical spiritual wisdom that lays out a step-by-step journey into personal transformation and wholeness, down to the very core of our being. It is a voyage of discovery to the Real Self through the layers of our defenses, denial and fear."
www.pathwork.org

Transpersonal Psychology- "Today, a more comprehensive view of human nature is developing… Based on observations and practices from many cultures, the transpersonal perspective is informed by modern psychology, the humanities and human sciences, as well as contemporary spiritual disciplines and the wisdom traditions."
(*www.atpweb.org/transperspect.asp*)

Family Constellation Healing- A Family Constellation is a 60-minute group process that has the power to affect generations of suffering and unhappiness. Bert Hellinger, the founder of this work, who studied and treated families for more than 50 years, observed that many of us unconsciously "take on" destructive familial patterns of anxiety, depression, anger, guilt, aloneness, alcoholism and even illness as a way of "belonging" in our families. Bonded by a deep love, a child will often sacrifice his own best interests in a vain attempt to ease the suffering of a parent or other family member.

Constellation Work allows us to break these patterns and reestablish our vital strength, tranquility and dignity.

www.hellinger.com - Bert Hellinger's official homepage, click on International Directories of Practitioners to find a local practitioner.

Other modalities can support the health of the body and emotions:

Reiki– "Reiki is one of the more widely known forms of energy healing. Energy Healing involves direct application of *Chi* for the purpose of strengthening the clients energy system (aura). Chi is the term used by the Chinese mystics and martial artists for the underlying force the Universe is made of."
(*reiki.7gen.com*)

Barbara Brennan Healing Science – "Brennan Healing Science is an enlightening system of healing that combines hands-on healing techniques with spiritual and psychological processes touching every aspect of your life."
(*www.barbarabrennan.com*)

Hakomi– Hakomi is a body-centered, somatic psychotherapy. The body's structures and habitual patterns become a powerful doorway to unconscious core material, including the hidden core beliefs which shape our lives, relationships, and self-images.

www.hakomiinstitute.com - International Headquarters of the Hakomi Institute

Alexander Technique– Alexander Technique is a method of mind/body integration, which leads to ease of movement and awareness. The Alexander Technique is usually taught in individual lessons, during which the student becomes aware of patterns of contraction in everyday activities such as walking, sitting, standing, bending and lifting.

www.alexandertech.com - The American Society for the Alexander Technique

Feldenkrais Method– The Feldenkrais Method is for anyone who wants to reconnect with their natural abilities to move, think and feel. Whether you want to be more comfortable sitting at your computer, playing with your children and grandchildren, or performing a favorite pastime, these gentle lessons can improve your overall well being. This a form of movement to promote healing and awareness.

www.feldenkrais.com - Feldenkrais Educational Foundation of North America

Rolfing– Developed over 50 years ago by Dr. Ida Rolf, Ph.D Rolfing structural integration works on the web-like complex of connective tissue (fascia) to release, realign and balance the whole body.

www.rolf.org - The Rolf Institute of Structural Integration

The Trager Approach– Utilizing gentle, non-intrusive, natural movements, The *Trager* Approach helps release deep-seated physical and mental patterns and facilitates deep relaxation, increased physical mobility, and mental clarity. These patterns may have developed in response to accidents, illnesses, or any kind of physical or emotional trauma, including the stress of everyday life.

www.trager.com - The Trager Approach

About The Price-Pottenger Nutrition Foundation

The Price-Pottenger Nutrition Foundation (PPNF) is completely independent of any commercial interest or government agencies. The foundation relies on the generous support of its members to be able to continue to make Dr. Price's research available. I encourage you to support the Price-Pottenger Nutrition Foundation. Your membership will help to support a future in which humankind enjoys optimal, vibrant health.

PPNF also has a great online bookstore with many high quality books about health and nutrition.

Contact them at:
Price-Pottenger Nutrition Foundation
P.O. Box 2614, La Mesa, CA 91943-2614
www.ppnf.org
info@ppnf.org
(619) 462-7600, 1-800-366-3748

About the Weston A. Price Foundation

The Weston A. Price Foundation is a nonprofit, tax-exempt charity, founded in 1999 to disseminate the research of nutrition pioneer Dr. Weston Price.

The Weston A. Price Foundation has local chapters to help support you in locating sources of nutrient-rich whole foods. E-mail chapters@westonprice.org, for more information about a local chapter near you. Chapters also provide advocacy to support small organic farmers and to help ensure access to whole foods throughout the world. The WAPF publishes a well-researched quarterly journal for members.

The Weston A. Price Foundation
PMB 106-380, 4200 Wisconsin Ave., NW, Washington DC 20016
Phone: (202) 363-4394 | Fax: (202) 363-4396
www.westonaprice.org

How to Order Additional Copies of Healing Our Children

Visit my website for easy online ordering:

www.healingourchildren.net

For bulk purchases please e-mail Golden Child Publishing

orders@goldenchildpublishing.com

References

[1] Pierrakos, Eva, International Pathwork Foundation *Pathwork Guide Lecture 171, Spiritual Laws,* http://www.pathwork.org/lecturesObtainingUnedited.html

[2] Bernardini, R. *The Truth About Children's Health.* Clifford, PRI Publishing, 2003: 282.

[3] Ibid., 287.

[4] Dr. Poehlman, K.H.. *Synthesis of the Work of Enderlein, Bechamps and other Pleomorphic Researchers,* Explore for the Professional, Vol. 8, No. 2, http://www.explorepub.com/articles/enderlein3.html

[5] BioMedix, *How We Rot and Rust: It all begins with pH* http://biomedx.com/microscopes/rrintro/rr1.html

[6] One video can be see at Grayfield Optical www.grayfieldoptical.com/humoral_pathology.html

[7] Bernardini, *The Truth About Children's Health,* 282.

[8] Vonderplanitz, A. *Recipe for Living Without Disease.* Santa Monica: Carnelian Bay Castle Press, 2002:171-172.

[9] Jensen, B. *Dr. Jensen's Guide to Better Bowel Care.* New York: Avery, 1999: 43.

[10] Jacob, S., and Francone, C. *Elements of Anatomy and Physiology.* Philadelphia: 1989: 27.

[11] Bieler, H. *Food is Your Best Medicine.* New York: Vintage Books, 1965: 15.

[12] Veith, I. *The Yellow Emperor's Classic of Internal Medicine.* Berkeley, 1966:97.

[13] Ibid., 98.

[14] Bieler, *Food is Your Best Medicine,* 40.

[15] Tilden, J. *Toxemia Explained.* Denver: 1926: 21.

[16] Ibid., 29.

[17] Bieler, *Food is Your Best Medicine,* Preface.

[18] Bieler, H. *Food is Your Best Medicine.* New York: Vintage Books, 1965: 8.

[19] Null, Dean G., C. Feldman, M. Rasio, D. *Death by Medicine,* Life Extension. http://www.lef.org/magazine/mag2004/mar2004_awsi_death_01.htm. For more research see: Iatrogenic Illness, http://www.garynull.com/Documents/Iatrogenic/Iatrogenic_index.htm.

[20] Ibid., http://www.lef.org/magazine/mag2004/mar2004_awsi_death_02.htm

[21] Complaint Text is located at: www4.dr-rath-foundation.org/The_Hague/complaint/

[22] Pierrakos, Eva, International Pathwork Foundation, *Pathwork Guide Lecture 17, Spiritual Laws.* http://www.pathwork.org/lecturesObtaining.html.

[23] Swami Vishwananda, http://www.vishwananda.org

[24] Pierrakos, Eva, International Pathwork Foundation. *Pathwork Guide Lecture 173, Basic Attitudes and Practices to Open the Centers.* http://www.pathwork.org/lecturesObtaining.html.

[25] Pierrakos, *Lecture 177, Pleasure - The Full Pulsation of Life,* http://www.pathwork.org/lectures/unedited/177.PDF

[26] Bieler, *Food is Your Best Medicine,* 39.

[27] Ibid.

[28] Ibid., 62.

[29] Ibid., 63.

[30] Ibid.

[31] Ibid., 64.

[32] Ibid., 72.

[33] Ibid., 73.

[34] Price, W. A. "Why Dental Caries With Modern Civilizations? I. Field Studies in Primitive Loetschental Valley, Switzerland," *Dental Digest,* (1933) March: 94.

[35] *National Health and Nutrition Examination Survey, 1999-2002.* National Center for Health Statistics, CDC. www.cdc.gov/nccdphp/publications/aag/pdf/oh.pdf.

[36] Price, "Why Dental Caries With Modern Civilizations? I. Field Studies in Primitive Loetschental Valley, Switzerland," 94.

[37] Ibid., 91.

[38] Ibid.

[39] Price, W. A. "Why Dental Caries With Modern Civilizations? IX. Field Studies Among Primitive Indians in Northern Canada," Dental Digest, (1934) April; 133.

[40] Ibid.

[41] Fallon, Sally. *The Right Price: Interpreting the Work of Weston Price*. Weston a Price Foundation http://www.westonaprice.org/basicnutrition/right_price.html,

[42] Ibid., 26.

[43] Price, W. *Nutrition and Physical Degeneration*. 6th Ed., 26.

[44] Price, W. *Nutrition and Physical Degeneration*. 6th Ed. La Mesa: Price-Pottenger Nutrition Foundation, 2004: 24.

[45] Price, W. *Nutrition and Physical Degeneration*. 8th Ed. La Mesa: Price-Pottenger Nutrition Foundation; 2008: 472.

[46] Ibid.

[47] Ibid., 27.

[48] Ibid,. 26-27.

[49] Ibid., 39.

[50] Ibid., 35.

[51] Ibid., 49.

[52] Ibid., 55-57.

[53] Ibid., 59.

[54] Ibid.

[55] Ibid., 164.

[56] Ibid., 171.

[57] Ibid.

[58] Ibid., 173.

[59] Ibid., 64.

[60] Ibid., 67.

[61] Ibid., 68.

[62] Page, M and Abrams, L. *Your Body is Your Best Doctor*. New Canaan: Keats Publishing Inc., 1972:188.

[63] Ibid., 170.

[64] Price, W. *Nutrition and Physical Degeneration*. 8th Ed., 274

[65] Ibid., 174.

[66] Ibid., 177.

[67] Ibid., 71.

[68] Ibid., 69.

[69] Bieler, *Food is Your Best Medicine* 15.

[70] Ibid., 65.

[71] Price, W.A. 7 Teaching Lessons. "Light From Primitive Races On Modern Degeneration, 4. Facial Beauty Lost in One Generation and Greater Injury to Later Born Children," La Mesa: Price-Pottenger Nutrition Foundation 2006: Slide 7.

[72] Ibid., Slide 8.

[73] Price, W.A. 7 Teaching Lessons. "Light From Primitive Races On Modern Degeneration, 1. A Sketch of the Primitive Races Studied," La Mesa: Price-Pottenger Nutrition Foundation 2006: Slide 35 & 37.

[74] Price, W.A. 7 Teaching Lessons. "Light From Primitive Races On Modern Degeneration, 2. How Primitive Races Have Prevented Tooth Decay," La Mesa: Price-Pottenger Nutrition Foundation 2006: Slide 59.

[75] Price, W.A. 7 Teaching Lessons. "Light From Primitive Races On Modern Degeneration, 7. Special Foods of Primitives for Parents-to-be and Race Regeneration," La Mesa: Price-Pottenger Nutrition Foundation 2006: Slide 8.

[76] Price, W. *Nutrition and Physical Degeneration*. 8th Ed. La Mesa: Price-Pottenger Nutrition Foundation; 2008: 463.

[77] Ibid., 192.

[78] Price, W.A. 7 Teaching Lessons. "Light From Primitive Races On Modern Degeneration, 2. How Primitive Races Have Prevented Tooth Decay," La Mesa: Price-Pottenger Nutrition Foundation 2006: Slide 39.

[79] Price, W. *Nutrition and Physical Degeneration*. 6th Ed., 198.

[80] Ibid., 174.

[81] Ibid., 332.

[82] Ibid., 71-72.

[83] Ibid., 92-93.

[84] Ibid., 49.

[85] Price, W.A. 7 Teaching Lessons. "Light From Primitive Races On Modern Degeneration, 4. Facial Beauty Lost in One Generation and Greater Injury to Later Born Children," La Mesa: Price-Pottenger Nutrition Foundation 2006: Slide 39.

[86] Ibid., 116.

[87] Dental Digest, 94 (March, 1936).

[88] Ibid., 76.

[89] Price, W. A. "Why Dental Caries With Modern Civilizations? XI. New Light On Loss of Immunity to Some Degenerative Processes Including Dental Caries," Dental Digest, 1934 July; 242.

[90] Price, W.A. "New Light Obtained on Dental Caries," *Dental Cosmos, a Monthly Record of Dental Science*. Vol. 78:866, http://www.hti.umich.edu/d/dencos/.

[91] Price, W. *Nutrition and Physical Degeneration*. 6th Ed., 77.

[92] Ibid., 84.

[93] Ibid.

[94] Ibid., 83.

[95] Ibid., 89.

[96] Ibid., 180.

[97] Ibid., 271.

[98] Price, W.A. 7 Teaching Lessons. "Light From Primitive Races On Modern Degeneration, 7. Special Foods of Primitives for Parents-to-be and Race Regeneration," La Mesa: Price-Pottenger Nutrition Foundation 2006: Slide 31.

99 Fallon, S. *Nourishing Traditions*. Washington, DC: New Trends, 1999: 24.

100 Price, W.A. 7 Teaching Lessons. "Light From Primitive Races On Modern Degeneration, 7. Special Foods of Primitives for Parents-to-be and Race Regeneration," 33.

101 Price, W. A. "Why Dental Caries With Modern Civilizations? XI. New Light on Loss of Immunity to Some Degenerative Processes Including Dental Caries," Dental Digest, (July, 1934): 242.

102 *New Childhood Arthritis Estimates,* National Center for Chronic Disease Prevention and Health Promotion., http://www.cdc.gov/arthritis/misc/childhood_arth_estimates.htm

103 Price, W. *Nutrition and Physical Degeneration*. 6th Ed 480.

104 Ibid., 482.

105 Ibid., 273.

106 Ibid., 483.

107 Pierrakos, E, International Pathwork Foundation, *Pathwork Guide Lecture 248, Three Principles of the Forces of Evil.* http://www.pathwork.org/lecturesObtaining.html.

108 Ibid.

109 Foresight: the Association for the Promotion of Preconceptual Care, http://www.foresight-preconception.org.uk/.

110 "Update on Overall Prevalence of Major Birth Defects --- Atlanta, Georgia, 1978—2005." MMWR Weekly, January 11, 2008 / 57(01);1-5. Centers for Disease Control and Prevention, http://www.cdc.gov/mmwr/preview/mmwrhtml/mm5701a2.htm

111 CIA World Factbook, United States. https://www.cia.gov/library/publications/the-world-factbook/print/us.html

112 Price, W. A., *Nutrition and Physical Degeneration,* 6th Ed. La Mesa: Price-Pottenger Nutrition Foundation; 2004: 174.

113 Ibid., 323

114 Ibid., 321

115 Ibid., 338.

116 Price, W. A., *Nutrition and Physical Degeneration,* 8th Ed La Mesa: Price-Pottenger Nutrition Foundation; 2004: 306.

117 Ibid.

118 Ibid., 309.

119 Ibid.

120 Price, W. *Nutrition and Physical Degeneration*. 6th Ed: 343.

121 Ibid., 341

122 Ibid., 340.

123 Ibid., 321.

124 Bieler, H. *Dr. Bieler's Natural Way to Sexual Health.* New York, Bantam Books: 1972: 26.

125 Bieler, H. *Dr. Bieler's Natural Way to Sexual Health.* New York, Bantam Books: 1972: 25-26.

126 Bieler, H. *Dr. Bieler's Natural Way to Sexual Health.* New York, Bantam Books: 1972: 25-26.

127 Ibid., 316

128 Ibid., 318

129 Price, W. A., 7 Teaching Lessons,. "Light From Primitive Races On Modern Degeneration, " 4. Facial Beauty Lost in One Generation and Greater Injury to Later Born Children," La Mesa: Price-Pottenger Nutrition Foundation 2006: Slide 44.

130 Price, *Nutrition and Physical Degeneration*. 6th Ed. 338.

131 Ibid., 316

132 Masterjohn, C. "Vitamins for Fetal Development: Conception to Birth." Wise Traditions: Volume 8 Number 4:24-35.

133 Price, *Nutrition and Physical Degeneration,* 6th Ed: 275.

134 Chart of Nutrient Intake Comparison, http://www.ers.usda.gov/briefing/dietandhealth/data/nutrients/tables.xls

135 Estimate done without clinical evidence

136 Micronutrient Information Center: Phosphorus, Linus Palding Institute, Oregon State University,.http://lpi.oregonstate.edu/infocenter/minerals/phosphorus/. Footnote from Dietary Reference Intakes: Calcium, Phosphorus, Magnesium, Vitamin D, and Fluoride, Food and Nutrition Board, Institute of Medicin:. Phosphorus Washington D.C., National Academy Press; 1997:146-189, (Averaged male and female intakes)

137 Price, W. A., "Why Dental Caries With Modern Civilizations? XI. New Light on Loss of Immunity to Some Degenerative Processes Including Dental Caries," *Dental Digest*, (July, 1934): 243.

138 Price, W. A., "Why Dental Caries With Modern Civilizations? V. An Interpretation of Field Studies Previously Reported," *Dental Digest,* (July 1933): 278.

139 Ibid., 278

140 Price, "Why Dental Caries With Modern Civilizations? "XI. New Light on Loss of Immunity to Some Degenerative Processes Including Dental Caries," 243.

141 Ibid.

142 Price, "Why Dental Caries With Modern Civilizations? "V. An Interpretation of Field Studies Previously Reported," 278.

143 Ibid.

144 Price, *Nutrition and Physical Degeneration,* 6th Ed, 269.

[145] Price, "Why Dental Caries With Modern Civilizations? V. An Interpretation of Field Studies Previously Reported," 278.

[146] Ibid.

[147] Price, "Why Dental Caries With Modern Civilizations? XI. New Light on Loss of Immunity to Some Degenerative Processes Including Dental Caries," 243.

[148] Ibid., 244

[149] Ibid.

[150] Fallon, S. *Nourishing Traditions*. Washington, DC: New Trends, 1999: 468-469.

[151] Price, "Why Dental Caries With Modern Civilizations? V. An Interpretation of Field Studies Previously Reported," 278.

[152] Price, *Nutrition and Physical Degeneration,* 6th Ed..48.

[153] Ibid., 51

[154] Ibid., 44

[155] Price, "Why Dental Caries With Modern Civilizations? V. An Interpretation of Field Studies Previously Reported," 278.

[156] Figures have been rounded up for simplicity

[157] Price, "Why Dental Caries With Modern Civilizations? XI. New Light on Loss of Immunity to Some Degenerative Processes Including Dental Caries," 243.

[158] Ibid.,

[159] Price, W. A., "Why Dental Caries With Modern Civilizations? IX. Field Studies Among Primitive Indians in Northern Canada," *Dental Digest,* (April, 1934): 133.

[160] Price, "Why Dental Caries With Modern Civilizations? XI. New Light on Loss of Immunity to Some Degenerative Processes Including Dental Caries," 243.

[161] Ibid.

[162] Ibid.

[163] Ibid.

[164] Price, *Nutrition and Physical Degeneration,* 6th Ed. 259.

[165] Price, "Why Dental Caries With Modern Civilizations? XI. New Light on Loss of Immunity to Some Degenerative Processes Including Dental Caries," 243.

[166] Ibid., 244

[167] Price, "Why Dental Caries With Modern Civilizations? XI. New Light on Loss of Immunity to Some Degenerative Processes Including Dental Caries," 244.

[168] Price, *Nutrition and Physical Degeneration.* 6th Ed, 260.

[169] Ibid., 258.

[170] Price, W. A., *Journal of the American Dental Association*, 1936: 888.

[171] Ibid., 8.

[172] Price, *Nutrition and Physical Degeneration,* 6th Ed. 148.

[173] God Gave us Cattle and Grass, Wild Watch, http://www.wildwatch.com/resources/other/maasai.asp,

[174] Cultures and Countries, Maasai, http://www.everyculture.com/wc/Tajikistan-to-Zimbabwe/Maasai.html,

[175] Price, *Nutrition and Physical Degeneration,* 6th Ed. 148.

[176] Ibid., 147.

[177] Ibid., 139.

[178] Price, *Nutrition and Physical Degeneration,* 6th Ed. 260.

[179] Pacific Islanders, Diet of, Internet FAQ archives, http://www.faqs.org/nutrition/Ome-Pop/Pacific-Islanders-Diet-of.html

[180] Dietary Reference Intakes, Institute of Medicine, http://www.iom.edu/Object.File/Master/21/372/0.pdf,

[181] 1. SUPPLEMENTARY DATA TABLES, USDA's 1994-96 Continuing Survey of Food Intakes by Individuals, Table Set 12, *US Department of Agriculture, Agricultural Research Service,* http://www.ars.usda.gov/SP2UserFiles/Place/12355000/pdf/Supp.PDF,

[182] Ibid.

[183] Ibid.

[184] Ibid.

[185] Third Report on Nutrition Monitoring in the United States, USDA. http://www.cdc.gov/nchs/data/misc/tronm.pdf

[186] Price, W. A. *Nutrition and Physical Degeneration,* 6th Ed. La Mesa: Price-Pottenger Nutrition Foundation; 2004: 399.

[187] Ibid., 401.

[188] Price, W. A. 7 Teaching Lessons. "Light From Primitive Races On Modern Degeneration: 7. Special Foods of Primitives for Parents-to-be and Race Regeneration," La Mesa: Price-Pottenger Nutrition Foundation 2006: Slide 13.

[189] Price, *Nutrition and Physical Degeneration,* 6th Ed.,400-401.

[190] Ibid., 397.

[191] Ibid., 401.

[192] Ibid., 400.

[193] Ibid.

[194] Ibid., 397.

[195] Price, 7 Teaching Lessons. "Light From Primitive Races On Modern Degeneration. 7. Special Foods of Primitives for Parents-to-be and Race Regeneration," Slide 8.

[196] Ibid., Slide 15.

[197] Price, *Nutrition and Physical Degeneration*, 6th Ed, 400-401.

[198] Price, W. A., "New Light Obtained on Dental Caries," *Dental Cosmos, a Monthly Record of Dental Science* Vol. 77:1040, http://www.hti.umich.edu/d/dencos/.

[199] Price, W.A. 7 Teaching Lessons. "Light From Primitive Races On Modern Degeneration: 7. Special Foods of Primitives for Parents-to-be and Race Regeneration," Slide 10.

[200] Ibid., Slide 11.

[201] Price, *Nutrition and Physical Degeneration*, 8th Ed, 465.

[202] Price, W. A., *Journal of the American Dental Association*, 1936: 888.

[203] Price, *Nutrition and Physical Degeneration*, 6th Ed, 401.

[204] Fallon, S., and Enig, M., *Guts and Grease: The Diet of Native Americans*. Weston A Price Foundation, http://www.westonaprice.org/traditional_diets/native_americans.html,

[205] Ibid.

[206] Ibid., 137

[207] Ibid., 401-402.

[208] Ibid., 402.

[209] Price, W. A. "Field Studies Among African Tribes." *Journal of the American Medical Association*, 1936:888.

[210] Diet for Pregnant and Nursing Mothers, Weston A Price Foundation. Available At: www.westonaprice.org/children/dietformothers.html, Accessed, March 10, 2007.

[211] For more about Bone Broth, Fallon, S. Broth is Beautiful, Available At: www.westonaprice.org/foodfeatures/broth.html, Accessed March 10, 2007.

[212] For more information about Lacto-Fermentation, Fallon, S. Lacto-Fermentation, Available At: www.westonaprice.org/foodfeatures/lacto.html

[213] For More Coconut Oil Information see, Enig, M. A New Look at Coconut Oil, www.westonaprice.org/knowyourfats/coconut_oil.html, Accessed March 10, 2007.

[214] For more Lard information – Forristal, L. Put Lard Back in Your Larder, Available At: www.westonaprice.org/motherlinda/lard.html, Accessed March, 10, 2007.
For more Vitamin D information – Sullivan, K. The Miracle of Vitamin D. www.westonaprice.org/basicnutrition/vitamindmiracle.html Accessed March 10, 2007.

[215] I cannot give an even approximate figure, but I suggest eating more than we currently are

[216] Sherman, H. C., "Positive Health Balances of Calcium and Phosphorus for Pregnancy," *Chemistry of Food and Nutrition*. MacMillian Company, Toronto: 470,

[217] Bieler, H. *Food is Your Best Medicine*. New York: Vintage Books, 1965: 186.

[218] Ibid., 196.

[219] Bieler, *Food is Your Best Medicine*, 190-191.

[220] Schmid, R., *Recovering from Vegetarianism*, Alternative Medicine Center of Connecticut, http://www.drrons.com/recovering-from-vegetarianism.htm,

[221] Fallon, S., *Nourishing Traditions*. Washington, DC: New Trends; 1999: 116.

[222] Ibid., 189-191.

[223] Price, *Nutrition and Physical Degeneration*, 6th Ed. 124.

[224] Ibid., 124.

[225] Ibid., 239.

[226] Fallon, S., and Enig, M., *Australian Aboriginies: Living Off the Fat of the Land.*, Weston A Price Foundation. http://www.westonaprice.org/traditional_diets/australian_aborigines.html

[227] Ibid.

[228] Price, *Nutrition and Physical Degeneration*, 6th Ed. 262.

[229] Fallon, S., and Enig, M., *Australian Aboriginies Living Off the Fat of the Land.* Weston A Price Foundation. http://www.westonaprice.org/traditional_diets/australian_aborigines.html

[230] Vonderplanitz, A. *We Want To Live*, 2005 Ed. Carnelian Bay Castle Press, Los Angeles; 2005:178.

[231] Bieler, *Food is Your Best Medicine*, 209.

[232] Fallon, S., and Enig, M., *Guts and Grease: The Diet of Native Americans*, Weston A Price Foundation, http://www.westonaprice.org/traditional_diets/native_americans.html

[233] Ravnskov, U. *The Cholesterol Myths*, www.ravnskov.nu/cholesterol.htm,

[234] Ravnskov, U. *The Benefits of High Cholesterol*, Weston A. Price Foundation http://www.westonaprice.org/moderndiseases/benefits_cholest.html.

[235] Fallon, *Nourishing Traditions*, 236. Excerpted from Forbes FYI pg

[236] Ibid., 4.

[237] Price, *Nutrition and Physical Degeneration*. 6th Ed. 109.

[238] Vonderplanitz, *We Want To Live,* 2005 Ed., 159-160.

[239] Pierrakos E, *Pathwork Guide Lecture 210: Visualization Process for Growing Into the Unitive State,* International Pathwork Foundation, http://www.pathwork.org/lecturesObtaining.html.

[240] Price, *Nutrition and Physical Degeneration,* 6th Ed., 422.

[241] Fallon, *Nourishing Traditions,* 37.

[242] Ibid., Also See: Fallon and Enig, *Vitamin A Saga,* Weston A. Price Foundation, http://www.westonaprice.org/basicnutrition/vitaminasag a.html

[243] Masterjohn, C. "Vitamins for Fetal Development: Conception to Birth." *Wise Traditions*: Volume 8 Number 4:29.

[244] Price, W. *Nutrition and Physical Degeneration, 8th Ed.* La Mesa: Price-Pottenger Nutrition Foundation; 2008: 253.

[245] Masterjohn, C. "Vitamins for Fetal Development: Conception to Birth." 28-29.

[246] Ibid., 335.

[247] Ibid., 480.

[248] Lee, R. Butter, Vitamin E and the 'X' Factor of Dr. Price, Price-Pottenger Nutrition Foundation. http://www.www.ppnf.org/catalog/ppnf/Articles/XFacto r.html

[249] Price, *Nutrition and Physical Degeneration.* 8th Ed. 133.

[250] Fallon, *Nourishing Traditions,* 618.

[251] Page, M., and Abrams, L., *Your Body is Your Best Doctor,* New Canaan: Keats Publishing Inc.;1972:129.

[252] *Mineral Primer,* Weston A Price Foundation, http://www.westonaprice.org/basicnutrition/mineralprim er.html,

[253] From a Realmilk presentation, *American Journal Public Health,* Vol 88., No 8, Aug 1998, http://www.realmilk.com/ppt/RawMilk.PPT

[254] From Realmilk presentation, US Census Bureau, 1997 (with population estimate 267,783,607) http://www.realmilk.com/ppt/RawMilk.PPT

[255] I recommend the Real Milk power point presentation if you want to learn the facts about the safety and health-promoting abilities of raw milk. www.realmilk.com/ppt/index.html.

[256] *Listeriosis and Pasteurized Milk,* MMWR Weekly, Centers for Disease Control, December 16, 1988 /37(49); 764-766, http://www.cdc.gov/mmwr/preview/mmwrhtml/000013 16.htm.

[257] *Division of Bacterial and Mycotic Diseases: Listeriosis,* Centers for Disease Control and Prevention.

http://www.cdc.gov/ncidod/dbmd/diseaseinfo/listeriosis g.htm,

[258] Ibid., 34.

[259] Bartlett, T. "The Raw Deal," Washington Post Magazine, October 1st, 2006, W18, http://www.organicconsumers.org/articles/article_3134. cfm

[260] Buttram, H. *For Tomorrow's Children.* Blooming Glen: Preconception Care Inc; 1990:Chapter 9.

[261] Price, *Nutrition and Physical Degeneration,* 6th Ed., 266.

[262] Ibid., 290.

[263] Ibid., 295.

[264] Ibid., 405, 408.

[265] Enig, M., *Gamma-Linolenic Acid.* Weston A Price Foundation. http://www.westonaprice.org/knowyourfats/gamma-linolenic.html,

[266] Gladstar, R., *Family Herbal,* Storey Books: North Adams, Massachussets, 2001:205.

[267] Wetzel, D., *Cod Liver Oil: Notes on the Manufacture of Our Most Important Dietary Supplement,* Weston A Price Foundation, http://www.westonaprice.org/modernfood/codliver-manufacture.html,

[268] Mercury Decision, May 16, 2006. The Center for Consumer Freedom, http://www.consumerfreedom.com/news_detail.cfm/hea dline/3033. The actual text can be read here: http://www.fishscam.com/downloads/060516_mercury_ p61_p62.pdf

[269] *Mercury,* Center for the Evaluation of Risks to Human Reproduction (CERHR), National Toxicology Program, http://cerhr.niehs.nih.gov/common/mercury.html

[270] Consumer Group, *Landmark Fish Study Should Put Mercury Fears To Rest,* The Center for Consumer Freedom. http://www.consumerfreedom.com/pressRelease_detail. cfm/release/192

[271] *Mercury,* http://cerhr.niehs.nih.gov/common/mercury.html,

[272] *Whale Meat,* Fishscam. http://www.fishscam.com/fwhalemeat.cfm,

[273] Consumer Group: *Landmark Fish Study Should Put Mercury Fears To Rest,* The Center for Consumer Freedom, http://www.consumerfreedom.com/pressRelease_detail. cfm/release/192

[274] Squires, S., "Pregnant? Say Yes to Seafood," Washington Post, Feb. 20, 2007, HE01.

http://www.washingtonpost.com/wp-dyn/content/article/2007/02/16/AR2007021602259.html

[275] Consumer Group, *Landmark Fish Study Should Put Mercury Fears To Rest*, The Center for Consumer Freedom. http://www.consumerfreedom.com/pressRelease_detail.cfm/release/192

[276] See: Wiley. H. *History of Crime Against the Food Law*. 1929.

[277] Starfield, B., MD, MPH, *The Journal of the American Medical Association* (JAMA) Vol 284, No 4, July 26th 2000. (Dr Starfield writes from the Johns Hopkins School of Hygiene and Public Health).

[278] Buttram, H. *For Tomorrow's Children*, 46.

[279] Hooton, Ernest A., *Apes, Men, and Morons*, Putnam: New York, 1937. (I removed a term that would now be considered inappropriate from this quote, but I wanted to use the quote)

[280] Bieler, H. *Food is Your Best Medicine*, 25.

[281] Fenske, Richard A., and others, *Environmental Health Perspectives*, Vol. 108, No. 6 (Jun., 2000), 515-520

[282] Fallon, S. *Nourishing Traditions*, 599.

[283] Ibid., 13-14.

[284] Ibid., 468-469.

[285] *Confused about Soy? Soy Dangers Summarized*, Weston A. Price Foundation, http://www.westonaprice.org/soy/index.html.

[286] Fallon, *Nourishing Traditions,* 51.

[287] *Ingredients of Vaccines - Fact Sheet,* Centers For Disease Control, http://www.cdc.gov/vaccines/vacgen/additives.htm

[288] Bieler, *Food is Your Best Medicine*, 202.

[289] *Radiation Ovens: The Proven Dangers Of Microwaves,* http://www.ecclesia.org/forum/uploads/bondservant/microwaveP.pdf

[290] Adapted from: *Dietary Dangers,* Weston A. Price Foundation http://www.westonaprice.org/basicnutrition/dietdangers.html

[291] Ibid., 397.

[292] Weschler, T. *Taking Charge of Your Fertility*. New York: Harper Collins, 2002:42.

[293] Buttram, H. *Our Toxic World*: *Who is Looking After Our Kids?,* http://www.healing.org/Child-chap%201.html

[294] Price, W.A., "New Light Obtained on Dental Caries," *Dental Cosmos, a Monthly Record of Dental Science."* Vol. 78:858, http://www.hti.umich.edu/d/dencos/

[295] Price, W.A. 7 Teaching Lessons. "Light From Primitive Races On Modern Degeneration, 4. Facial Beatuy Lost In One Generation and Greater Injury to Later Born Children," La Mesa: Price-Pottenger Nutrition Foundation 2006: 2.

[296] Price, W. *Nutrition and Physical Degeneration,* 8th Ed. La Mesa: Price-Pottenger Nutrition Foundation; 2008: 275.

[297] Price, W. *Nutrition and Physical Degeneration.* 8th Ed., 274

[298] Ibid., 308

[299] Ibid., 363.

[300] Ibid., 414.

[301] Price, W.A., "New Light Obtained on Dental Caries," 858

[302] Price, W. *Nutrition and Physical Degeneration.* 6th Ed., 324, cited in Brown, G., *Melanesians and Polynesians*. London: Macmillan, 1910.

[303] Ibid., 323 cited in Baden, G. T., *Among the Ibos of Nigeria*. Philadelphia: Lippincott, 1921.

[304] Ibid,. 323 cited in Wiffen, T., *North-West Amazons*. N. Y: Duffield, 1915.

[305] Ibid., 398

[306] Ibid., 398.

[307] Foresight, http://www.foresight-preconception.org.uk/

[308] Ibid., 403

[309] Ibid., 403.

[310] Fallon, S. *Nourishing Traditions*., Washington, DC: New Trends, 1999:235. from Health Freedom News

[311] Vonderplanitz, A. *We Want To Live,* 2005 Ed. Los Angeles: Carnelian Bay Castle Press, 2005:278.

[312] Bieler, H. *Dr. Bieler's Natural Way to Sexual Health.* New York: Bantam Books, 1972: 206.

[313] Bieler, H. *Food is Your Best Medicine.* New York: Vintage Books, 1965: 172.

[314] Price, "New Light Obtained on Dental Caries," 858.

[315] I cannot give an even approximate figure, but I suggest eating more than we currently are

[316] Fallon, S. *Nourishing Traditions.* Washington, DC: New Trends; 1999:598.

[317] Price, *Nutrition and Physical Degeneration*, 6th Ed. 401.

[318] Price, W.A. 7 Teaching Lessons. "Light From Primitive Races On Modern Degeneration, 7. Special Foods of Primitives for Parents-to-be and Race Regeneration," La Mesa: Price-Pottenger Nutrition Foundation 2006: Slide 23.

[319] Fallon, S. and Enig, M., *Vitamin B12: Vital Nutrient for Good Health*, Weston A. Price Foundation, http://www.westonaprice.org/basicnutrition/vitaminb12.html,

[320] Ibid.

[321] Buttram, H. *For Tomorrow's Children.* Blooming Glen: Preconception Care Inc; 1990:172-173.

[322] Ibid., 172.

[323] Crewe, J.R., *Real Milk Cures Many Disease,* http://www.realmilk.com/milkcure.html

[324] Bieler, *Food is Your Best Medicine,* 183.

[325] Vonderplanitz, A. *Recipe for Living Without Disease,* Santa Monica: Carnelian Bay Castle Press, 2002:10.

[326] Price, *Nutrition and Physical Degeneration,* 6th Ed. 107.

[327] Christopher, J., *Herbal Home Health Care.* Springville: Christopher Publications, 1976:84.

[328] Ibid.

[329] Ibid.

[330] Bieler, *Dr. Bieler's Natural Way to Sexual Health,* 12-14.

[331] Ibid.

[332] Judd, G., *Good Teeth Birth to Death,* Glendale: Research Publications, 1997: 39.

[333] Hirzy, W., "Why EPA's Headquarters Professionals' Union Opposes Fluoridation," May 1, 1999. Fluoride Action Network, May 1, 1999, http://fluoridealert.org/hp-epa.htm.

[334] Buttram, *For Tomorrow's Children,* 43.

[335] Ibid., 44.

[336] Ibid.

[337] Garrison, K., *What's In Your Nail Polish and Shampoo? The safety of cosmetics & personal care products.* http://www.ema-online.org/greenlight_2004_fall_personal_care_products.htm,

[338] Buttram, *For Tomorrow's Children,* 113.

[339] *Mercury Free and Healthy,* DAMS Inc, http://www.amalgam.org/#anchor67472

[340] Buttram, *For Tomorrow's Children,* 171.

[341] Ibid., 172.

[342] Ibid., 90.

[343] Ibid., 122.

[344] Singer, K., *Rethinking Reproductive Health,* http://www.westonaprice.org/women/reprod-health.html

[345] Buttram, *For Tomorrow's Children,* 175

[346] Nagda, B.L., "Tribal Population And Health In Rajasthan," Population Research Center, Mohanlai Sukhadia University, India, http://www.krepublishers.com/02-Journals/T%20&%20T/T%20&%20T-02-0-000-000-2004-Web/T%20&%20T-02-0-001-076-2004-Abst-PDF/T%20&%20T-02-1-001-008-2004-Nagda-001/T%20&%20T-02-1-001-008-2004-Nagda.PDF

[347] Campbell-McBride, N., *Gut and Psychology Syndrome,* United Kigndom: Medinform Publishing, 1994:31.

[348] Ibid., 32.

[349] Buttram, *For Tomorrow's Children,* 131.

[350] Ibid., 133.

[351] Ibid., 135.

[352] "Stop the Indiscriminate Spraying of 'Friendly Fire' Pesticides," An Open Letter by Concerned Physician and Scientists Page 4.

[353] Glenville, M., *Health Professionals' Guide to Preconception Care,* Foresight, http://www.foresight-preconception.org.uk/booklet_healthproguide.htm.

[354] Buttram, *For Tomorrow's Children,* 121.

[355] Glenville, *Health Professionals' Guide to Preconception Care,*

[356] Matthews, R., *Ultrasound Scans Linked to Brain Damage in Babies,* http://www.mercola.com/2001/dec/19/ultrasound.htm,

[357] BMJ, 17 July 1993 and BMJ, 3 July 1993,, Quotation from BMJ, July 3rd, http://www.foresight-preconception.org.uk/booklet_prepforpreg.htm,

[358] Ibid.,

[359] Klotter, J. *Cesarean Deliveries,* Townsend Shorts, Townsend Letter for Doctors and Patients, http://www.townsendletter.com/Nov2006/shorts1106.htm,

[360] Ibid.

[361] Glenville, *Health Professionals' Guide to Preconception Care*

[362] Pierrakos, E., Pathwork Guide Lecture 101: The Defense., International Pathwork Foundation, http://www.pathwork.org/lecturesObtaining.html.

[363] Pierrakos, E., Pathwork Guide Lecture 17: The Call – Daily Review, International Pathwork Foundation, http://www.pathwork.org/lecturesObtaining.html

[364] Pierrakos, E., Pathwork Guide Lecture 14: The Higher Self, The Lower Self and the Mask, International Pathwork Foundation, http://www.pathwork.org/lecturesObtaining.html

[365] Pierrakos, E., Pathwork Guide Lecture 83: The Idealized Self-Image, International Pathwork Foundation, http://www.pathwork.org/lecturesObtaining.html

[366] Weschler, T., *Taking Charge of Your Fertility.* New York: Harper Collins, 2002:XIX.

[367] Ibid., 4.

[368] Singer, K., *Fertility Awareness, Food, and Night-Lighting,* Weston A Price Foundation, http://www.westonaprice.org/women/fertility.html

[369] Weschler, *Taking Charge of Your Fertility,* 50.

[370] Ibid., 57.

371 Ibid., 355.

372 *Protective effect of a thermoreversible gel against the toxicity of nonoxynol-9*, Center for National Scientific, http://cat.inist.fr/?aModele=afficheN&cpsidt=1701663

373 Weschler, *Taking Charge of Your Fertility*, 354.

374 Ibid., 350.

375 *Surveillance for Pregnancy and Birth Rates Among Teenagers*, by State, Centers for Disease Control, United States, 1980 and 1990, http://www.cdc.gov/mmwr/preview/mmwrhtml/000315 62.htm#00000536.htm,

376 Ibid.

377 *Teenagers in the United States: Sexual Activity, Contraceptive Use, and Childbearing, 2002*, Centers for Disease Control, http://www.cdc.gov/nchs/data/series/sr_23/sr23_024Fac tSheet.pdf.

378 Pierrakos, E., Pathwork Guide Lecture 34: Preparation for Reincarnation, International Pathwork Foundation http://www.pathwork.org/lecturesObtaining.html

379 Ibid.

380 Eckhart, T. The Power of Now, New World Library; 1997.

381 Eckhart, T. The True Nature of Space and Time The Power of Now, New World Library; 1997.

382 Price, W. *Nutrition and Physical Degeneration*. La Mesa: Price-Pottenger Nutrition Foundation; 2004: 398.

383 Ibid., 398.

384 Ibid., 83-84. Birth of Canadian Indians near Brantford, Ontario.

385 Ibid., 336.

386 Price, W.A. Dental Cosmos, a Monthly Record of Dental Science. "New Light Obtained on Dental Caries" Vol. 78:861 Available At: http://www.hti.umich.edu/d/dencos/. Accessed February 27, 2007.

387 Ibid., 334-335.

388 Ibid., 403.

389 Vaughan, K.O. *Safe childbirth: the three essentials*. London: Baillière, Tindall and Cox, 1937.

390 Price, W. *Nutrition and Physical Degeneration 6th Edition*. La Mesa: Price-Pottenger Nutrition Foundation; 2004: 412.

391 Tully, G. What to Do in Pregnancy Spinning Babies.http://www.spinningbabies.com/index.php?option= com_content&task=category&sectionid=1&id=1&Itemi d=2

392 Ibid., 413.

393 Price, W. *Nutrition and Physical Degeneration*. La Mesa: Price-Pottenger Nutrition Foundation; 2004: 315.

394 Ibid., 365.

395 Tully, G. Will Baby Fit? Spinning Babies. http://www.spinningbabies.com/index.php?option=com _content&view=article&id=76:will-baby-fit- &catid=35:to-do-in-labor&Itemid=2

396 Ibid., 379.

397 Tully, G. Activities to help a fetus into a good starting position before labor , Spinning Babies http://www.spinningbabies.com/index.php?option=com _content&task=category&sectionid=1&id=1&Itemid=2 (link may not go to exact page)

398 Ibid.,

399 Will Baby Fit, http://www.spinningbabies.com/index.php?option=com _content&task=view&id=33&Itemid=32

400 Batt, M. Natural Prenatal Care & Childbirth Education, Unpublished, 14.

401 Price, W. *Nutrition and Physical Degeneration*. La Mesa: Price-Pottenger Nutrition Foundation; 2004: 411.

402 Bieler, H. *Dr. Bieler's Natural Way to Sexual Health*. New York, Bantam Books: 1972: 18-19.

403 Ibid.,

404 Ibid.,

405 Vonderplanitz, A. *We Want To Live, 2005 Edition*. Carnelian Bay Castle Press, Los Angeles; 2005:328.

406 Vonderplanitz, A. *Recipe for Living Without Disease*. Santa Monica; Carnelian Bay Castle Press; 2002:146.

407 Vonderplanitz, A. E-mail Eonversation, pain reducing formula

408 Sullivan, K. Great Pains: Tips for Having an Easy Childbirth, Weston A Price Foundation. Available At: http://www.westonaprice.org/women/great_pains.html Accessed March 28.2007.

409 Obermeyer, C. *Cultural Perspectives on Reproductive Health*. Oxford University Press, 2001: 51.

410 Bieler, H. *Dr. Bieler's Natural Way to Sexual Health*. New York, Bantam Books: 1972: 18.

411 Bieler, H. *Dr. Bieler's Natural Way to Sexual Health*. New York, Bantam Books: 1972:19

412 Ibid., 18.

413 Fallon, S. Enig, M. Inside Japan: Surprising Facts About Japanese Foodways, Weston A Price Foundation, Available At: http://www.westonaprice.org/traditional_diets/japan.ht ml Accessed March 28, 2007.

414 Ibid.

415 Price, W. *Nutrition and Physical Degeneration*. La Mesa: Price-Pottenger Nutrition Foundation; 2004: 407-408.

416 Ibid., 408.

[417] Ibid., 408.

[418] Johnson, K. Daviss, B. "*Outcomes of planned home birth with certified professional midwives: large prospective study in North America.*" British Medical Journal, 2005;330:1416 (18 June).

[419] "*Midwifery care, social and medical risk factors, and birth outcomes in the USA. MacDorman MF, Singh GK. J Epidemiol Community Health 1998 May;52(5):310-7.* Available At: http://www.garynull.com/Documents/Iatrogenic/Wome n/Pregnancy.htm, Accessed March 28,2007.

[420] *Mothering the Mother* by Klaus, Kennel, and Klaus, Da Capo Press 1993.

[421] "Supportive nurse-midwife care is associated with a reduced incidence of Cesarean section. Butler J, Abrams B, Parker J, Roberts JM, Laros RK Jr. Am J Obstet Gynecol 1993 May;168(5):1407-13. Available At: http://www.garynull.com/Documents/Iatrogenic/Wome n/Pregnancy.htm, Accessed March 28,2007.

[422] Null, G. Dean, C. Feldman, M. Rasio, D. Death by Medicine, *Life Extension.* March, 2004: Available At: http://www.lef.org/magazine/mag2004/mar2004_awsi_ death_01.htm, More Research, Iatrogenic Illness, Available At: http://www.garynull.com/Documents/Iatrogenic/latroge nic_index.htm. Accessed Jan, 19, 2007.

[423] Mehl-Maddrona, L. Medical Risks of Epidural Anesthesia During Childbirth. http://www.healing-arts.org/mehl-madrona/mmepidural.htm.

[424] Klotter, J. Cesarean Delivery, Townsend Letter for Doctors and Patients, Available At: http://www.townsendletter.com/Nov2006/shorts1106.ht m, Accessed July 1, 2007.

[425] *Source: Cesarean section: medical benefits and costs. Shearer EL. Soc Sci Med 1993 Nov;37(10):1223-31, Referenced from Gary Null's Health Website,* http://www.garynull.com/Documents/Iatrogenic/Wome n/Pregnancy.htm

[426] *Source: Cesarean section: medical benefits and costs. Shearer EL. Soc Sci Med 1993 Nov;37(10):1223-31, Referenced from Gary Null's Health Website,* http://www.garynull.com/Documents/Iatrogenic/Wome n/Pregnancy.htm

[427] *Obstet Gynecol.* 2000;95:589-595

[428] Gifford, D. "Lack of Progress in Labor" Obstetrics and Gynecology, Available At: http://www.greenjournal.org/cgi/content/full/95/4/589, Accessed July 1, 2007.

[429] Cesarean, A Life Saver, Not a Lifestyle, http://www.spinningbabies.com/index.php?option=com _content&task=view&id=19&Itemid=32

[430] Online at, http://www.blackwell-synergy.com/doi/abs/10.1111/j.1523-536X.2006.00102.x, *BIRTH 33:3 September 2006)*

[431] Vonderplanitz, A. *We Want To Live, 2005 Edition.* Carnelian Bay Castle Press, Los Angeles; 2005:329.

[432] *Source: Cesarean section: medical benefits and costs. Shearer EL. Soc Sci Med 1993 Nov;37(10):1223-31, Referenced from Gary Null's Health Website,* http://www.garynull.com/Documents/Iatrogenic/Wome n/Pregnancy.htm.

[433] International Pathwork Foundation. Pierrakos E, Pathwork Guide Lecture 140, Conflict of Positive Versus Negative Oriented Pleasure as the Origin of Pain. Available At: http://www.pathwork.org/lecturesObtaining.html. (unedited)Accessed February 27, 2007.

[434] International Pathwork Foundation. Pierrakos E, Pathwork Guide Lecture 140, Conflict of Positive Versus Negative Oriented Pleasure as the Origin of Pain. Available At: http://www.pathwork.org/lecturesObtaining.html. Accessed February 27, 2007.

[435] Max, J. Interview with Eckhart Tolle, Available At: http://themaxes.blogspot.com/2005/11/interview-with-eckhart-tolle.html, Accessed March 28, 2007.

[436] International Pathwork Foundation. Pierrakos E, Pathwork Guide Lecture 23,Questions and Answers, vailable At: http://www.pathwork.org/lecturesObtaining.html. Accessed February 27, 2007.PGL 23

[437] Romm, A. *Natural Health After Birth: The Complete Guide to Postpartum Wellness*, Healing Arts Press; 2002.

[438] Bauer, I. *Diaper Free:The Gentle Wisdom of Natural Infant Hygiene.* Natural Wisdom Press, Saltspring Island: 2001:211.

[439] Pierrakos, E., International Pathwork Foundation, Pathwork Guide Lecture 134, The Concept of Evil. http://www.pathwork.org/lecturesObtaining.html.

[440] Pierrakos, E., International Pathwork Foundation, Pathwork Guide Lecture 255, The Birth Process – Cosmic Pulse. http://www.pathwork.org/lecturesObtaining.html.

[441] Bert Hellinger, How Love Works, http://www.hellinger.com/international/english/hellin-ger_lectures_articles/how_love_works.shtml

[442] Eckhart, T., The Power of Now. New World Library, 1997.

[443] Pierrakos, E., International Pathwork Foundation. Pathwork Guide Lecture 73, Compulsion to Recreate and Overcome Childhood Hurts, http://www.pathwork.org/lecturesObtaining.html.

[444] Pierrakos, E., International Pathwork Foundation, Pathwork Guide Lecture 207, The Spiritual Symbolism and Significance of Sexuality. http://www.pathwork.org/lecturesObtaining.html.

[445] The Liedloff Society for the Continuum Concept, http://www.continuum-concept.org/cc_defined.html

[446] Price, W. *Nutrition and Physical Degeneration.* 6th Ed. La Mesa: Price-Pottenger Nutrition Foundation; 2004: 399.

[447] Pierrakos, E., International Pathwork Foundation. Pathwork Guide Lecture 192, Real and False Needs. http://www.pathwork.org/lecturesObtaining.html.

[448] The Liedloff Society for the Continuum Concept

[449] Ibid.

[450] Stuart-Macadam, P., and Dettwyler, K., *Breastfeeding Bicultural Perspectives*, Aldine Transaction; 1995: 43. Excerpted from Clellan Ford, Human Relations Area Files (Ford, 1964:78-79)

[151] Ibid., 49.

[452] Price, W. *Nutrition and Physical Degeneration.* 6th Ed: 65.

[453] Stuart-Macadam, P., and Dettwyler, K., *Breastfeeding Bicultural Perspectives*: 4

[454] Ellis, H., *Studies in the Psychology of Sex.* http://www.psyplexus.com/ellis/78.htm .

[455] Palmer, B., The Importance of Breastfeeding as it Relates to Total Health. http://www.brianpalmerdds.com/bfing_import.htm

[456] Price, W., *Nutrition and Physical Degeneration.* 6th Ed :182-183.

[457] Christopher, J., *School of Natural Healing.* Christopher Publications, Springville; 1976:xxii.

[458] Collins, H., "Indian feeding cup may help babies learn to breast-feed." Milwaukee Journal Sentinel, May 30, 1999, http://findarticles.com/p/articles/mi_qn4196/is_19990530/ai_n10522551

[459] Pierrakos, E., International Pathwork Foundation. Pathwork Guide Lecture 17, Spiritual Laws. http://www.pathwork.org/lecturesObtaining.html.

[460] Pierrakos, E., International Pathwork Foundation. Pathwork Guide Lecture 169 The Masculine and Feminine Principles in the Creative Process. http://www.pathwork.org/lecturesObtaining.html.

[461] Ibid.

[462] Ibid.

[163] Ibid.

[464] Bauer, I., Natural Infant Hygiene - A Gentle Alternative to Long-Term Diapering. Gentle Parents. http://www.gentleparents.com/bauer.html,

[465] Bauer, I., Diaper Free. The Gentle Wisdom of Natural Infant Hygiene, http://www.natural-wisdom.com/,

[466] Pierrakos, E., International Pathwork Foundation. Pathwork Guide Lecture 119, Movement, Consciousness, Experience: Pleasure, the Essence of Life. http://www.pathwork.org/lecturesObtaining.html.

[467] Ibid.

[468] Ibid.

[469] Ibid.

[470] Ibid.

[471] Circumcision Resource Center, Summary of General Circumcision Information, http://www.circumcision.org/information.htm, Accessed April 9, 2007.

[472] Goldman, R. Questioning Circumcision, A Jewish Perspective, http://www.jewishcircumcision.org/book.htm, Accessed April 9, 2007.

[473] ⎯⎯⎯

[474] Amma, Embracing the World, Available At: http://www.amma.org,

[475] Price, W. *Nutrition and Physical Degeneration,* 6th Ed.: 170.

[476] Pierrakos, E., International Pathwork Foundation. Pathwork Guide Lecture 204, What is the Path? http://www.pathwork.org/lecturesObtaining.html.

[477] Pierrakos, E., International Pathwork Foundation. Pathwork Guide Lecture 191, Inner and Outer Experience. http://www.pathwork.org/lecturesObtaining.html.

[478] Thesenga, S. *The Undefended Self.* Pathwork Press; Delmar,1994:150.

[479] Pierrakos, E., International Pathwork Foundation. Pathwork Guide Lecture 145, Responding to the Call of Life. http://www.pathwork.org/lecturesObtaining.html.

[480] Pierrakos, E.,International Pathwork Foundation. Pathwork Guide Lecture 160, Conciliation of the Inner Split. http://www.pathwork.org/lecturesObtaining.html.

[481] Pierrakos, E., and Thesenga, D., *Fear No Evil* Pathwork Press, Madison, 1993:139.

[482] Ibid., 140, 141

[483] Pierrakos, E., International Pathwork Foundation., Pathwork Guide Lecture 154, Pulsation of Consciousness. http://www.pathwork.org/lecturesObtaining.html.

[484] Pierrakos, E., International Pathwork Foundation. Pathwork Guide Lecture 197, Energy and Consciousness in Distortion, Evil. http://www.pathwork.org/lecturesObtaining.html.

[485] Ibid.

[486] Pierrakos, E., International Pathwork Foundation. Pathwork Guide Lecture 248, THREE PRINCIPLES OF THE FORCES OF EVIL; PERSONIFICATION OF EVIL. http://www.pathwork.org/lecturesObtaining.html.

[487] Rappoport, J., "Vaccine Dangers and Vested Interests" *Nexus Magazine*, Volume 13, Number 2 http://www.nexusmagazine.com/articles/VaccineResearcher.html,.

[488] http://en.wikipedia.org/wiki/Koch's_postulates

[489] http://www.neue-medizin.com/lanka2.htm

[490] http://www.klein-klein-aktion.de/contents/Bird_Flu/bird_flu.html

[491] http://en.wikipedia.org/wiki/Plural_of_virus

[492] Bieler, H. *Food is Your Best Medicine*. New York: Vintage Books, 1965: 40.

[493] Tilden, J. *Toxemia Explained*. Denver: 1926: 19

[494] Buttram, H., Letter to British Medical Journal, October 4, 2004. http://www.bmj.com/cgi/eletters/325/7373/1134/a, Reference from Whale. http://www.whale.to/a/buttram9.html

[495] Incao, P., Hepatitis B Vaccination Testimony in Ohio, March 1, 1999, http://www.whale.to/m/incao.html

[496] Rappoport, J. "Vaccine Dangers and Vested Interests" *Nexus Magazine*.

[497] Ibid.

[498] Ibid.

[499] Francis, R. "What About Vaccinations." Beyond Health, http://www.beyondhealth.com/Articles/vaccinations.asp

[500] Journal of the American Medical Association July 3, 1926, p.45, www.deathbyvaccination.com

[501] Ibid.

[502] VAERS Reports, Whale, http://whale.to/v/vaers_reports.html

[503] Ibid.

[504] Bernardini, R. *The Truth About Children's Health*. Clifford, PRI Publishing, 2003:249.

[505] Morbidity and Mortality Weekly Report, Surveillance Summaries, January 24, 2003, Vol. 52 No.SS-1 CDC, http://www.cdc.gov/mmwr/PDF/ss/ss5201.pdf

[506] Kessler JAMA 1993

[507] Surveillance for Safety After Immunization: Vaccine Adverse Event Reporting System (VAERS) --- United States, 1991—2001, CDC. http://www.cdc.gov/MMWR/preview/mmwrhtml/ss5201a1.htm

[508] Ibid.

[509] Vaccine-Preventable Diseases and Specific Vaccines CDC. http://www.cdc.gov/node.do/id/0900f3ec8005df1f

[510] Some information hiding and Supression has been documented in *Deadly Immunity* by Robert Kennedy http://www.rollingstone.com/politics/story/7395411/deadly_immunity/,

[511] Chickenpox from 1894-2000. Whale, http://www.whale.to/v/chicken1.html,

[512] MMWR Weekly, May 28, 1999, Prevention of Varicella Updated Recommendations of the Advisory Committee on Immunization Practices (ACIP), http://www.cdc.gov/mmwR/preview/mmwrhtml/rr4806a1.htm,

[513] Romm, A., *Vaccinations, A thoughtful Parent's Guide*. Rochester; Healing Arts Press; 201:67.

[514] Thompson, J., "Should I Vaccinate My Child?" *Well Being Journal*, http://www.wellbeingjournal.com/index.php?option=com_content&task=view&id=34&Itemid=58,

[515] Flu vaccination quotes, Whale, http://www.whale.to/v/quotes3.html,

[516] Tilden, J.H., *Children Their Health And Happiness*, http://www.whale.to/a/tilden3.html,

[517] Francis, R., "What About Vaccinations." *Beyond Health*, http://www.beyondhealth.com/Articles/vaccinations.asp

[518] National Vital Statistics Reports, Volume 52, Number 3, September 18, 2003, On Table 10. page 31. http://www.cdc.gov/nchs/data/nvsr/nvsr52/nvsr52_03.pdf,

[519] http://www.medalerts.org, (Search 2002: death - yes)

[520] Romm, A. *Vaccinations, A thoughtful Parent's Guide*: 59.

[521] Measles. Whale, http://www.whale.to/vaccines/measles.html,

[522] Thompson, J., "Should I Vaccinate My Child?" *Well Being Journal*

[523] Bieler, H. *Food is Your Best Medicine*. New York: Vintage Books, 1965: 104.

[524] *The Vaccine Reaction*, National Vaccine Information Center, http://www.apfn.org/apfn/vaccine.htm,

[525] Ibid.

[526] Letter to the editor of The Sheridan Press, Sheridan, WY, Vaccine Liberation Information, http://www.vaclib.org/chapter/wypress.htm,

[527] *Hepatitis B, the Untold Story*, 909 Shot, http://www.909shot.com/Diseases/hepbnlr.htm,

[528] Francis, R. "What About Vaccinations." *Beyond Health*,

[529] Bieler, H. *Food is Your Best Medicine*: 47.

[530] The U.S. Government's VAERS Database, http://www.medalerts.org, (Search Terms: Hib & 2005 & Died).

531 Romm, A. *Vaccinations, A thoughtful Parent's Guide.* Rochester: 63.
532 Bieler, H. *Food is Your Best Medicine*: 195.
533 West, J., *Polio in the United States* http://www.geocities.com/harpub/pol_all.htm.
534 Francis, R. "What About Vaccinations." *Beyond Health*
535 Nkuba, K. *Polio vaccine genocide in Uganda.* Whale, http://www.whale.to/a/nkuba.htm.
536 Romm, A. *Vaccinations, A thoughtful Parent's Guide*: 65.
537 Ibid.
538 Rubella Quotes, Whale, http://www.whale.to/v/rubella9.html.
539 Kalokerinos, A. and Dettman, G. "Does Rubella Vaccination Protect?" *Australian Nurses Journal*, reprinted in *The Dangers of Immunization* page 54, Whale, http://www.whale.to/v/rubella9.html
540 Thompson, J. "Should I Vaccinate My Child?" *Well Being Journal.*
541 The U.S. Government's VAERS Database, http://www.medalerts.org, (Search Terms: MMR & 2005).
542 Thompson, J. "Should I Vaccinate My Child?" *Well Being Journal.*
543 Romm, A. *Vaccinations, A thoughtful Parent's Guide*: 12.
544 Ibid., 74.
545 Petek-Dimmer, A. *Does systematic Vaccination give health to people?* Aegis Switzerland. http://www.whale.to/a/petek.html.
546 American Life League, Whale, http://www.whale.to/vaccines/tetanus18.html.
547 Petek-Dimmer, A. *Does systematic Vaccination give health to people?* Aegis Switzerland.
548 Francis, R. "What About Vaccinations." *Beyond Health.*
549 Romm, A. *Vaccinations, A thoughtful Parent's Guide*: 71.
550 Thompson, J. "Should I Vaccinate My Child?" *Well Being Journal,*
551 Mendesohn, R. *The Medical Time Bomb of Immunization Against Disease, The greatest threat of childhood diseases lies in the dangerous and ineffectual efforts made to prevent them,* Whale. http://www.whale.to/vaccines/mendelsohn.html#WHOOPING%20COUGH.
552 Thompson, J. "Should I Vaccinate My Child?" *Well Being Journal.*
553 *Vaccine Side Effects*, CDC. http://www.cdc.gov/nip/vaccine/side-effects.htm.
554 *Surveillance for Safety After Immunization: Vaccine Adverse Event Reporting System (VAERS)* --- United States, 1991—2001, CDC, http://www.cdc.gov/MMWR/preview/mmwrhtml/ss5201a1.htm.
555 Rappoport, J. "Vaccine Dangers and Vested Interests" *Nexus Magazine*
556 Fisher, L. *Opening Statement, Vaccine Safety Forum at the Institute of Medicine*, May 13, 1996. http://www.909shot.com/Loe_Fisher/blfrighttoinformed.htm.
557 Price, W.A. "Contributing Factors to the Degenerative Diseases" *Dental Cosmos, A Monthly Record of Dental Science*. Vol. 72:1123. http://www.hti.umich.edu/d/dencos/.
558 Price, W. *Nutrition and Physical Degeneration*, 6th Ed. La Mesa: Price-Pottenger Nutrition Foundation; 2004:190.
559 Price, W.A. "New Light Obtained on Dental Caries" *Dental Cosmos, a Monthly Record of Dental Science* Vol. 78:859. http://www.hti.umich.edu/d/dencos/.
560 Thompson, J. "Should I Vaccinate My Child?" *Well Being Journal*
561 *Vaccination Hoax*, Whale. http://www.whale.to/a/hoax.html#6.%20%20Contaminants.
562 Di. Fabio, A. "Universal Oral Vaccine: The Immune Milk Saga!" *Townsend Letter for Doctor's and Patients.* http://www.tldp.com/ & http://www.tldp.com/New%20Articles/Universal%20oral%20vaccine%20Part%201.htm.
563 Vonderplanitz, A., *We Want To Live,* 2005 Ed. Carnelian Bay Castle Press, Los Angeles; 2005:319.
564 Howenstine, J. "Vaccines Cause Cancer" Letter to the Editor. *Townsend Letter for Doctors and Patients*, Feb-March, 2004 http://findarticles.com/p/articles/mi_m0ISW/is_247-248/ai_113807035,
565 *Cancer*, Think Twice Global Vaccine Institute. http://thinktwice.com/s_cancer.htm.
566 *Vaccines Cause Immune Supression* Mercola.Com http://www.mercola.com/article/vaccines/immune_suppression.htm.
567 Ibid.
568 *Nobel Winner: Aids a WMD*, News 24, http://www.news24.com/News24/Africa/News/0,,2-11-1447_1602547,00.html.
569 *AIDS*, Animal Research Takes Lives, http://www.health.org.nz/aids2.html.
570 *AIDS,* Think Twice Global Vaccine Institute, http://thinktwice.com/s_aids.htm.

[571] Kalokerinos, A. "Dr Archie Kalokerinos MBBS PhD FAPM." *International Vaccine Newsletter,* June 1995. Whale, http://whale.to/vaccines/kalokerinos.html.
[572] Bishop, D. "The Dirty Needle Scam." Whale, http://whale.to/v/needle.html.
[573] Ibid.
[574] Pierrakos, E., Pathwork Guide Lecture 244, *Be In the World But Not Of the World, The Evil of Inertia,* International Pathwork Foundation, http://www.pathwork.org/lecturesObtaining.html.
[575] Ibid.
[576] Ibid.
[577] U.S. Department of Justice - Office of Justice Programs Bureau of Justice Statistics, Correctional Surveys, http://www.ojp.usdoj.gov/bjs/glance/tables/corr2tab.htm
[578] Walmsley, R. *World Prison Population List* (fourth edition), http://www.homeoffice.gov.uk/rds/pdfs2/r188.pdf.
[579] Montessori, M., *The Montessori Method*, trans. George, A. New York: Frederick A. Stocks Company 1912:1-27.
[580] Ibid.
[581] Bryson, C., and Griffiths, J., *Flouride, Teeth, and the Atomic Bomb,* Flouride Action Network, http://www.fluoridealert.org/WN-414.htm.
[582] Ibid. 26.
[583] Scharzer, D., and Conrad, L., and Braynt, E., "The Legality of Homeschooling: Complying with California Law," *Home School Association of California,* http://www.hsc.org/chaos/legal/compulsory_attendance.php.
[584] Farris, M. "Has America Abandoned Parental Rights?" *The Home School Court Report,* July/August 2006. http://www.hslda.org/courtreport/V22N4/V22N401.asp.
[585] "Our History," *Home School Legal Defense Fund.* http://www.hslda.org/about/history.asp.
[586] Walker, C. "Waking Up To The Holographic Heart, Staring Over With Education" *Wild Duck Review,* http://www.ratical.org/many_worlds/JCP98.html.
[587] Ibid., 224.
[588] Pierrakos, E., Pathwork Guide Lecture 174, Self-Esteem, International Pathwork Foundation. http://www.pathwork.org/lecturesObtaining.html.
[589] Pierrakos, E., Pathwork Guide Lecture 49, Obstacles on the Path: Old Stuff, Wrong Guild, and Who, Me? International Pathwork Foundation, http://www.pathwork.org/lecturesObtaining.html.
[590] Price, W. *Nutrition and Physical Degeneration. 6th* Ed: 353.
[591] Price, W. *Nutrition and Physical Degeneration. 6th* Ed: 360, 362.
[592] Ibid., 359.
[593] Ibid., 488.
[594] Jensen, B., *Dr. Jensen's Guide to Better Bowel Care.* New York: Avery; 1999: 38.
[595] Fallon, S., *Nourishing Traditions*, Washington, DC: New Trends, 1999: 601.
[596] Bieler, H., *Food is Your Best Medicine.* New York: Vintage Books, 1965: 198.
[597] Allbriton, J. *Growing Wise Kids, Nourishing a Growing Baby,* Weston A. Price Foundation, http://www.westonaprice.org/children/nourish-baby.html.
[598] Ibid.
[599] Nagel, R., *Cure Tooth Decay: Heal and Prevent Cavities With Nutrition.* Golden Child Publishing, 2009.
[600] Price, W. A. "Why Dental Caries With Modern Civilizations? IX. Field Studies Among Primitive Indians in Northern Canada," *Dental Digest,* 1934 April; 131.
[601] Ibid.
[602] Fallon, S., *Nourishing Traditions*: 600.
[603] Price, W.A., "Light From Primitive Races On Modern Degeneration: 2. How Primitive Races Have Prevented Tooth Decay," *7 Teaching Lessons* La Mesa: Price-Pottenger Nutrition Foundation 2006: Slide 19.
[604] Allbriton, J., *Growing Wise Kids, Nourishing a Growing Baby.*
[605] Fallon, S., and Enig, M., *Why Butter is Better*, Weston A. Price Foundation.
[606] Ibid.
[607] Ibid.
[608] Bieler, H. *Food is Your Best Medicine*: 198.
[609] Allbriton, J., *Growing Wise Kids, Nourishing a Growing Baby.*
[610] Bieler, H. *Food is Your Best Medicine*: 198.
[611] Price, W. *Nutrition and Physical Degeneration. 6th* Ed. La Mesa: Price-Pottenger Nutrition Foundation; 2004: 260.
[612] Price, W. *Nutrition and Physical Degeneration. 6th Ed*: 403.
[613] Ibid., 70.
[614] Price, W.A., "Light From Primitive Races On Modern Degeneration: 7. Special Foods of Primitives for Parents-to-be and Race Regeneration," *7 Teaching Lessons,* La Mesa: Price-Pottenger Nutrition Foundation 2006: Slide 21.
[615] Ibid., 401-402.
[616] Price, W.A., "South Sea Islanders and Florida Indians" *Dental Cosmos, a Monthly Record of Dental Science.* Vol. 77:1040, http://www.hti.umich.edu/d/dencos/.

[617] Price, W.A., "New Light Obtained on Dental Caries" *Dental Cosmos, a Monthly Record of Dental Science,* Vol. 78:858, http://www.hti.umich.edu/d/dencos/.

[618] Price, W. *Nutrition and Physical Degeneration.* 6th Ed:137.

[619] Ibid., 99.

[620] Price, W.A., "New Light Obtained on Dental Caries" Vol. 78:871.

[621] Price, W. *Nutrition and Physical Degeneration.* 6th Ed: 470.

[622] Price, W. *Nutrition and Physical Degeneration.* 6th Ed: 274.

[623] Ibid., 270-271.

[624] Price, W.A., "Light From Primitive Races On Modern Degeneration: 7. Special Foods of Primitives for Parents-to-be and Race Regeneration," *7 Teaching Lessons,* La Mesa: Price-Pottenger Nutrition Foundation 2006: Slide 3.

[625] Foresight, the Association for the Promotion of Preconceptual Care, http://www.foresight-preconception.org.uk/.

[626] Sprott, J., *Look at Cots to Isolate Possible Cause of SIDS* http://www.pnc.com.au/~cafmr/sprott/sids-gas.html.

[627] Ibid.

[628] Schetchikova, N., *Truth in Science: the Right to Know and the Freedom to Decide* –3rd International Public Conference on Vaccination. Whale, http://www.whale.to/a/pdf/vaccinations.pdf#search=%22hepatitis%22.

[629] Mehl-Madrona, L., Forum on Alternative and Innovative Therapies, http://www.healing-arts.org/children/index.htm.

[630] Ferrie, H., "Autism, Causes Known and Cures Possible," *Vitality*, May 2003, http://www.kospublishing.com/html/children.html.

[631] Olmsted, D., *The Age of Autism: The Amish Elephant* http://www.upi.com/archive/view.php?archive=1&StoryID=20051024-095736-4490r.

[632] Ellwood-Mielewski, D., *A Young Boy's Amazing Recovery From PDD and Autism-Like Symptoms*, Mercola.com, http://www.mercola.com/2004/apr/24/autism_recovery.htm.

[633] Fallon, S., *Nourishing Traditions:* 24.

[634] Christopher, J., *Herbal Home Health Care.* Springville: Christopher Publications, 1976: 113

[635] Price, W. *Nutrition and Physical Degeneration.* 6th Ed: 415.

[636] Ibid., 297.

[637] Riordan, H., *Overcoming Depression,* Orthomolecular.org, http://www.orthomolecular.org/library/articles/ocdepression.shtml.

[638] Bieler, H., *Dr. Bieler's Natural Way to Sexual Health,* New York, Bantam Books: 1972: 26.

[639] Buttram, H. *For Tomorrow's Children.* Blooming Glen, Preconception Care Inc., 1990:16.

[640] Ibid.

[641] Price, W., "New Light Obtained on Dental Caries" Vol. 78: 865.

[642] Price, W., *Nutrition and Physical Degeneration.* 6th Ed: 295.

[643] Conrad, D., *The Great American Tragedy,* quoted in Fallon, S. *Nourishing Traditions:* 301

[644] Ibid., 494.

[645] Silkman, R. *Is it Mental or is it Dental?-- Cranial & Dental Impacts on Total Health* http://www.westonaprice.org/healthissues/facial-development.html

[646] Buttram, H. *For Tomorrow's Children.* Blooming Glen, Preconception Care Inc; 1990:16.

[647] Christopher, J., *Herbal Home Health Care*: 1.

[648] Tilden, J., *Toxemia Explained.* Denver, 1926:13.

[649] Bieler, H. *Food is Your Best Medicine*: 39, 198.

[650] Ibid., 40.

[651] Ibid., 39.

[652] Ibid., 81.

[653] Bieler, H. *Food is Your Best Medicine.* New York: Vintage Books, 1965: 15.

[654] Bieler, H. *Dr. Bieler's Natural Way to Sexual Health*: 61.

[655] Ibid., 64.

[656] Pierrakos, E., International Pathwork Foundation., Pathwork Guide Lecture 250, INNER AWARENESS OF GRACE -- EXPOSING THE DEFICIT. http://www.pathwork.org/lecturesObtaining.html.

A

awareness, 7, 9, 40, 108, 128, 143, 144, 149, 150, 151, 177, 179, 183, 195, 214, 224, 225, 227, 231, 236, 238, 239, 240, 255, 257, 260, 265, 286, 288, 297, 317, 322, 330, 346, 354, 357
Azomite, 82, 100

B

babies, Bone marrow, 322, 324, 333
babies, Foods to avoid, 323
babies, special foods, 322
bacteria, 2, 4, 5, 10, 48, 97, 134, 135, 264, 275, 322, 339, 343, 345
bagels, 67, 83
barefoot, 127, 342, 343
Beaufort d'Alpage, 68
beef, 70, 81, 82, 85, 86, 87, 95, 96, 99, 100, 119, 123, 124, 126, 167, 319, 320, 326, 338
Being a Positive Role Model, iii, 257
belief system, 3, 2
Bernard Jensen, 125, 314, 355, 388
Beyond FAM
    SFAM, 153
Bioenergetics, 149, 356
birth, vii, 13, 14, 20, 29, 31, 48, 51, 52, 53, 58, 59, 66, 73, 75, 93, 94, 99, 103, 112, 117, 118, 119, 120, 121, 122, 124, 129, 131, 133, 134, 135, 137, 139, 140, 141, 144, 147, 149, 150, 151, 152, 153, 154, 157, 159, 160, 161, 162, 163, 164, 165, 166, 167, 168, 169, 170, 171, 172, 173, 174, 175, 176, 177, 179, 180, 181, 182, 185, 188, 190, 196, 202, 203, 205, 208, 213, 217, 232, 236, 237, 273, 281, 282, 320, 329, 331, 334, 336, 339, 340, 343, 347, 354, 355
Birth , A Child-Centered Birth, 180
birth control pills, 119, 120, 122, 124, 131, 134, 137, 150, 152, 153, 163, 177
Birth control pills, 124, 134
birth defects, 29, 31, 51, 52, 53, 58, 59, 66, 73, 93, 94, 112, 133, 139, 159, 172, 329, 334
Birth Defects a Response to the Environment, 58
Birth Defects and, 51
Birth Defects from Nutrient Deficiencies, 53
Birth Defects from the Father, 53
Birth Defects in Humans from Modern Foods, ii, 55
Birth Position, 166
Birth Scenario, modern, 173
birth, 5 days prior, 167
birth, diet, 166
birth, diet after, 167
birth, Preparing the Physical Body, 164
birth, rapid, 159, 160, 163
Birth, unassisted, iii, 173
biscuits, 67
Blame, iii
bloating, 11
blood sugar, 82, 84, 87, 98, 106, 107, 241, 327, 328, 340
bloodstream, 10, 124, 263, 267, 337

boasting civilization, 40, 46
body care products., 133
body chemistries, 59
body chemistry, 23, 84, 106, 140, 322, 328, 342, 355
Body Work, 166
bone broth, 82, 85, 280, 322
bone marrow, 81, 82, 85, 100, 126, 319, 322, 323, 324, 326
bone soup, 81
boundaries, 160, 189, 191, 218, 231, 256, 257, 302
brain, 11, 67, 69, 99, 117, 138, 140, 181, 196, 254, 269, 273, 276, 279, 284, 327, 335, 336, 337, 339, 341, 342, 354
bread, 17, 65, 68, 83, 98, 100, 103, 166, 208, 326, 333, 343
breakfast cereal, 46, 67, 71, 83, 103, 107, 321
breast feeding, 338
breastfeeding, 86, 173, 177, 183, 198, 199, 202, 210, 211, 212, 213, 231, 280, 321, 324, 335, 337, 338, 339
breastmilk, 75, 86, 88, 91, 106, 194, 197, 203, 211, 212, 219, 225, 251, 259, 320, 321, 323, 338, 341, 342, 343, 347
Breastmilk Alternative, 321
broccoli, 81, 96, 99
brotherhood, 59, 310, 349
butter, 15, 16, 17, 53, 68, 78, 80, 81, 82, 83, 85, 86, 87, 88, 89, 92, 93, 94, 95, 100, 101, 106, 108, 118, 122, 124, 125, 126, 127, 162, 167, 168, 235, 280, 281, 283, 299, 319, 320, 322, 323, 325, 326, 327, 328, 332, 333, 337, 341, 343
butter fat, 15, 16

C

cake, 46, 67, 107, 131
cakes, 67, 106
calcium, 17, 64, 65, 69, 72, 73, 79, 82, 95, 96, 97, 99, 101, 106, 107, 108, 325, 327, 333, 338, 341
calories, 64, 65, 66, 67, 68, 69, 84, 87, 89, 108, 121
Can You Hike Carrying 300 pounds?, 31
Canada Indians, 13, 14, 39, 64, 70, 80
candy, 67, 107, 138, 189, 304, 342
candy bars, 67, 107, 304, 342
Car Seats, iii, 232
carrots, 53, 81, 82, 100, 125, 126, 328
castor oil, 127
cattle, 53, 71, 91, 107
Cattle tribes in Africa, 118
Cause of Disease, 3, 1
cavities, 3, 19, 22, 23
celery, 81, 82, 86, 107, 109, 125, 126, 212, 323, 328
Centers for Disease Control, 44, 51, 97, 271, 276
Centers of Disease Control, 337
cereals, 71, 79, 82, 107, 108, 319, 333
Cesarean Delivery, iii, 174
Cesarean Delivery, preventing harm, 176

cheese, 15, 16, 17, 68, 78, 80, 81, 82, 83, 85, 87, 89, 93, 95, 96, 97, 107, 119, 124, 167, 323, 325, 326, 327, 328, 341
Chicken Pox, 3, 346
Child Spacing, 117
Children Want to participate and Be treated As Equals, 229
children's health, 346
Chinese medicine, 8, 9, 353
chocolate, 22, 46, 67, 69, 103, 299
cholesterol, 87, 88
Chromium, 99
cigarettes, 83, 121, 132
Circumcision, iii, 231
civilization, 10, 28, 47, 133, 312
clams, 68, 71, 78, 81, 85, 87, 94, 99, 100, 119, 123, 319, 325
Clay, 100
cleaning products, 131, 133
cleansing, 10, 63, 87, 90, 119, 120, 125, 128, 129, 131, 133, 137, 263, 280, 334, 340, 346, 353, 355
Cleansing and Healing, ii, 120, 124
clothing, 132, 141, 172, 218, 226, 255, 284
clubbed feet, 53, 57, 58
coconut oil, 81, 82, 83, 84, 85, 87, 88, 106, 127, 323, 327
Coconut Oil, 127
Coercion, 296
coffee, 19, 67, 100, 132
cold, 3, 87, 126, 128, 129, 144, 180, 188, 250, 274, 277, 297, 299, 342, 346
colds, 48, 272, 273, 321, 343
commercial foods, 46, 105, 321
Common Confusion, iii, 219
compassion, 1, 4, 5, 7, 15, 46, 48, 49, 64, 91, 131, 143, 150, 172, 179, 185, 191, 214, 216, 219, 222, 225, 227, 228, 236, 237, 246, 251, 260, 261, 279, 286, 297, 301, 309, 310, 317, 330, 342, 350
compressed, 24
conception, vii, viii, 24, 46, 52, 69, 75, 76, 79, 92, 95, 111, 112, 119, 122, 123, 126, 128, 134, 144, 150, 151, 153, 154, 159, 181, 334, 336
Concluding Words on the Disease Of, 59
Conclusion about Birth, iii, 182
consciousness, 3, 9, 11, 46, 47, 48, 49, 59, 128, 129, 150, 183, 191, 197, 199, 203, 232, 237, 248, 254, 257, 260, 261, 285, 289, 309, 311, 330
Consequence of Distorted Father Energies, 215
Continuum Concept, 202
Continuum of Care, 203
cookies, 67, 71, 83, 103, 106, 228, 257, 328
Copper, 99
Core Energetics, 149, 240, 356
cosmetics, 131, 133, 138
crab, 122
crackers, 67, 83, 103, 106, 166, 299, 326

cream, 78, 81, 83, 86, 87, 89, 93, 97, 98, 122, 124, 125, 126, 133, 212, 274, 320, 322, 323, 325, 326, 327, 328, 333, 337
Creating Physical Health, ii, 120
Creating Physical Health — 3.5 months to one year prior to conception, 121
Creator, 29, 48, 184, 233, 278, 295, 297, 301, 309, 312, 334, 349, 350, 351
CRT, 140
cry, why, iii, 226
cucumber, 82, 125
curing disease, 3

D

Daily Guidelines, 81
Daily Review, 145
Daily Review, sample, 146
dairy, 18, 19, 34, 65, 68, 71, 81, 82, 83, 92, 95, 96, 97, 121, 280, 320, 321, 323
Dancing, 149
Dark Forces, 137
David Whyte, 6, 11, 270, 301
Deadly Food, ii, 105
death, 4, 5, 7, 10, 13, 20, 36, 37, 40, 41, 47, 48, 50, 59, 64, 73, 91, 133, 134, 137, 140, 171, 173, 174, 232, 270, 271, 272, 276, 277, 279, 280, 281, 288, 308, 313, 329, 333, 335, 348, 388
Death by Western Medicine, 7
defensive posture, 142, 143, 238, 242, 246
degenerative disease, 3, 41, 48, 59, 112, 276, 331
Degenerative Diseases Were Found at the Point of Contact with, 39
Dental Arch, 18
dentist, 13, 134, 354
Destroying the bond, 297
Detoxification, 103
deva, 104, 135, 136, 138, 148, 160, 169, 176, 179, 195, 233, 237, 254
Devas, 136
developed faces, 24
diabetes, 3, 7, 48, 71, 120, 276
diapers, 191, 225, 226
diarrhea, 7, 10, 87
diet, 3, ii, iv, 3, 23, 32, 43, 68, 69, 71, 84, 95, 166, 319, 323
Diet for Children 5 months to 6 Years, iv, 319
Diet for One year, 323
Diet of Healthy Indigenous Canadian Indians, 69
Diet of Healthy Indigenous Eskimos, 69
Diet of Healthy Indigenous People in the Outer Hebrides, 68
Diet of Healthy Indigenous People in the Swiss Alps, 68
diet, 4 Months, 322
diet, 6 months, 119, 122, 123, 212, 321, 322, 323
diet, 8 months, iv, 128, 205, 323
diet, 9 months +, 323

Tragic Child Raising Practices of the West, 207
Transcending Negativity, 195
transform our world, 199
Traumatic separation, 208
Tuberculosis, 37, 40, 41, 276
two brothers, 3, 19

U

U.S. diet, 64
Uffe Ravnskov, 87
Ultrasound, 140
Unassisted Birth, iii, 173
unconscious, 31, 59, 88, 89, 90, 142, 145, 154, 171, 172, 185, 198, 218, 224, 230, 240, 257, 262, 289, 356
Undefended Mother, 246
unhealthy, 3, 4, 5, 10, 11, 13, 29, 58, 63, 64, 80, 83, 103, 105, 107, 108, 109, 117, 120, 126, 129, 131, 176, 184, 192, 195, 211, 212, 216, 257, 276, 278, 313, 319, 328, 330, 343, 346
United States, 2, 7, 45, 47, 51, 55, 59, 64, 72, 91, 97, 138, 142, 231, 271, 272, 275, 278, 286, 295, 335, 348
unitive, 48, 90, 157, 173, 183
unitive perspective, 90
Universe, iii, 9, 17, 29, 49, 58, 64, 157, 198, 199, 201, 202, 294, 297, 330, 352, 356
Unpastuerized, 97
Unrealistic Boundaries, iii, 254
urination, 11

V

Vaccinations Do Not Protect Against Disease, 272
Vaccinations, Tools of Genocide, iv, 283
Vaccine Adverse Event Reporting (VAERS), 269, 270, 272
Vaccine Final Words, iv, 289
Vaccine Induced Diseases, 271
Vaccines are Government Sponsored Medical Bioterrorism & Institutionalized Murder, 269
vaccines, developing natural immunity, iv, 280
Vaccines, diseases caused by, 276
vaccines, don't work, 280
vaccines, genocide, iv, 283
vaccines, poisons, iv, 278
Vanadium, 100
vegan, 90, 355
vegetable juice, 81, 82, 83, 84, 103, 125, 213, 283, 320, 323, 336
vegetable oil, 3, 67, 83, 87, 88, 106, 320, 327
vegetables, 3, 19, 22, 53, 67, 68, 69, 70, 81, 82, 83, 84, 85, 86, 87, 88, 91, 93, 96, 97, 98, 99, 100, 101, 103, 106, 108, 121, 125, 126, 166, 168, 213, 283, 299, 319, 320, 321, 322, 323, 327, 328, 333, 336, 340
Vegetables and Fruit, 98
vegetarianism, ii, 89, 90

Viera Scheibner's, 267
virus, 3, 47, 139, 263, 264, 265, 266, 274, 275, 277, 279, 284, 313, 343, 345
viruses, 2, 3, 4, 47, 48, 264, 265, 275, 278, 284, 345
vis medicatrix naturae, 6
vital, 5, 7, 85, 92, 98, 132, 134, 175, 210, 237, 246, 319, 338, 340, 341, 348, 356
vitamin A, 52, 53, 54, 55, 58, 72, 93, 94, 97, 120, 124, 281, 344
vitamin B, 64, 99, 118, 119, 124
vitamin B1, 124
Vitamin B-12, 99, 123
vitamin B2, 124
vitamin B3, 124
vitamin B6, 119, 124
vitamin E, 79, 93, 94, 106, 119, 281, 335
vitamins, 16, 17, 24, 55, 58, 64, 65, 67, 68, 70, 72, 73, 76, 81, 84, 86, 87, 89, 90, 92, 93, 94, 95, 98, 99, 101, 103, 104, 107, 108, 109, 111, 112, 118, 120, 124, 126, 127, 133, 280, 281, 282, 313, 325, 328, 333, 340, 345
Vitamins Lost from Contraceptive Use, 124

W

Walter R. Hadwen, 5, 272
water, 4, 17, 24, 33, 58, 63, 64, 65, 70, 82, 85, 86, 97, 100, 101, 120, 126, 127, 128, 131, 132, 133, 139, 142, 167, 193, 229, 250, 251, 255, 284, 298, 299, 314, 317, 320, 323, 325, 336, 337, 342
water fluoridation, 132
Water Hyacinth, 79
western medicine, 6, 7, 8, 11, 13, 48, 173, 270, 283, 288, 294, 314, 345
Weston A. Price, 6, vii, viii, 13, 14, 15, 16, 17, 18, 19, 20, 21, 22, 23, 25, 26, 27, 28, 29, 30, 31, 32, 33, 34, 35, 36, 37, 38, 39, 40, 41, 42, 43, 45, 46, 51, 52, 53, 54, 55, 56, 57, 58, 64, 66, 70, 72, 76, 77, 80, 84, 90, 92, 93, 94, 95, 96, 98, 100, 101, 108, 111, 112, 113, 114, 115, 116, 117, 127, 134, 154, 159, 160, 162, 164, 166, 168, 205, 212, 236, 280, 313, 314, 324, 326, 331, 332, 335, 341, 343, 347, 355, 357, 388
Weston A. Price Quotes
    Aborigine Supreme Force, 24
    Aborigines & Whites suffering, 20
    away from modern contact, 36
    bedfast child, 46
    bedridden or coughing children, 40
    birth was an insignificant experience, 159
    child's health influenced by parents., 52
    decline of modern civilization, 331
    diet of Canadian Indians, 69
    diet of Eskimos, 69
    diet of Outer Hebrides, 68
    dietary suggestions, 100
    discouragement and a longing for death, 36
    distress of a group of primitive people, 43

Lightning Source UK Ltd.
Milton Keynes UK
UKOW040707101011

180060UK00004B/8/P